Cancer
Care
Nursing

Cancer
Care
Nursing

MARILEE IVERS DONOVAN, R.N., M.N.

Clinical Specialist in Oncology;
Instructor, Medical-Surgical Nursing
School of Nursing
University of Pittsburgh
Pittsburgh, Pennsylvania

SANDRA GIRTON PIERCE, R.N., M.N.

Assistant Professor, Oncologic Nursing
Medical-Surgical Nursing
School of Nursing
University of Pittsburgh
Pittsburgh, Pennsylvania

APPLETON-CENTURY-CROFTS / New York
A Publishing Division of Prentice-Hall, Inc.

Library of Congress Cataloging in Publication Data

Donovan, Marilee Irvers.
    Cancer care nursing.

    1. Cancer nursing. I. Pierce, Sandra Girton,
joint author. II. Title. [DNLM: 1. Neoplasms—
Nursing. WY156 D687c]
RC266.D66   610.73'6   75-14042
ISBN 0-8385-1031-0

Copyright © 1976 by APPLETON-CENTURY-CROFTS
A Publishing Division of Prentice-Hall, Inc.

77 78 79 80 / 10 9 8 7 6 5 4 3

Prentice-Hall International, Inc., London
Prentice-Hall of Australia, Pty. Ltd., Sydney
Prentice-Hall of India Private Limited, New Delhi
Prentice-Hall of Japan, Inc., Tokyo
Prentice-Hall of Southeast Asia (Pte.) Ltd., Singapore ·

PRINTED IN THE UNITED STATES OF AMERICA

Dedicated to

NELLIE KUHTIK ABBOTT, R.N., Ph.D.

Our former mentor, motivator, and reinforcer, who, in ways too numerous and pervasive to mention, made this project possible.

and

JOAN ALTREE PIEMME, R.N., M.N. Ed.

Our former instructor and continuing friend, whose enthusiasm and excitement about cancer nursing attracted us into this field.

Preface

The idea for this book has been germinating in the minds of the authors for several years. It originated when they were classmates in graduate school studying oncologic nursing as their clinical specialty in a master's program in medical-surgical nursing. It grew when one went on to function as a clinician working exclusively with cancer patients and the other went on to teach oncologic nursing in a master's program. Throughout these experiences, both had felt a need for a book written about cancer for nurses working or studying within the field of cancer. Much information was always available, but little of it was aimed at nursing problems, and what was written for nurses did not often convey the attitudes and information believed by the authors to be essential for working with cancer patients. With proper preparation, nurses may play a role in educating their colleagues, in improving public education, possibly in assisting with some research projects, and in improving patient services and patient care. Since the volume of data needed to adequately handle all these areas in one work is unmanageable, the authors have chosen to concentrate on the last area, believing that this aspect should provide some groundwork for the others.

One of the main goals of this work is to influence the philosophy of nurses who work with cancer patients. The aim is to promote a more positive orientation to the difficulties encountered. Something can be done for all cancer patients. We should not feel useless or helpless just because every patient is not cured. We must learn to accept those problems for which there are no solutions, while concentrating on areas where improvements or alternatives are possible and available. The mere fact that some burdens can be lightened and that an aggressive attack is planned is often enough to reengage a depressed patient in the act of living, particularly if the patient is actively included and participates in the goals. Every human being must have some hopes and something to which he can look forward. Nursing care planning may be able to provide or support some hopes and some tangible goals. Perhaps the patient with lung cancer may be incurable, but if he can be relieved of a constant cough, he may be able to eat, sleep, and enjoy some of the pleasures of life. Persons who choose to become involved with the cancer patient's problems must be prepared, however, to face some issues which are not easy to handle: the meaning of life, death, disfigurement, the predictability or unpredictability of events, the "why" of things. Patients pose questions which may make one extremely uncomfortable. If one views this as a challenge rather than a defeat, much can be done; the risks are often many, but then so too are the rewards.

The approach of this work is to outline a course of actions appropriate to problems presented by cancer patients. The rationale for both the problems and the approaches is detailed only enough to permit nurses to comprehend the mechanisms involved. When dealing with cancer, this becomes a sizable task, as every cell, tissue, and organ in the body may be affected by cancer, and nearly all physiologic and pathologic processes may be involved. However, only by attempting to understand some of this will the practitioner be able to make judgments, draw parallels, adjust plans, and apply knowledge from one situation to another. The sequence of topics hopefully lends itself to a logical progression.

The authors are acutely aware of the amount of information which is excluded in this approach. However, to ease the guilt of omission, we remind the reader that there are countless volumes and journals which deal with other broad and esoteric aspects which cannot be included here.

M.I.D.
S.G.P.

Contents

**Cancer
Care
Nursing**

1
Introduction

The decade of the 1970s might fittingly be called the decade of the crab in American medicine. It is the decade in which much money, effort, and attention began to be devoted to solving some of the problems and remaining mysteries of cancer. The effects of cancer are certainly monstrous enough to justify this intensified focus.

Cancer has long been recognized as one of the major health problems in this country. A few statistics, some economic considerations, and an awareness of other, more nebulous aspects of the price of these diseases bear testimony to this statement.

Cancers are second only to cardiovascular-renal diseases as causes of death in the United States. As other illnesses become curable or controllable, people are more likely to develop and die from the prevalent serious ailments which cannot yet be treated very successfully, mainly heart diseases and cancers. The overall incidence of cancer has shown a slight, steady increase over the years. Even with allowances made for more accurate diagnosis and better reporting of cancer cases, some of this is probably a true increase. Much of this true increase can probably be attributed to the lengthening life expectancy of the population. Since many types of cancer appear mostly in older age groups, an expanding aged population group would help to account for the rise in numbers of cancer cases. If one adds to this the possibility that heavier environmental pollutants are also affecting cancer incidence, it can readily be seen that cancer may well become an even larger problem unless measures are discovered to reduce its impact.

The financial aspects of cancer are staggering. Vast sums of both government and private monies are spent on numerous varieties of research, public and professional education, development and implementation of preventive and diagnostic measures, treatment, and other areas. Treatment and loss of earnings are economic burdens usually borne by individual families, often with devastating results. Treatment frequently involves very expensive procedures, drugs, and supplies. It may involve lengthy and repeated hospitalizations. Rehabilitation may be costly and prolonged. The monetary cost of cancer to individuals and to society as a whole is prodigious.

Then, too, there are immeasurable prices in the costs of cancer, for we have not yet been able to quantify mental anguish. Anguish takes many forms and occurs in a variety of situations. We see all of these in the problems related to cancer. We see dread, fear, anxiety, hopelessness-depression-despair, loneliness, bereavement, and numerous other kinds of suffering. While some of these reactions are normal and unavoidable, a few of them could be and should be eliminated or reduced.

Cancer is seen by many people in a way that harbors the above feelings. It may still be viewed as a stigma: a disease of the unclean, the lower classes; a retribution by a supernatural or subconscious power for wrongdoing; an unspeakable, mysterious horror. Many firmly believe it to be uncontrollable and thus nearly synonymous with death, and that death is seen as a painful, ugly, prolonged, and lonely one. All of these attitudes combine to make the majority of the population cancerophobic and extremely denial-prone regarding the possibility of developing cancer. As long as the existing attitudes prevail, denial will remain firm, and efforts to promote prevention, early detection, and early treatment will continue to be hampered.

It seems that the best ways to alter the faulty connotations of cancer are through sound education, dissemination of accurate information, alleviation of the secrecy and mystery surrounding cancer, and aggressive management of problems attendant in cancer patients. Obviously, health professionals must lead the way. If they cannot alter their feelings to a more optimistic approach, the lay public can hardly be expected to do so. Health professionals will not be fighting the battle with the weapons already available if they are unaware that there are as many types of cancer as there are types of divisible cells in the body, that each type behaves differently, that many are curable, that many of the incurable ones can be controlled for many years, and that even those which are incurable or uncontrollable need not result in a painful, lonely, or needlessly prolonged death.

Those knowledgeable about the elusiveness and the complexity of the riddles pertaining to cancer do not expect any basic solutions quickly. In fact, there is much evidence to support the belief that the discoveries elucidating the unknowns of cancer will be the foundations of the mysteries of life itself. Since major breakthroughs may not come for years, the great amount of information presently available must be used to maximum benefit. While waiting for new advances, we must work with the tools at hand. One of the purposes of this text is to translate some of this information into a tool for nurses.

2
The Meaning of Cancer

The magnitude of the problem of cancer in our society is only partially indicated by the statistics on mortality and morbidity. Morbidity figures do not tell of the panic inherent in the mere thought of cancer, the role changes and conflicts which may arise when cancer is treated, or the dozens of other problems encountered by the persons who face the diagnosis of cancer. The patient with cancer, because of the meaning of cancer in our society, faces one of the greatest stress situations known to man. Since cancer is frequently a chronic disease with periods of acute intensive illness interwoven with the constant threat of death, the patient with a diagnosis of cancer must face the problems of each of these kinds of illnesses. Often he must do all of this simultaneously.

THE PATIENT AND CANCER

It is generally agreed that cancer is unique among diseases in the degree of anxiety it evokes. Despite one's education and knowledge, the word "cancer" is usually synonomous with death. One remembers the friend who survived several heart attacks or the neighbor who returned to work less than six months after a stroke. At the same time, one remembers the aunt who died of brain metastases only a year after her physicians told her that the radical mastectomy they had performed had "taken care of her problem." The cancer victims who are cured are forgotten. Only the misery of those who have died stands out in the memory. Despite an even poorer prognosis, chronic glomerulonephritis or recurrent congestive heart failure does not elicit the fatalistic response characteristic of a patient with carcinoma.

Equally as stressful as a confrontation with mortality are the other threats that

3

cancer holds. The individual fears the loss of usefulness or more precisely the loss of his ability to produce. American culture may be viewed as a blending of three ethics.[1] Rural America and the older population of most areas of the country follow the rigid rules and norms of the Protestant ethic. Included among these norms are hard work, self-reliance, and industry. For the past half-century, the young and the educated have ascribed to a Freudian-oriented ethic. It is more flexible, but the norms of service and kindness to others as well as development of one's potential demand as much productivity as does the more rigid Protestant ethic. The newer experiential movement is oriented toward doing and experiencing everything and actively changing society. Productivity and independence are essential in all of these forces. Thus the threat of dependency causes conflicts of a very basic nature. The prospect of losing self-determination, of being totally dependent, and of being nonproductive can be more anxiety producing than the prospect of death itself.

Physical attractiveness is more openly threatened by cancer than by most diseases. The mention of malignancy evokes visions of mutilated faces, nauseous odors, and dehumanized and emaciated bodies. Even when the tumor is not visible, an individual must cope with these threats and with a self-image no longer in accord with the values of youth and beauty.

To a great degree the fear generated by various diseases and their treatment is related to the hostile or unresolved feeling associated with the body parts involved. Fear is increased as the significance of the organ to the individual increases. Three of the five leading sites of cancer involve organs which are important for their valued functions and also because of the degree of ambivalence related to them: breast, uterus, colon/rectum. Sexually-oriented and excretory organs are associated with one's earliest confrontations with cultural restrictions. The fear, ambivalence, and guilt thus relating to these organs and to their continued normal functioning are great.

One may also fear that his disease, the results of the treatment, or the status changes which he presumes will result will cause others to flee from him. His own belief that cancer is a visible punishment for specific evils in his past, that cancer is contagious, or that cancer causes strange changes in people may be projected onto those about him. The patient's own natural inclination to flee from those who have cancer makes it difficult for him to believe that others will not abandon him. Too often the patient's fears are realized, as others do leave him. If not from fear of contagion or from judgment, they leave from an inability to confront the anxieties that cancer evokes in them.

Cancer is probably one of the lowest status diseases on record, with the possible exception of tuberculosis and venereal diseases. (Even the latter are becoming quite acceptable among the more liberated and younger segments of the population.) Cancer, however, is still often considered a disease of the unclean and thus a social stigma. Combining this with all the other taboo aspects of cancer, one finds cured cancer patients much less likely to mention, and almost never likely to freely discuss, their previous illness, as opposed to former victims of high status diseases, such as coronary artery disease or hypertension. These diseases we associate with power, aggressiveness, and the good life. The taboos regarding body parts affected by cancer also contribute to the secrecy surrounding this disease. A lady does not speak of her breasts, her uterus, or her rectum, nor does a gentleman mention his prostate, his testicles, or his colon. Hearts, kidneys, stomachs, and nerves are more acceptable topics for conversation. Since it is human nature to value social acceptance and to avoid offending or making others uncomfortable, cancer patients are hardly allowed any forum to share their experiences. Somehow the public must be desensitized to permit a more open, frank, and honest approach to the problems of cancer. Recently television, in such popular shows as *All in the Family* as well as in specials, has begun to deal realistically with the problems of cancer.

More than any other disease, people equate cancer with severe pain. The cardiac patient is seen as lucky because he is struck down quickly with short-lived pain. The person with cancer is pitied for what is considered an inevitably prolonged death dominated by pain which is refractory to all current methods of relief.

When one looks at some of the norms proposed by one authority as representative of our society, a broad view of the meaning of cancer emerges. These norms include (1) monogamy, (2) a family unit composed of parents and children, (3) a mother who provides comfort and care in the home, (4) toilet training by the age of 2, (5) obedience assured by reward and punishment, (6) relationships between sexes mediated by sexual intercourse, (7) religious training, and (8) visible success, measured by wealth, power, and acceptance.[2] Even in this day of rapid change, an individual feels pressures to marry and have children and to conform to the role of wife-mother or husband-father. One feels somehow rewarded when things go well and punished if difficulties arise. Even in this age of nonconformity, an individual measures his worth in some degree through the eyes of his reference groups. Does he meet their standards? Does he follow the rules of the group? The person with cancer faces the possibility of never being able to conform to these norms. "Will I, a breastless woman, ever be able to marry?" "What will our life be like without children?" "What did I do to have to endure this?" "How can I ever go out again with this colostomy?" "What kind of man am I to have my wife providing for and taking care of me?" "Will my wife leave me now that I'm impotent?" These and many more questions besiege the person with cancer.

Cancer is frequently a chronic illness. Even when the treatment is curative, the person's reaction to the disease can result in a chronic psychologic handicap. Studies of the reactions of chronically ill individuals have been done for the most part with patients suffering from tuberculosis. Experience seems to substantiate the assumption that these observations are valid for the cancer patient as well. The chronically ill person is a socially displaced person. He is suspended between life and the future. Prolonged hospitalization intensifies this isolation from life. He feels he is no longer master of his life and his body; they are being controlled by forces external to him and beyond his understanding. A deranged sense of time, value changes, and a multitude of emotional responses are the logical sequelae. The exact emotional response depends on many subjective factors. If one believes that there is a cancer personality, be it causative or incidental, the majority of these responses will be fatalistic and depressive in nature. Some of the more subjective factors which influence how an individual perceives the intrusion of cancer into his life and his reaction to this perception include (1) his premorbid personality (his norms, values, conflicts, and coping mechanisms), (2) his concept of self, (3) his feelings about health and illness, (4) his previous experiences with illness and with cancer specifically, (5) the reactions of those whose opinions he values (reference groups), and (6) his perception of the consequences of the disease.

Coping Behaviors

A variety of defense mechanisms are employed in dealing with the threat of cancer. The degree of anxiety inherent in such a diagnosis elicits more primitive defenses than do other less basic threats. All persons facing death, a change in health or status, or any significant loss go through a series of stages in coping with and adjusting to this reality. Engel's model of adaptation to loss provides a framework upon which to hang the variety of reactions one sees in the oncologic patient. The four stages of adaptation are (1) disbelief, (2) developing awareness, (3) reorganization, and (4) resolution.[3]

DISBELIEF. In the stage of disbelief, the person attempts to postpone the impact of the diagnosis with (1) avoidance, where he does not notice the symptom, (2) suppression, where the symptom is recognized but dismissed, or (3) denial, where the significance is suspected but dismissed. The individual cannot as yet openly face the reality of the situation. A person may not block the entire situation but may isolate the emotional component from his consciousness—dissociation. It is amazing that a patient can talk of his illness and even handle the prosthesis which will be needed after radical surgery and yet remain emotionally detached. One can only assume that self-preservation allows the person to dissociate in this way to facilitate the necessary activity while preventing emotional overload. Denial over a period of time is a poor outlet for anxiety. The patient must continually expend ever increasing amounts of energy to prevent progress to the next stage.

DEVELOPING AWARENESS. The actions characteristic of the stage of developing awareness are considerably more varied than those in the stage of denial. Anger is the predominant emotion. The dependency resulting from the diagnosis and therapy makes the patient extremely vulnerable. This vulnerability elicits intense anxiety and a desire to flee or attack the object feared. However, in our culture there are taboos controlling the expression of anger. This is especially true when the object of the anger is important to the patient's well-being, as is the physician. Some express anger at God, luck, life, their poor health practices, or previous doctors. Others may displace this anger onto objects in the environment. The object of displacement is most often the individual or group with whom the patient feels safest, the family or strangers. This hostility can seldom be openly and fully expressed but manifests itself in irritable and demanding behaviors. The patient receives very little relief, feeling that he has been unable to blow up, yet his hostility is apparent to all. Internalized anger, in the form of depression and withdrawal, is also common. The major goal at this time is to assure the patient of his value and promote his own self-worth. The patient hates and rejects his body, which is so defective. He expects others will feel the same. His hostile or withdrawn behavior makes it difficult for his family and those involved in his care to show him that he remains a worthwhile, loved person. One technique to reinforce a patient's individual worth is the prompt resolution of physical needs. Relief of the feelings of isolation, guilt, and rejection is an essential step. And actions speak when words fall on deaf ears.

REORGANIZATION. It is only as the person begins the process of reorganization that he can openly discuss his illness. Some of the behaviors of the previous stages continue into this stage. Even blatant denial recurs periodically as the patient needs relief from the stresses of coping. Dependency and aggression are seen most often as the principal behaviors of this stage. Dissociation, identification, and depressive and paranoid reactions also occur. The need to talk is great, but since anger and withdrawal may alternate with dependency, aggression, and a desire to talk, the need for continual evaluation of the patient's needs is of paramount importance. A good listener will be able to gauge the situation and act as a safety valve as well as teacher, counselor, and care-giver.

RESOLUTION. The stage of resolution implies a positive adjustment to the illness. It is hoped that the modifications the patient makes in his way of perceiving self, life, and his environment and his reaction to these modifications will be beneficial and realistic. Unfortunately this is not always the case, and one must realize the limits of the situation. Not all people have healthy ways of coping with day-to-day stresses. We can hope to help these patients cope with the adjustments necessitated by the diagnosis of cancer, but we are foolish to expect optimal functioning from all. There are those individuals who find it so difficult to cope with life on a daily basis that the additional stress of a diagnosis of cancer may be the license to assume a pattern of behavior that they feared to assume before, eg, extreme dependency or withdrawal. There are the positive examples as well: the shiftless person who finds direction in facing this threat; the depressive who finds life is worth living when faced with the prospect of losing it. As nurses we must be acutely aware that we can act as guides through the process of adjustment, but we cannot make people adjust nor can we alter very significantly their patterned ways of adjusting.

Crises

The impact of the diagnosis of cancer is not a single traumatic experience. The person faces a number of crises: (1) fear of the meaning of the symptoms, (2) diagnosis, (3) treatment, (4) metastasis, (5) dying. As symptoms develop, one becomes more uneasy, and most often the dread of cancer soon crosses the mind. A study conducted in the early 1960s in California noted that nearly 7 percent of the population studied delayed in seeking treatment.[4] The major factor in this delay was fear of the diagnosis and its implications. Only when the symptoms themselves cause more anxiety than the prospect of treatment does the person seek medical aid. The magnitude of the symptoms which must occur to force some individuals to seek medical help is astounding. One must be careful not to assume that the person who delays seeking medical attention for obvious disease does not value health or that he is stupid or self-destructive. The person himself may be unable to understand the full motivation which prompted such a delay. Frequently he will exhibit a great deal of guilt. Like anger, one cannot talk a person out of guilt. Actions of acceptance must do the speaking.

The person who has been confronted with distressing symptoms may have already begun coping with the diagnosis of cancer. The person whose disease is discovered at routine examination has had no such opportunity and may initially have a more intense reaction to both the diagnosis and the treatment. Both the diagnosis and the proposed treatment may seem out of proportion to the person who has had no cues to tell him he is sick.

The admission to the treatment center is another crisis. Soon thereafter the patient must face another threat, treatment. Be it radiation, chemotherapy, or surgery, the prospect of treatment poses a myriad of problems for the patient. If the patient is cured, the crises of the malignancy end here. But as soon as the first signs of metastasis occur, the patient must begin to face two new crises: (1) recurrence, and (2) the final crisis for the patient, death. As one faces each of these periods of crisis, anxiety levels are high, defenses are at their ebb, and the opportunity for therapeutic intervention is at its peak.

Hope

Hope is the key word. As long as there is life, there is hope. This is needed whether the patient's prognosis is excellent or poor. Patients who know or suspect a malignancy are very fatalistic. Whether they know their diagnosis or not, whether they are curable or not, they share a common preoccupation with death, bereavement, and a detachment from the future. The well-meaning attitudes of doctors, nurses, and family, intended to spare the patient from the diagnosis, often intensify this fatalism. Suddenly there occur perceptible changes in established relationships, and suspicion is generated. The patient asks himself, ''What is it that they can't talk to me about?'' He soon finds an answer within himself which may be more or less frightening than the truth.

How each person around the patient feels about and reacts to him has a definite effect on the maintenance of a hopeful environment. Far too often one of the following two approaches prevails. (1) The patient who consistently seeks information about his disease, its treatment, and his progress usually finds an answer. What he is told are often the negative aspects, the side effects, the anxieties of the informant. What he is usually not told is what he can do to help himself, the support he will receive from others, and the other hope-maintaining aspects. Presented under the banner of honesty, the fears of the informant may be preventing hope from tempering honesty. (2) The opposite approach is to tell the patient nothing—one cannot lie if one is silent. This approach fails to consider the patient's imagination and the answers it is providing for his unanswered questions. The question need not be to tell or not to tell, but rather by whom should what be told and when. Each patient provides the information by which to formulate the answers to these questions.

Some factors about hope vary within the stage of the illness. Initially one hopes that the symptoms are not serious, are not cancer. Then one hopes that the treatment is curative. In this stage the foremost need is for information, and the patient needs to be informed and assured in the way he is able to hear and accept. No text can tell exactly what to tell an individual. Only his questions and his responses to each increment of information provided can be the guide. All patients need positive information. They need a positive approach by which it is conveyed that help is available, that treatment is effective, and that those about them are hopeful. Anything less allows anxiety and imagination to lead the patient into expectations of metastasis, pain, and death.

If there is a recurrence the meaning of hope changes for the patient and usually for the family as well. They hope for more time to finish things that need to be finished. They continue to hope for cure, but need to be helped to see that there is hope in control as well. The diabetic may wish there were a cure, but realism limits his hopes to adequate control with diet and medications. For some cancer patients a chronic illness controlled by regular doses of medication is also a realistic goal.

At this time the relationship with the physician is paramount. He is a symbol of hope. It is only through his continued interest that the patient need not despair. The fear of being abandoned by this *hope-person* becomes overpowering. Patients protect their physicians by not questioning, by limiting their complaints, and by treating the physician as they wish to perceive him, as the miracle worker. Because the patient relates to the physician in this manner, the physician is not honestly appraised by the patient of his needs and fears. Also, there may be little emotional energy left to develop a worthwhile relationship with other health personnel. However, a therapeutic relationship developed between patient and health worker at an earlier stage may be maintained throughout this period. This is a difficult time in which to promote hope. The person who has already proven himself to the patient can evaluate the most appropriate way to assist this particular individual. Many people cannot fill this role. The ill person's ability to relate is limited by the demands of this stage of his illness and by his physical and emotional reserves.

The patient's self-worth is repeatedly threatened as the malignancy progresses. It is difficult to maintain hope when one perceives the fatalism of others. As a result he requires ongoing reassurances that he remains a worthwhile, loved human being. Prompt physical care and frequent verbal contacts along with and supplemental to the physical care are means of providing this hope-maintaining environment.

The patient also needs limits. Family and friends, more so than medical personnel, often are of the opinion that if the person is so sick let him have his way. Nothing is more defeating to the maintenance of a functioning individual. What is given out of love is easily taken for hopelessness, lack of interest, fear, or rejection. The patient sees that he is no longer required to adhere to the laws of his society. This is interpreted as no longer being a functioning member of that society. It would seem that life separated from the values of usefulness, order, productivity, and expectations for the future becomes a kind of nonexistence. Hope in this context has little meaning.

Prolonged hospitalization with its isolation from life makes it more difficult for the patient to maintain hope, activity, life patterns, beneficial coping mechanisms, and a positive attitude toward treatment, the environment, and the people about him. Mere recreation will not suffice to fill the many empty hours. What constitutes true diversional activity is very individual. Television, reading, and knitting generally do not qualify. Activities that busy the mind as well as the body and provide a sense of accomplishment and usefulness can assist in developing a hopeful environment. Eating in a common dining room, half-completed crossword and jigsaw puzzles, and groups engaged in a common project are appropriate for some patients. When uselessness is a major component, involvement according to the patient's ability in a community volunteer program, such as dictating books for the blind, can help.

THE FAMILY AND CANCER

The meaning of cancer to the family members is not much different from the meaning of cancer to the patient. They fear that the loved one will die, will be mutilated, will suffer. Not all of their fears and concerns are totally for the patient. The shock of the diagnosis of cancer elicits many coping patterns, but present in all is an increased awareness of self and one's functioning. Like the ill person himself the family member may become symptom-conscious and very aware of every change in his body. The family members see more clearly the relationship of the cancer patient to the family and the implications that disease and death have for the family unit. The threatened loss of the individual or the changes necessitated by the illness or treatment require many adjustments within the family. Some of the changes envisioned by the family are realistic, many are unrealistic. Members dependent on the sick individual fear abandonment and that they cannot go on without the customary support given by the patient.

Role Changes

Anticipated role changes are a further cause of anxiety. The changes anticipated or necessitated may directly oppose personal or cultural patterns. The wife may wonder if she has the capacity to support a family. A husband may question whether he can be both mother and father to young children. Most individuals find that filling their own roles and doing what is expected of them is taxing at times. It is no wonder that the prospect of assuming the role of another elicits feelings of fear, anger, jealousy, and personal injury. The willingness of the participants to assume new roles is not the only variable to be considered in measuring the effect of the anticipated or real role changes. View the current struggle in our society for both men and women to be free to engage in those endeavors, to perform those tasks, and to develop those roles that appeal to them as individuals. To gain satisfaction and not guilt in the process is more difficult. Much has been written about and by people claiming to be free of cultural stereotypes. If such were true on a large scale, it probably would not be newsworthy. Even those who staunchly support the idea are not oblivious to the many social pressures and internalized norms which make these changes difficult to attain and uncomfortable to maintain. Even without strong personal or cultural taboos it is extremely difficult to effectively fill a role not normally assumed in one's culture. There are few if any good role models.

Conflicts

Also of concern are the functional changes resulting from the disease or its treatment. Due to anxiety and/or lack of knowledge, patients and families often misinterpret or assume facts regarding the disease and its treatment. For example, many couples assume that after a hysterectomy for carcinoma of the cervix (Wertheim hysterectomy) sexual relationships will be impossible. On the other hand it is equally as likely that a woman having an anterior exenteration for carcinoma of the bladder will not even suspect that it would affect sexual functioning.

One often neglects to consider the additional conflicts which may arise among society's expectations of sick members, the goals of the sick person, the family, and the restrictions of the disease itself. A sick person is dependent, inactive, trusting, and grateful. The sick person who is to be rehabilitated does not benefit from these traits. He needs to seek independence whenever possible, challenge the idea and fact of invalidism, find ever expanding activities within his abilities, and maintain relationships based on respect and sharing, not on fear or gratitude. When the defect is obvious, society expects that the individual will conform to the accepted definition of a sick person. Often great pressures are exerted to force compliance. When the defect is not obvious, society may not accept the above traits in a person. Simultaneously, the family and friends who know the diagnosis are likely to expect or even force the patient to accept his role as a sick person. In any given instance, the family and friends may be working with society against the patient or with the patient against society, or both society and the family may be pulling in different ways against the patient. An example may clarify this point.

> LV is a 26-year old female who is engaged to be married. She is one year post radical mastectomy. Metastasis to the skull has occurred, and treatment has begun, including bilateral oophorectomy, 5-fluorouracil (5-FU), and radiation. She looks like a healthy, vivacious, intelligent, and happy young woman. Society expects what one would expect of any happy, healthy young lady. She will marry her fiancé on the previously arranged date, bear children, live for the future, be carefree and not too serious. Family and friends look at her with her prognosis paramount in their minds. They condemn any plans for marriage, weep that her love for children is to go unrequited, and consistently avoid all references to the future. LV herself is trying to cope with the reality of a life which includes her love for and reliance on her fiancé, her values regarding the quality of life, the magnitude of what has happened to her in the past year, and much more. She is also called upon to cope with the pressures exerted upon her by those in the environment in which she must live.

Finances

Another honest concern of families is finances. The mere mention of cancer calls forth visions of never ending hospitalizations, innumerable medications, repeated consultations, increasingly more specialized care, and rapidly waning funds. The cost of cancer care is not to be minimized. However, for some the fear of financial ruin or fear that care may not be available because of limited funds is a source of worry out of proportion to the reality of the situation.

Guilt

The less often discussed concerns of the family of a patient with cancer include contagion, heredity, and guilt. For years people have associated cancer with a given area, a certain house, a certain family, a certain set of actions. At various times the health professions have given silent support to these beliefs because of insufficient data to refute them. With time most of these associations have proven to be unfounded in fact. The tenacity with which people cling to these beliefs attest to the magnitude of the need to find some answer to the question, "Why me?" If one can find a cause, one can feel safer by avoiding the cause. One can even be secure in his inevitable doom if the cause is unavoidable. This gives the person some sense of control. (More than any other disease, cancer leaves one feeling totally devoid of control.) With the current emphasis on viruses and cancer, the fear of contagion will undoubtedly loom larger. An individual seeking to find some rational basis for the cancer is easily attracted to the idea of contagion. This reduces his fears regarding the unknown qualities of cancer, but the fears associated with being with the patient or caring for the patient with cancer become overwhelming at times. The fear of a hereditary influence is closely linked to the fear of contagion. Families view it as a curse upon the family, an unavoidable foe stalking its prey. Often this leads to a cancerophobia which prevents them from seeking care for any ailment because they might discover cancer. It also can lead family members to guilt, especially that having given the disease to their child, their other children will also develop it.

Throughout this chapter it should be evident that the fatalism produced by the identification of cancer with pain and inevitable death plays a major role. Even the problems associated with fears of contagion and heredity would be no more than minor problems if the principals did not react as if it were useless to diagnose or treat cancer because of its universally fatal outcome.

THE NURSE AND CANCER

As health professionals we often think of ourselves as insulated from the many pressures that we see reflected in our patients. Cancer is a threat to the nurse as well as to the patient. Knowledge may alter our responses to various stimuli, but we cannot ignore completely the culture in which we live and its subtle influences upon us. That anxiety can interfere with the assimilation and use of knowledge is an accepted fact. When one discusses cancer with many nurses, it is astounding how very little they know of this disease which they see so much and of which they are so frightened. The very knowledge that could help them cope with some of these anxieties is denied them by the fear of cancer that prevents them from learning. Nurses and physicians are more acutely aware of the failures in cancer care than is the lay public. This serves to reinforce the innate fears previously discussed. At present most deaths in the United States continue to take place in institutions providing nursing care. It is understandable then that nurses would associate cancer with death at least as strongly as the public. The patients who are curable occupy little nursing time. They are fleeting faces in the masses of suffering humanity that comprise a nurse's day. The patient who is not cured, who faces the very things that we fear at the mention of the word cancer, returns many times to imprint his sorrowful tale on the memories of those who render him care.

Stresses

Since most nurses are young, relatively healthy individuals, it is difficult for them to see that what is so terribly important now may not seem as important when one is very ill. The problem of dependence or hope or hospitalization must seem more ominous to the healthy person trying to imagine how it would feel than to the sick individual who has been adapting to each change as it has occurred. Trying to imagine what the patient is going through can be very worthwhile if one recognizes the limits of such a fantasy. Not only must one be aware of the differences from one individual to another, but one must also be cautious not to assume that Patient X's perception of his environment and his reactions to it are the same as those of Mr. X, the same person before his illness. The transition from health to illness produces many changes.

Many of the threats of cancer are universal. Being a nurse does not isolate one from these stresses; it may actually intensify many of the threats. A nurse is a helping person hired to do a particular job. Helpers must help, and if the nurse defines helping in terms of cure, she is frequently seeing herself as a nonhelper. The family wants to help the patient because they love him (or a variety of other personal motives). The nurse needs to help the patient for at least two reasons: (1) she cares for the patient, and (2) nursing means helping—it is part of her image as a nurse. To not help is to lose a portion of oneself. So the nurse who measures her helpfulness, her success, by cure rate frequently faces threats to her individual integrity that are alien to the patient and the family members. She faces further problems because of her role as a nurse. The family has a deep attachment for the loved one who is sick. Their fears are primarily based on the relationship which exists with the sick person. The nurse is less deeply attached to each patient, but she has varying degrees of relationship with many patients. Inherent in these relationships are many of the problems mentioned previously: dependency-independency, loss of control, helping, success. The number of times that a nurse must cope with these stresses is another factor. Varying amounts of emotional energy are required in caring for patients, in grieving for the dying, and in handling one's role in the process. The sum total of this for a given nurse may at times be emotionally exhausting. Believing that good nurses ''don't get involved'' or ''don't cry'' or ''can take it'' can add guilt feelings to all the other feelings with which she is desperately trying to cope.

Each person has imbedded in his personality certain characteristics and experiences which affect the meaning of cancer for him. This was mentioned in reference to the patient; it is equally true for the nurse. The number of experiences with cancer that a nurse has increases the likelihood of poor experiences having become part of the total meaning of cancer for her. The possibility also exists that she will develop ways of coping with the problems of cancer that reinforce her beliefs about the disease and its effect on people. For instance, the nurse who has had previously poor experiences with pain and its alleviation and who feels that cancer is inherently painful may find it very difficult to spend much time with the patient in pain. This isolation with its possible resulting delay in administration of analgesics decreases the analgesic effect. The patient's unrelieved pain will reinforce said nurse's idea that cancer is inherently a disease of intractable pain.

We have been looking at just one of the limits—that of one's own personality and life experiences. Another limit is that of time. The hurried nurse seldom has the time to do all she wishes for a given patient, and priorities must be set. One needs to be cautious that the priorities are not a reflection of nurse preference rather than patient need. Still other limits are those of knowledge and ability. One needs to recognize these limits in order to function safely and as a motivation to continue learning. In striving to expand one's limits by increasing one's knowledge and skills, it is important not to lose sight of the fact that there are continually changing limits imposed by numerous factors in the environment. Personal problems, sickness, and interpersonal relationships on the job can all impose limits on the functioning of a nurse. If she is recovering from an illness or concerned about a hospitalized spouse, she will be less receptive, less observant, less understanding, less organized, and more distractable. Feelings of guilt and fear of reprisal frequently compound the problem. Recognition of all the identifiable limits in a given situation allow one to set goals and to define approaches in tune with reality.

Over the years nursing literature has examined the various techniques employed in coping with anxiety-producing situations, which are an integral part of dealing with the basic facts of life. The majority of these techniques involve flight of some form. Some nurses avoid the situations by leaving nursing entirely or by finding areas which are safe for them. Even in these safe areas it is difficult to avoid all threats. Finding this true, nursing has found ways of remaining emotionally and verbally isolated despite physical proximity. This may be defined as emotional detachment, professionalism, or not getting too involved. In an area in which patient-centered care is becoming a norm rather than a phrase on paper, this detachment is more difficult but not impossible to maintain. By using various communication-blocking techniques, a nurse can interview patients and sit and talk with them without fear of being confronted by anything too unsettling. Most of the time she is totally unaware that she is maintaining an effective emotional barrier between herself and those patients who might possibly pose a threat to her emotional equilibrium.

Anger and blatant anxiety are seldom seen in routine nursing functioning. Both are perceived as uncontrolled emotion, and, as such, would elicit more discomfort in the form of guilt than the discomfort caused by the initiating' situation. Psychosomatic types of illness are common. One would suspect that there exists a relationship between the inability to become angry or anxious or flee and the number of somatic complaints seen in nurses caring for cancer patients.

There is obvious safety in routines and policies. When all else fails, a nurse can always seek the shelter of hospital policy, higher priorities, or procedural con-straints.

All persons need to succeed. In medicine success has been measured by cure rate or improvement in the patient's condition. In nursing we have assumed the same criteria. If the patient improves and goes home, we win; if he dies, we lose. However, nurses are not physicians. Except for the areas of prevention and detection, nurses have little to do with the cure process. If the goal of nursing is meeting patients' needs, success needs to be measured in terms of this goal. The surgeon's ability or inability to remove the tumor need have no bearing on nursing's success with the same patient. The physician is at the disadvantage—his goal is set for him by convention. Nursing has the option to set more flexible goals and therein to find their successes. Only occasionally does a nurse have the right to feel successful because a patient lived. Only occasionally need she feel guilty because a patient died. Hour by hour patients are satisfactorily achieving goals, the attainment of which is directly attributable to nursing care. In this area as in many others it is time to stop walking in the shadow of the physician, time to find the realm of nursing.

Coping with Cancer Nursing

What a horrible picture! Patient, family, and medical personnel all over-whelmed by anxieties, milling about employing mechanisms which isolate them from one another and prevent resolution of the conflicts precipitating their be-haviors. Is there an answer? How does one cope with these problems? If man were not capable of the courage, the adaptability, and the motivation to face and conquer adversity in his life, this would indeed be a bleak picture. Man has the capacity not only to face physical and emotional stresses in his own life but also to reach out a helping hand to another human being along the way. The oncologic nurse needs to be more than an experienced technician. She needs to be a human being reaching out to her fellow man and offering herself with her knowledge, her skills, and her humanity. To be able to do this the oncologic nurse needs four things (1) knowledge, (2) a philosophy of life compatible with cancer nursing, (3) satisfaction (positive reinforcement), and (4) supportive guidance (peer support).

KNOWLEDGE.   A sound knowledge of the problem is basic. What is cancer? What are its causes? What can be done? These questions must have answers. The answers provide a basis for a realistic appraisal of the problem, the basis for a sound philosophy of cancer nursing, and the basis for realistic nursing care. This text does not propose to cover the allied subjects of anatomy, physiology, and pathology. The authors at times regret that this is so but intend to keep to their original purpose of providing a guide to nursing approaches to the problems of the cancer patient. However, at this time it seems appropriate to point out the need to have knowledge and understanding of information in all these areas. The purpose of this section is to enumerate the kinds of facts about cancer which the authors think are essential to the nurse if she is to circumvent the mysticism which surrounds cancer and to face realistically the processes of identifying the patient care problems, instituting nursing measures to deal with these problems, evaluating the results, and obtaining positive reinforcement.

Cancer is a group of diseases characterized by disordered growth. Much is known about some of these diseases, and very little is known about others. An ever increasing knowledge of cancer in general and knowledge of the pathology and natural history of the various tumors encountered in daily practice is essential. Some are rapidly growing, some pose a serious threat to life, some are slowly growing, and some become life-threatening only because of neglect. Some are easy to diagnose, and some are easy to treat. One type of cancer may be no more like another than the common cold is like gram-negative septicemia. Both the cold and septicemia are infections. Both a basal cell carcinoma and melanoma are skin cancers. The differences outnumber the similarities.

Equally as important to know is the stage of the tumor. Stage I carcinoma of the cervix and Stage IV carcinoma of the cervix present totally different management problems. This is true of most malignancies. The in situ or Stage I tumor is usually asymptomatic and presents primarily teaching and psychosocial care problems for nursing. On the other hand, the Stage IV lesion is attended by multiple physical problems and a growing threat of death. Knowledge of the pathology of cancer, the natural history of various tumors, staging, and grading provide the nurse with the facts by which she can give honest reassurance and assist the patient in setting and attaining realistic goals. The nurse who has this knowledge and understanding can say to the patient with Stage I Hodgkin's disease that radiation will very likely cure his disease, that he has no reason to limit his plans for the future, that regular appointments with his physician are important but not to further treat the disease, and that there is no reason for fatalism. Her approach to this patient must be drastically different from her approach to a patient with a modified Dukes' classification Type C lesion of the colon. What is realistic skepticism in the latter would be unrealistic fatalism in the former. Lack of this type of knowledge supports the inclination to view all cancer as hopeless and inevitably painful and terminal.

In addition to increased knowledge of various malignancies, one must know various prevention/detection measures. The American Cancer Society estimates that 75 percent of the lung cancer in the United States would not exist if cigarette smoking were eliminated. Even a cursory look at mortality statistics makes it obvious that detection of an early-stage lesion is definitely worthwhile. We currently have the means of detecting and curing nearly all of the colon-rectal and cervical cancers. Yet the death rate does not proportionately decline. The means of accomplishing this reduction in cancer mortality must be made available. Nurses are in a position to spearhead this drive in their occupation, in their social life, and in their personal life. The prudity which prevents people from actively seeking examination and even treatment of symptoms of genital organs and organs of elimination must be dispelled. Innovative ways of bringing these detection measures to the population must be implemented, and nurses must be familiar with the factors involved. According to Rosenstock[5], in order for people to avail themselves of screening or early detection measures, they must, first of all, see themselves as susceptible to the disease. The average person sees himself roughly as susceptible to cancer as to death. Fear is so great that denial runs rampant, and the fear must be diminished before denial will wane. A slight threat is usually useful in arousing motivation, but extreme threat interferes with adaptive action, so there is a delicate balance to be maintained between anxiety arousal and anxiety reduction. Secondly, people must believe that courses of action are open to them which, in their view, would reduce the likelihood of occurrence of the disease or reduce the seriousness of the problems should the disease occur. In addition, they must believe that taking the proposed action would not in and of itself lead to or entail greater threats than the health threat they are attempting to diminish. One need only consider the embarrassment, cost, inconvenience, and sometimes discomfort of detection measures to see the problems inherent here, not to mention the extreme threats of available treatment methods (mutilation, pain, cost, and so on). Obviously people must also know where and how to obtain services, and unfortunately services are not always readily available. Last, the health motive must be seen as important and must not be less of a priority than other needs which may be competing for resources. Two other needs often seem to overshadow health needs: finances and social approval. As long as physicians belittle patients who appear for minor complaints (physicians are high-status citizens whose disapproval is hard for many people to confront), as long as housing and food are poor and scanty, as long as neighbors and friends reinforce the attitude "if it doesn't bother you, don't worry about it," we will be fighting a losing battle in the promotion of early detection of cancer. Sadly, the prevalence of many types of cancer is highest in lower socioeconomic groups where many of these competing needs are greatest. It is difficult to convince a poor, ghetto-dwelling mother of six that she should be concerned about having an annual Pap test when she is trying to cope with getting enough bread on her table. She will tell you to come back some other time, and who can blame her?

The rationale for and effects of various treatment modalities must be understood. The nurse will never need to decide which treatment to institute, but she is constantly called upon to clarify and reiterate and support what the physician has told the patient is the preferred treatment. She is called upon to instill or increase a patient's faith in and acceptance of the treatment plan. She must deal with the patient's reaction, physical and psychologic, to the treatment. And she must face, recognize, analyze, and resolve her own reactions to radical treatment, radiation, palliation, and multiple therapy regimens. How one can expect to do any of this without a sound theoretical basis is inconceivable.

Information does not alter attitudes. The facts about the cancer problem serve as the basis upon which one builds a philosophy of working with cancer patients. An unrealistically fatal idea of cancer assures an unrealistic and fatalistic approach to the cancer patient and his problems. A realistic theoretical base does not assure a hopeful supportive approach. Knowledge of oneself is also essential: knowledge of what fears lie beneath the fatalism one feels, knowledge of the threats cancer and cancer care pose for oneself in an individual, unique way. When one's secret fears, motivation, and defenses are examined and understood, their irrational control of behavior is diminished. Their influence does not cease because one recognizes their existence, but recognition provides the first step to rational control. If one knows what interferes with his reaching out to a cancer patient in a helpful manner and one has a philosophy which is compatible with patient care, one will have the motivation to find the ways of dealing with his personal deficiencies/obstacles in the nursing situation.

Knowledge of the numbers of nursing measures which can be employed to relieve and assist a patient and skill in applying these measures does much to increase a nurse's composure in the situation. A large repertoire of skills assures fewer situations in which the frustration of "nothing one can do" predominates. Increasing competence brings increasing confidence to try new measures which, in turn, further increases competence.

PHILOSOPHY.   Philosophy has been mentioned many times. What kind of philosophy is meant? What kind of philosophy is compatible with cancer nursing? Certainly many different ways of looking at life, self, living, giving, doing, and other people support one in the day-to-day caring for a person with cancer. The authors can only say that they have found their philosophies capable of doing this and present a philosophy as an example. Life is worth living, but what is life and what is living can only be answered by the individual involved. The patient who is willing to submit to mutilative surgery does not necessarily value life more than the patient who refuses such treatment. They may only define life and living in radically different ways. Death is inevitable, it is the culmination of every life. It can be made easier, less fearful, and postponed, but it cannot be forever prevented. The meaning of death, like the meaning of life, has no universals. Each individual sees it in his own unique way. Every person has fears, concerns, and needs which make his disease, his treatment and his situation different for him. Each person also has strengths and resources possibly never before evidenced which can give him the courage, adaptability, and motivation to face and conquer adversity in his life. The helping hand of another is one of these resources which can help to conquer the problems of living. Despite our cultural norm somewhat to the contrary, an individual has the right to expect that others will come to his aid in times of need. And as important as all of the preceding is the personal belief that "I, all that I am, all that I know, and all that I can do can be of help to this other person."

POSITIVE REINFORCEMENT.   The problem of grieving for so many patients simultaneously and the effect that this has on the nurse have been discussed.

Knowledge and philosophy do not prevent this. Ambivalence, guilt, and frustration intensify the work of grieving. Much of the guilt and frustration come from identifying and striving for unachievable goals or from abandoning the patient because of fear of failure. This fear of failure even affects the care of the patient with a curable malignancy. Need one fail so often? One step in the solution involves setting realistic patient-centered goals. If, based on knowledge of the patient and his disease, cure is unlikely, then the goals set are not cure related. On the other hand, if cure is highly probable, whether or not the patient is cognizant of this, the goals are very cure oriented. The goals of nursing care must be attainable by nursing measures. Then nursing can devote itself to attaining the goal and in the attainment derive much satisfaction.

We hesitate to talk of the rewards of nursing. Self-sacrifice and altruism are seen as the ideal. One is to forget oneself in devotion to the patient. Impossible for the most part! If one receives nothing in return for the effort expended, one soon expends less effort. It is as if one has a certain complement of emotional energy. Some have more; some have less. If it is continually given away and never restored, it is eventually depleted. The debits are there, they have been enumerated in various ways; the credits are also there, they are the successes one attains. Pain relief sufficient to allow the patient to continue relating to his wife, minimal transient nausea and vomiting after chemotherapy, self-assurance with an ileal bladder, a peaceful death—these are all goals for a specific patient which are realistic and attainable through concerted nursing care. In none of these instances is the goal cure related, but the patient's life will be better, more meaningful, and more real because of nursing care directed toward these goals. The nurses involved will have the satisfaction of goal achievement even in the face of declining health and approaching death. The rewards, the reenergizers, are there. Someone needs only to structure the situation so that they are attainable.

Another method which is effective in dealing with the fatalism is to seek follow-up on patients. The traditional maxim against involvement makes many nurses hesitant to call upon a patient after discharge or even after transfer to another unit. What other investment of nursing time can so clearly identify for a nurse her strengths and weaknesses and perpetuate a hopeful outlook as a postdischarge call to a patient in whom the nurse has invested a great deal of her time, energy, and commitment? A call to a patient six months after radiation for early Hodgkin's disease will acquaint the nurse with those areas in which the patient faced difficulty in adjustment and rehabilitation so that she can consider these in preparing future patients. It will also be encouraging and emotionally invaluable to hear of the patient's successes, continued good health, and readjustment. Both the problem of universal fatalism and the problem of emotional depletion are dealt a blow by a single conversation.

In order to provide this type of feedback on a large scale, patient's names could be added to a list kept by each unit. This list could be submitted after a period of time to the tumor registry or the physician's office for follow-up information on these patients. An effort may need to be made to assure that patients with curable malignancies are included as well as those patients who elicit concern because of advancing disease.

PEER SUPPORT. Having attained a working knowledge of cancer and the implications for prevention, diagnosis, and treatment, developed a philosophy compatible with cancer care, and learned to find successes by realistic goal definition, one can begin to cope with the anxieties of cancer nursing. When a favorite patient dies, when a person's pain is out of control, when one knows she cannot really give of herself that day for personal reasons, when a patient rejects the offer of help, an additional method of help is frequently beneficial. An asset which complements all the other measures is the support and assistance of a kindred spirit. At times this is an indispensable component, as in the initial experiences with committing oneself to the cancer patient. To risk this, despite all the self-protective instincts which say "flee," is aided greatly by the encouragement and interest of one who shares this commitment.

The group dynamics of a given setting can contribute to or impede nursing care. Where norms exist which strictly define how involved one gets with patients, how much time and effort is expended, and that nursing consists of procedures to carry out physician's orders, implementing the ideas in this chapter will be difficult. Motivation of the group leader and a change in her attitudes and behavior is often a prerequisite. Increasing knowledge by conferences, seminars, and readings and emotional support and guidance may be sufficient to spark the interest and provide the challenge sufficient to initiate this change. In other cases the services of a person qualified in group process may be needed to help the group deal with the complex pressures which chain them to a set of behaviors which interfere with maximal patient care and with their own job satisfaction. Then if one can guide the motivated learner through a single experience of full commitment, self-knowledge, realistic goal setting, success, and emotional satisfaction, it will be difficult for this person to return to previous methods of coping which provide fewer rewards.

SUMMARY

Cancer poses one of the greatest anxiety-producing threats in our society. Cancer nursing is not an easy specialty. One cannot deny the multiple stresses resulting for patient, family, and health workers. One can recognize and accept these and learn to cope with them. One can apply one's knowledge of cancer, prevention/detection, therapy, and care in the framework of a compatible philosophy to setting and meeting realistic goals. At times the price is high, but the rewards seem to more than compensate.

References

1. Folta JR, Deck ES (eds): A Sociological Framework for Patient Care. New York, Wiley, 1966
2. Garner HH: Psychosomatic Management of the Patient with Malignancy. Springfield, Ill, Thomas, 1966
3. Engel G: Grief and Grieving. Am J Nurs 64:93–98, September 1964
4. A Study of the Needs of Cancer Patients in California. San Francisco, American Cancer Society, 1962
5. Rosenstock IM: Public response to cancer screening and detection programs. J Chronic Dis 16:407–418, 1963

Bibliography

Abrams RD: The patient with cancer—His changing pattern of communication. N Engl J Med 274:317–322, 1966
Ackerman LV, DelRegato JA (eds): Cancer: Diagnosis, Treatment, and Prognosis, 4th ed. St. Louis, Mosby, 1970
Aiken L, Aiken JL: A systematic approach to the evaluation of interpersonal relationships. Am J Nurs 73:863–867, May 1973
Allen W: Possible hazards in estrogen administration. Cancer 24:1137–1139, 1969
American Cancer Society, Inc.: 1973 Cancer Facts and Figures. New York, American Cancer Society, 1974
———: Proceedings of the Sixth National Cancer Conference, Denver, Colorado, September 18–20, 1968. Philadelphia, Lippincott, 1970
———: Cancer Management. Philadelphia, Lippincott, 1968
Ammon LL: Surviving enucleation. Am J Nurs 72:1817–1821, October 1972
Ashley D: An Introduction to the General Pathology of Tumors. Baltimore, Williams & Wilkins, 1972
Bahnson CB (ed): Second conference on psychophysiological aspects of cancer. Ann NY Acad Sci 164:307–634, 1969
Bard M: The psychologic impact of cancer. Ill Med J 118:155–159, 1960
Beland I: Clinical Nursing: Pathophysiological and Psychosocial Approaches, 2nd ed. New York, Macmillan, 1970
Berni R, Fordyce WE: Behavior Modification and the Nursing Process. St. Louis, Mosby, 1973
Bouchard R: Nursing Care of the Cancer Patient, 2nd ed. St. Louis, Mosby, 1972
Brauer PH: Should the Patient Be Told the Truth? Nurs Outlook 8:672–676, December 1960
Burch PRJ: New approach to cancer. Nature 225:512–516, 1970
Cameron CS: The Truth About Cancer. New York, Collier Books, 1967
Cancer Facts and Figures, 1973. New York, American Cancer Society, 1973
Chase BA, Robbins GF: Guidelines for Comprehensive Nursing Care in Cancer. New York, Springer, 1973
Christopherson V: Role modifications of the disabled male. Am J Nurs 68:290–293, February 1968
Cowdry EV: Etiology and Prevention of Cancer in Man. New York, Appleton, 1968
Crary WG, Crary GC: Depression. Am J Nurs 73:472–475, March 1973

Crate M: Nursing functions in adaptation to chronic illness. Am J Nurs 65:72–76, February 1965

Craytor JK, Fass ML: The Nurse and the Cancer Patient. Philadelphia, Lippincott, 1970

Day E: The patient with cancer and his family. N Engl J Med 274:883–886, 1966

Epstein SS: Chemical hazards in the human environment. CA 19:276–281, 1969

Francis GM: Cancer: The emotional component. Am J Nurs 69:1677–1681, August 1969

Goldsborough J: Involvement. Am J Nurs 69:66–68, January 1969

Green HN, Anthony HM, Baldwin RW, et al: An Immunologic Approach to Cancer. London, Butterworths, 1967

Harris JE, Sinkovics JG: The Immunology of Malignant Disease. St. Louis, Mosby, 1970

Hugos R: Living with leukemia. Am J Nurs 72:2185–2188, December 1972

Keough G, Niebel HN: Oral cancer detection—A nursing responsibility. Am J Nurs 73:684–687 April 1973

Klagsburn SC: Cancer, emotions and nurses. Am J Psychiatry 126:71–78, 1970

Klagsburn SC: Communication in the Treatment of Cancer. Am J Nurs 71:944–948, May 1971

Koenig R, Levin SM, Brennan MJ: The emotional status of cancer patients as measured by a psychological test. J Chronic Dis 20:923–930, 1967

Leighton J: The Spread of Cancer: Pathogenesis, Experimental Methods, Interpretations. New York, Academic, 1967

Le Shan L: An emotional life-history pattern associated with neoplastic disease. Ann NY Acad Sci 125:780–793, 1966

Luckmann J, Sorensan KC: What Patients' Actions Tell You About Their Feelings, Fears, and Needs. Nurs 75 5:54–61, February 1975

Lunceford JL: Leukemia. Nurs Clin North Am 2:635–647, 1967

Mangen St. FX: Psychological aspects of nursing the advanced cancer patient. Nurs Clin North Am 2:649–658, 1967

Market CL: Neoplasia: A disease of cell differentiation. Cancer Res 28:1908–1914, 1968

Parets AD: Emotional reactions to chronic physical illness. Med Clin North Am 51:1399–1408, 1967

Payne EC, Krant MK: The psychological aspects of advanced cancer. JAMA 210:1238–1242, 1969

Peck A: Emotional reactions to having cancer. CA 22:284–291, 1972

Proceedings of the National Conference on Cancer Nursing. American Cancer Society, 1973

Robinson L: Psychological Aspects of the Care of Hospitalized Patients. Philadelphia, Davis, 1972

Rosenaw W: The nature and mechanism of metastasis. Oncology 24:21–25, 1970

Ross WS: The Climate is Hope. Englewood Cliffs, NJ, Prentice-Hall, 1965

Rubin P (ed): Clinical Oncology for Medical Students and Physicians. Rochester, NY, American Cancer Society, 1970

Schwartz LH, Schwartz JL: The Psychodynamics of Patient Care. Englewood Cliffs, NJ, Prentice-Hall, 1972

Shand HC, Finesinger JE, Cobb S, Abrams RD: Psychological mechanisms in patients with cancer. Cancer 4:1159–1170, 1951

Shepardson J: Team approach to the patient with cancer. Am J Nurs 72:488–491, March 1972

Sorenson KM, Amis DB: Understanding the world of the chronically ill. Am J Nurs 67:811–917, April 1967

Sutherland AM: Psychological impact of cancer surgery. Public Health Rep 67:1139–1143, 1952

———, Orback CE: Psychological impact of cancer and cancer surgery: II Depressive reactions associated with surgery for cancer. Cancer 6:958–962, 1953

The Developmental Biology of Neoplasia. Symposium sponsored by the American Cancer Society, Cherry Hill, NJ, September 11–13, 1967. Cancer Res 28:1797–1914, 1968

Travelbee J: To find meaning in illness. Nurs 72 2:6–8, 1972

Vaillot MC Sr.: Hope: The restoration of being. Am J Nurs 70:268–273, February 1970

Veninga R: Communications: A patient's eye view. Am J Nurs 73:320–322, February 1973

Wu R: Behavior and Illness. Englewood Cliffs, NJ, Prentice-Hall, 1973

3
Dying

That death is synonomous with cancer is a belief far out of proportion to reality. Thus, for the nurse caring for a cancer patient, death is an unavoidable component of every relationship. The cured and curable are called upon not to experience death but to confront it. The cancer nurse must listen to, support, and guide the fearful curable as well as the stoic dying. Unacceptable mutilating surgery and unremitting pain are probably the only other areas eliciting feelings which approach the magnitude of those evoked by the confrontation with death.

A THEORETICAL FRAMEWORK

Dying can be viewed in a variety of ways, and the many current books and articles on the subject have dealt with it in almost every conceivable fashion. It is difficult to feel that one can add anything of significance to this volume of material. The contribution the authors hope to make is the practical application of existing principles and theories in the day-to-day functioning of an oncology nurse. To do so, an attempt has been made to summarize the ideas of those experts whose works have formed a basis for this daily practice, and from this base to look at the process of dying and the people involved from the unique vantage point of the bedside nurse.

Glaser and Strauss

It has been ten years since Glaser and Strauss conducted their historic sociologic study of the process of dying.[1] The situation they described has changed little in the interim. Trajectory and awareness were among the factors they described. Trajectory refers to the pattern of decline by which the process of dying may be identified. It has shape and occurs over time so that it can be graphed. The stresses and the reactions to these stresses vary with the trajectory. The lingering trajectory (including lingering beyond the expected time of death) and the unexpected quick decline are common courses followed by the dying cancer patient.

The most important factor studied by Glaser and Strauss was the degree of awareness of the realities of the situation possessed by each of the persons involved in the process of dying. Four types of awareness were identified. The characteristic patterns and tactics for maintaining relationships within each framework are relevant to the current discussion. In *closed awareness,* the dying person is kept totally unaware of the reality of his impending death. The likelihood of maintaining such a lack of awareness constantly decreases as more people are involved and as patients become more sophisticated. Far more likely to exist is *suspected awareness* or *mutual pretense.* The suspicious patient engages in repeated attempts to validate internal or external cues regarding the likelihood of his demise. This leads to a situation resembling a battle between patient (trying to reveal) and the rest of the world (trying to conceal). As a patient's suspicions are verified sufficiently for him to be sure that he is dying, the game of mutual pretense begins. This is a serious game with rules which include restrictions on topics of conversation, controlled shows of emotions, and efforts to maintain things as normal. Much of what is considered appropriate behavior in the presence of a person with a terminal illness is based on the necessity of playing mutual pretense.

When both the patient and those around him acknowledge that he is dying, *open awareness* exists. Because each person has an idea of the manner in which a person should die, this level of awareness is not without its problems. Divergent opinions among patient, staff, and family can create a stressful atmosphere filled with defensive rather than therapeutic behaviors. An excellent illustration of the variety of problems possible despite open awareness is the story of 23-year-old Lyn Helton *(The Lyn Helton Story,* popularized by the CBS movie, *Sunshine).*[1] Tactics of limiting involvement by talking rather than listening, discussing only safe topics, total avoidance of dying patients, and insistence on approved dying patterns exist despite the awareness level of patient or family. Despite the trajectory or the awareness level, the patient and his family are often left alone without allies, traveling a strange and fearful road in a strange and fearful place.

Glaser and Strauss, among others, have concluded that involvement of health care personnel with a terminal patient, indeed the care he receives, is proportional to various personal and social characteristics of the patient. These include age, financial status, physical attractiveness, repulsive aspects of the disease, optimism or pessimism concerning the outcome of the disease, therapeutic enthusiasm of the primary physician, attitudes toward euthanasia, and the group mood concerning talking with those who are dying (open awareness).[1,2]

Jeanne Quint Benoliel, who was a member of the Glaser-Strauss investigating team, has applied their work to nursing. A relationship needs to be established with a dying person which provides continuity of contact over time, opportunity for active involvement, confidence, and trust. To provide this for many instead of a few, it is essential to establish a working climate based on the projected trajectory of decline for the specific group of patients involved. This climate should be geared to meet patient needs, family needs, and staff needs. For as Jeanne Quint Benoliel so clearly illustrates in her book *The Nurse and the Dying Patient*, it is extremely difficult to continue to care for dying patients without the addition of some compensatory social relationships for the caretaker.[4]

Avery Weisman

The process of dying viewed as a psychologic event has been dealt with by a number of authors. Various stages of adaptation and their inherent coping behaviors and conflicts have been identified. Drs. Elisabeth Kubler-Ross and Avery Weisman are among the more notable figures who have described the psychologic steps taken by an individual who is approaching death. According to Dr. Weisman three stages may be identified as occurring over time. Stage I exists from the time the person begins to notice some stressful symptoms until the diagnosis is confirmed. At this time efforts to protect the status quo by denial, rationalization, and seeking reassurances are evident. Stage II encompasses all the time between diagnosis and the point of final decline.* Dr. Weisman agrees with Glaser and Strauss when he states that the reaction to the loss called death cannot begin until that death is seen as inevitable. As succinctly expressed by Glaser and Strauss, certainty must precede preparation.[2]

Having allowed for confrontation with this inevitability, be it immediate or indeterminant, the patient faces conflicts in four areas: (1) impaired self-esteem, (2) feelings of endangerment (fear of pain), (3) fear of annihilation (fear of cessation of self), and (4) fear of alienation (fear of losing relationships with others).[3] The dying individual reacts to these four basic fears throughout both Stage II and Stage III, the stage of final decline. The threats to self-esteem seem to be most basic. A person who feels worthless rather than worthwhile has greater fears of endangerment, annihilation, and alienation. Respect for the individual by perceptive humane care, including consistent adequate pain control, allows him to maintain sufficient self-respect to confront the other fears and reach that point where he can "die his own death."[6] Though Dr. Weisman gives some specific rules for therapists, he hastens to add that technique and credentials are less important than the ability to be alert, compassionate, available, and responsive.[5,6]

Since this chapter is discussing dying patients, those patients who are treated and cured are not even being considered.

Elisabeth Kubler-Ross

Dr. Ross's five stages of dying have been well known since the publication of her book, *On Death and Dying*. Having discussed with over 400 dying patients what they were experiencing, Dr. Ross identified the following stages: (1) denial—"No, not me . . ." (2) anger—"Why me?" (3) bargaining—"Yes, me, but . . . ."(4) depression—"Yes, me . . . ." and (5) acceptance.[7] Dr. Ross has shown by her method that learning the needs of dying patients from those who are dying is therapeutic as well as informative. Her transcribed conversations illustrate that even when facing the ultimate crisis, man has the capacity to adapt and that this adaptation is an evolving process. It was evident in a number of her examples that health professionals may join with the family and friends in an unrecognized attempt to impede the dying person's coping behavior. Dr. Ross noted that the single most important factor throughout this process of adapting is hope. However, she proceeds to clarify that hope is not a static state but an everchanging, multifaceted component which each person must define for himself at a given moment in time.

George Engel

As Dr. Ross's stages of dying have become the acceptable framework within which to view the dying patient, George Engel's stages of grieving are the usual framework within which one views the response of the bereaved. Grief is seen as a wound, a gaping hole in an individual's psyche. Grieving or bereavement is the healing process. Initially shock, disbelief, and denial predominate as the bereaved seek to minimize the assault by recognizing the reality gradually. As awareness develops, anger, anguish, and crying mediated by cultural mores become evident. The work of grieving is intimately bound to the funeral rituals which emphasize the reality of death, the need for help, group support, and identity with the deceased. The psychologic work of bereavement is to resolve the loss, abandon the dependence on the deceased, and begin new relationships. The success of this process can be assumed when the bereaved has the ability to remember comfortably and realistically both the pleasures and the disappointments of the lost relationship."[8]

Colin Parkes

As a result of his studies of bereaved individuals, Dr. Parkes has identified symptoms which are associated with pathologic, delayed, or prolonged resolution of the grieving process. These include (1) extreme expressions of guilt, (2) assumption of the symptoms of the deceased, (3) delay of the onset of grief for longer than two weeks, (4) additional crises in close temporal relationship with this loss, (5) previous excessive grief and depression, (6) a high degree of psychologic reliance on or ambivalence toward the deceased, (7) unexpected, untimely death, and (8) a culture which prevents expression of the multitude of feelings elicited by this event.[9]

PRINCIPLES APPLIED TO CARE OF THE DYING

Many other qualified authors have written of the process of dying, and the selection of those summarized and listed in the references attests to the bias of the authors as well as to their objective merit. It is from the works summarized that the authors have gained insight into their own behavior and that of their patients, and it is from this base that practice was begun and is continued.

The Patient

Counseling or nursing the dying patient/family cannot occur without caring. Caring about the patient as an individual human being worthy of the investment of oneself is prerequisite to the development of a beneficial relationship. Only in proportion to what the nurse is willing to give of herself to the patient can the patient safely give of himself into the nurse's hands. Dying is a unique and frightening experience, and an individual is not likely to derive much comfort or direction from one whom he cannot trust. It is often not appreciated that in a relationship with a dying patient, the contract between the patient and the nurse assumes that the nurse-therapist will act as protector and guide on this last and most unique journey of the patient's life. If the patient is to confront and solve the problems attending the dying process, including increasing dependence and decreasing autonomy, he must feel safe in surrendering varying amounts of himself. Only in an atmosphere of trust and caring where he is assured that his worth is a reflection of his humanity, not of some unpredictable external characteristic, can this be encouraged and facilitated.

So closely linked to caring that it is difficult to relegate it to second place is continuity of care. Ruth Abrams has written that during the stage of progression of his illness, the patient is unable to relate to anyone other than the physician—the healer.[10] It is the authors' belief and observation that this need not be true. The patient who is dealing with the fact of progression of his illness, increased symptomatology, and the commencement of decline often lacks the emotional resources and energy to engage in the testing process which precedes the development of a therapeutic relationship. He does, however, have the need and the ability to continue an already tested and trusted supportive relationship. It is therefore a high priority that patients whose cancer is not cured be followed from hospital to home and back to the hospital or clinic by a single caring person with whom the patient can continue to interact. The physician frequently cannot assume this role. Time, education, the need to maintain some distance from the person to whom he must do objectionable things, and accepted doctor-patient roles all impede this type of relationship. By means of a system which brings the visiting nurse into the hospital to become part of a relationship already established between the clinical nursing specialist and the patient and which continues the contacts among these three individuals whether the patient is hospitalized or at home, a relationship can be maintained throughout that period previously considered not amenable to therapeutic intervention. At this time, as at any time in the patient's illness, good physical care is the best psychologic care. Possibly the prepared nurse has an advantage over the psychologist or social worker because she is in a position to relieve pain, change position, alter the environment, or change an ostomy appliance while assessing, teaching, counseling, supporting, or listening. An example of one such patient may clarify this point.

Mrs. K, a young mother of six, entered the hospital in hepatic coma from metastatic reticulum cell sarcoma, which had previously been diagnosed as psychosomatic arthritis. Mr. K was angry—very angry! Initiation of chemotherapy produced amazing improvement. After two months of hospitalization, Mrs. K was to return home. She had talked of dying, of the care of her children, of her feelings of inadequacy, and of her inability to cope with altered self-image. Her family remained angry. Mrs. J, the visiting nurse who was to assume responsibility for nursing care of Mrs. K after discharge, visited her in the hospital before discharge. During these visits, she was able to talk with Mrs. K and Mr. K within the framework of a relationship which they had developed with the clinical nursing specialist. They already accepted this relationship as caring, understanding, accepting, and beneficial to them. Problems and questions regarding the need for visits, the functions of the nurse, and finances were discussed and clarified.

Following discharge Mrs. K stopped talking about cancer and dying and became withdrawn and depressed over the loss of her hair, weakness, and her inadequacies as a wife and mother. She could neither tolerate her dependency nor mobilize enough strength to exert herself independently. Mr. K's anger persisted. It now focused on her current physician and what Mr. K perceived as the absence of both quantity and quality in his wife's remaining life. The physician, in response to this constant barrage of hostility, considered referring the patient to another oncologist.

The visiting nurse, the clinical specialist, Mr. K, and Mrs. K developed a plan to begin to deal with these interacting problems. The clinical specialist was present for Mrs. K's biweekly visits for chemotherapy. The visiting nurse arranged one of her visits for the afternoon following chemotherapy. This assured Mrs. K the presence of a supportive person during the stressful event of receiving the hated medication without the angry outburst precipitated when Mr. K tried to stay with her. The home visit after chemotherapy allowed Mr. and Mrs. K to ventilate their fears, angers, and frustrations, and specific measures to control nausea, vomiting, and pyrexia were initiated and evaluated. Information and alterations in the therapeutic regimen were transmitted to Mrs. J, the visiting nurse, who in turn clarified and helped implement these over the following two weeks. Mrs. J and the clinical specialist compared observations weekly as needed, and with the help of Mr. and Mrs. K revised the plan of care as indicated. For six months this routine continued. Except for the outpatient visits, Mrs. K related exclusively to Mrs. J. Mr. K's angry outbursts decreased. Mrs. K became involved once again in some of her prized activities. The subject of dying, the quality of life, and the care of her children again became major topics of conversation between Mrs. K and Mrs. J.

Suddenly Mrs. K was hospitalized with hematemesis and melena. The bleeding could not be controlled, since once again there were gross hepatic metastases. Much of what happened the last week of Mrs. K's life was relevant only in the context of the conversations she had had with Mrs. J over the previous months. Mrs. J visited Mrs. K and her family in the hospital during that last week. The primary relationship, however, was between Mrs. K and the clinical specialist, and between Mr. K and the clinical specialist. The emphasis at this time was on helping Mr. K find some measure of the acceptance that Mrs. K had achieved. The day before Mrs. K died, Mr. K was able to say he sought no revenge, he thanked all who had loved and helped his wife, and he was content to sit quietly by her side holding her hand until she slipped from a coma into death. Mrs. J visited Mr. K several times later. There are many problems in raising a young family without a mother, but the prospects for the future are far better than anyone would have predicted.

Not every hospital can arrange this degree of continuity, nor does every patient require it. This was an extremely difficult family. Their total rejection of all health-related personnel combined with simultaneous high dependency needs created a situation which demanded a conscious effort to remain caring, to listen in order to meet their needs as they perceived them. The results when this degree of communication and coordination have been required have surpassed expectations. It seems that the patient fuses the person of the visiting nurse with that of the hospital-based clinical specialist, saving immeasurable effort in having to relate to two different persons. In response to this, the two nurses must exert every effort to assure consistency, to enhance this phenomenon, and to minimize the demands on the patient so that he can use his waning energies to deal with the problems of living until death.

How a given institution or a given nurse is extended to provide this kind of continuity must vary with the situation. Essential is that these facts are recognized and an effort made to allow for their implications: (1) one cannot assess the home environment from the hospital setting, (2) patients who are very ill have limited ability to develop even those relationships which are in their own best interest, and (3) fear of abandonment (alienation) is often a fear greater than the fear of death itself.

Assignment of a primary-care nurse or nurses has been proposed as a method of assuring caring and continuity in the hospital setting. Return of a chronically ill patient to the same unit and the same primary nurse(s) would be one way of capitalizing on an already existing relationship. Certainly one of the merits of an oncology unit is that patients return to a familiar setting which they know is supportive. Experience has shown that giving a patient or family a phone number and a name (in writing) to contact with any questions, fears, successes, or just to talk has immense value. Most never use the number. Those who do so use it judiciously.

Jeanne Quint Benoliel has summarized what the authors have been trying to say.

> As a result of my work with patients facing death, I have come to define personalized care as having three components. First, each patient has *continuity of contact* with at least one person who cares for him as a human being. Second, the individual is provided with *opportunity to know* what is happening and to *participate in decisions* affecting how he will live and how he will die. Third, the recipient of services has confidence and trust in those who are providing care.[11]

Knowledge and skill play a major role in the relationship between a nurse and a dying patient. Not only is it necessary to know what the physician has told the patient, but the nurse must also have a good working understanding of the natural history of various types of cancer. In some settings a comatose hypercalcemic woman with multiple sites of osseous metastases, might be considered terminal. Yet the nurse with knowledge of the natural history of breast cancer, the available therapies, and the information from the patient's history that this lady had never received any treatment beyond mastectomy five years previously could hardly consider that she was working with a terminal patient. To help a patient and his family cope with the reality of a terminal illness, the nurse needs to know how to differentiate chronic illness from terminality. If the patient and his family are encouraged to begin the final process of decathexis too soon, the problem of a patient who is socially dead while very much physically alive can occur. This may seem to be a radical example, but with cancer, where death is instantaneously associated with the diagnosis but where the disease is characterized by remissions and exacerbations, the likelihood that either the patient will live beyond his social death or that denial of terminality will develop is high.

Basic nursing skills are necessary to minimize symptoms and to allow the patient the atmosphere and the time in which he can complete his unfinished business. Pain should never be allowed to intrude, nor should indignities against the person assault this progressively more helpless human being. Control of pain, control of elimination, control of odor, cleanliness, and rest equal basic humane care. The rights of a dying patient are clearly outlined in ''The Dying Person's Bill of Rights'':

The Dying Person's Bill of Rights*

I have the right to be treated as a living human being until I die.

I have the right to maintain a sense of hopefulness however changing its focus may be.

I have the right to be cared for by those who can maintain a sense of hopefulness, however changing this might be.

I have the right to express my feelings and emotions about my approaching death in my own way.

I have the right to participate in decisions concerning my care.

I have the right to expect continuing medical and nursing attention even though ''cure'' goals must be changed to ''comfort'' goals.

I have the right not to die alone.

I have the right to be free from pain.

I have the right to have my questions answered honestly.

I have the right not to be deceived.

I have the right to have help from and for my family in accepting my death.

I have the right to die in peace and dignity.

I have the right to retain my individuality and not be judged for my decisions which may be contrary to beliefs of others.

I have the right to discuss and enlarge my religious and/or spiritual experiences, whatever these may mean to others.

I have the right to expect that the sanctity of the human body will be respected after death.

I have the right to be cared for by caring, sensitive, knowledgeable people who will attempt to understand my needs and will be able to gain some satisfaction in helping me face my death.

*This Bill of Rights was created at a workshop on ''The Terminally Ill Patient and the Helping Person,'' in Lansing, Mich., sponsored by the Southwestern Michigan Inservice Education Council and conducted by Amelia J. Barbus, associate professor of nursing, Wayne State University, Detroit.

Each individual has certain strengths which can be drawn upon even during the process of dying. So often emphasis is placed on losses, weaknesses, and deficits to the exclusion of the inherent strengths. At times it is very difficult to identify any positive aspect or strength in the situation, but seldom is there no such aid available. The family may be rejecting, the outlook may be bleak, and physical symptomatology may be difficult to control, but the patient's religious beliefs may be a potential source of strength and consolation. In this age where many reject established religion, we often fail to recognize the value which traditional religious beliefs have for some individuals at times of crisis. Often just listening is sufficient to allow a patient to draw on his own deep faith and beliefs. At other times praying with a patient or reading appropriate religious materials may help a person whose faith is currently insufficient to provide much support and comfort but who indicates a need and desire to rely on this aspect of his life. For some, life after death, union of their suffering with the suffering Christ, or growth and purification through suffering answer the question "Why me?" and lead to peaceful acceptance. However, this is a process within an individual and not something which can be imposed from without. Despite her own convictions, a nurse should have minimal difficulty supporting a person's need for religion, beliefs, and strengths if the principles of individualized assessment and capitalizing on assets are remembered. And in the words of the Reverend Trevor Baskerville,

> When you feel that you have provided all the spiritual consolation you can, when you have listened as long as you can, when your sensitivity to the patient's feelings have grown dull, when you feel that acceptance of the patient is beyond you, do not hesitate to call the chaplain or the patient's minister, who, perhaps, is more skilled and experienced.[12]

The Family

Throughout the following section, reference is repeatedly made to the family or to the family member. Who is this family? Obviously a family may be composed of any number of individuals from the elderly childless couple to Grandma Smith, the matriarch of a closely knit clan of 10 children, 50 grandchildren, and 22 great-grandchildren. What of the retired railroad conductor whose dog, King, is his constant companion and guardian? What of Miss Jones' college roommate of three years who has enjoyed a relationship equal to that of sister? It has been proposed that with increased social and geographic mobility and the subsequent reduction in the size of the basic family unit, friend-friend relationships have developed to the point where they must often be considered equal in magnitude to traditional intrafamily relationships. Certainly the legal relationship among relatives is different from that among friends, but grief is not proportional to legal ties but to psychic and emotional bonds. It behooves the nurse who relates to the families of dying patients to recognize the existence and magnitude of a variety of relationships. In the following paragraphs, when referring to family, the authors also refer to these special friends who are emotionally if not biologically related.

One biologic relative who, though not forgotten, is often specifically excluded is the child. Children are barred from the hospital to protect them from pathogens and to shelter them from the sights of illness and death. The closer they are emotionally to the dying person the more strict is their exclusion by the family. How irrational is all this well-meant protection! It is recognized that an adult may need to vent his feelings about the death of his friend or relative. How much more is this needed by a child who has less sophisticated defenses, more vivid imagination, and more dependent ties to the dying patient? This well-meant protection of the child does him no favor—soon reality will thrust the facts upon him. To whom will he turn then—those who lied to him, those who could not help him? What will they say to him now? Far better that he be prepared, that he understand with as few irrational fears as possible, and that he be part of a caring, compassionate group whose common bond is love for the deceased and a need for the help of one another.

Knowledge of the patient and his family, their concerns, fears, needs, and their relationships with one another are the guideposts which define the nurse's role with a given dying patient. Unresolved guilt, fears, promises, previous experiences, and interactions affect how each person views what is happening. In order to help the patient and his family it is necessary to begin to see the total situation as each of them sees it. The patient, his wife, his son, and his friends may have very different perceptions of what is transpiring. Because of these different perceptions, they possess different goals and different expectations. To assist them to draw closer to one another, to help one another, and to comfort one another requires respect for and understanding of these differences. That one can never completely understand as another person understands does not free one from the responsibility for trying. The error of prejudging the patient or his family members is often prevented simply by listening quietly while they express their feelings about what they are experiencing.

> Mr. T, who visits his dying wife for only five minutes a day when he has no other commitments, who flirts with the nurse, and who shows no signs of grief, can easily be judged as an unloving, uncaring, and unfaithful husband. This judgment, in turn, elicits anger from the staff in proportion to their positive feelings for his dying spouse. A brief conversation may reveal a totally different story. Mr. T cannot bear to look at his once beautiful wife now emaciated and jaundiced. The guilt generated by this revulsion makes each visit more difficult. Mrs. T does not want him to see her as she is and constantly tells him to leave. Each visit is torture for both and endured only for appearances. Mrs. T's withdrawal from the family had precipitated their grieving several months earlier, and Mr. T already accepts his wife as "gone."

To fail to assess these factors would lead to setting unrealistic goals, choosing inappropriate interventions, inflicting unnecessary stress on the patient and her family, and frustrating everyone concerned.

The needs of the people involved with dying patients are diffuse. Only by eliciting their individual evaluation of what is happening, what will happen, what they want, and what they fear can realistic plans be drawn. Is it more traumatic for a mother to watch a son convulse from hypoxia secondary to lung metastases or to stand in the hallway alone while strangers rush in and out of his room? Is there a way to make even such a traumatic death less mechanistic? Are the procedures of suction, sedation, and oxygenation worthwhile for the family if not for the patient? Is it better for the elderly gentleman to stay in the room with the body of his wife to await the funeral director, personally handing over his spouse of 30 years, or to leave her to be cleaned, wrapped, and taken to the morgue? Training, hospital policy, and personal sentiment are resorted to in answering these questions. Seldom is the mother asked which actions she would prefer or the elderly spouse asked his preference. Can these situations be handled in such a way that the final moments need not be a set of prearranged procedures and techniques? There are no universal answers. The patient and the family have the right and often the need to make these decisions with all of the knowledge, counseling, and help that can be provided.

What do families need at this time? How can a nurse hope to be of help at such a time? The situation itself is catastrophic. The outcome cannot be changed. What can a nurse contribute which would be more than insignificant? Most often it is not the total crisis to which the bereaved are reacting. It is often the very insignificant which matters. The isolation, this moment's unspoken fear, an unanswered question, guilt, exhaustion, hunger, pain, boredom, or frustration—these are the factors which contribute to the catastrophe of dying. These are some of the problems that a prepared nurse can help the family cope with on a day-to-day basis. At the same time, the relationships which develop aid in dealing with the more pervasive problems of grief, loneliness, and the practical problems of adjusting to a new life after the patient dies.

Being there, saying only what another human being prompts one to say, or saying nothing communicates a great deal. The extreme isolation imposed on the dying patient is imposed on the family as well. Rather than physical withdrawal, the family will likely be inundated by well-meaning friends and professionals seeking to "take their mind off it." The presence of one kindred spirit who can quietly and courageously confront the dying experience with the family can do more than a million well-meant distractions. At times compassionate presence is all that is required. However, the nurse needs to be attuned to the fact that most families are experiencing generalized anxieties, specific fears, or unanswered and often unanswerable questions. Expressing these fears and questions helps to rid them of some of their terror and aids in developing a perspective or philosophy which is appropriate to the individual at this time. The nurse needs to be cautious that she does not project her concept of the questions and fears the family *should* have. On the other hand, she should not hesitate to discuss the range of normal fears, the universality of ambivalence, and common questions in the course of a conversation with the family if she perceives that they may be reticent to acknowledge such feelings and are suffering an additional burden because of this reticence.

Realistic guilt is another matter. It is not the province of the nurse to minimize or dismiss a person's feelings of guilt. What she can do is to help the individual look at the guilt as objectively as possible and then to help him explore acceptable methods of resolving the guilt if this is feasible. Often a frank conversation between the patient and the family member can relieve much realistic and unrealistic guilt on both sides. Though one often thinks of this kind of encounter in terms of an open awareness framework, even the patient and family who cannot confront the reality of death may be able to be honest with one another in terms of "the changes in our lives," "this sudden illness," or "seeing you sick has caused me to think about. . . ."

Despite the fact that the authors previously criticized the practice of trying to divert the family, diversion does have an important role to play. No family member can sit at the bedside of a dying relative 24 hours a day. A method for assuring regular reprieve from this intense situation needs to be discovered. At times this may mean that a nurse volunteers to sit with the patient or give care usually given by a member of the family. This provides the family with the opportunity to get away, to breathe freely, to recharge their emotional batteries, and to talk with one another. This time is especially important if children are involved. The relative needs to have time to relate to the child and to help the child begin to understand what is happening. Children are brave and wise when given the chance. Kept uninformed and protected, their imagination and guilt can paint a more terrifying picture than any reality. Parents are uncomfortable trying to prepare a child for the acceptance of death, and their reticence is reinforced by societal mores. The nurse can be helpful to parents by (1) encouraging them to express their feelings, (2) acquainting them with information regarding the value and necessity of preparing the child, (3) assisting them in finding ways to tell the child, even by role playing, and (4) being available to the parent and the child for further support.

It is important to recall that family members have needs which have nothing to do with the patient and which the devoted relative may be ignoring. These can include the need for nourishment, rest, medication, special diet, activity restrictions, or medical supervision. The nurse can help the family members as individuals and the family as a group to acknowledge not only the existence but the acceptability of these many needs. She may also be of assistance in formulating a plan to meet these needs. Obviously what are realistic solutions when a patient is deteriorating rapidly from cerebral metastases are not viable solutions when the patient's dying is prolonged. The family needs to be recognized as the client also. Every effort should be exerted to identify, plan, implement, and evaluate care in terms of their individual physical, psychologic, spiritual, educational, social, and financial factors as well as those of the patient. The exact method of intervention depends on many variables. For hospital nurses, the most difficult (and the crucial) step is recognizing the family as a valid client with a right to service and care.

In the hospital all family members are outsiders. This fosters frustration—the frustration of helplessly watching a loved one die without being able to do a single thing while strangers bustle efficiently about doing many things. Even in the home, where the care of the sick is woman's work, men are frequently prevented from actively engaging in caring for the dying person. Both in the hospital and at home, all interested parties—male, female, child—can have their need to do something recognized and at least partially met. Each is a unique person whose merit lies in his unique capabilities. A man can often lift, turn, and move a patient more easily than can a smaller woman. He can engage in the diversion of a man-to-man conversation with the male patient. A child can help change a bed, draw a picture, or give a big hug. Even the family who perceives the role of the nurse doing all for the patient may find it to their own benefit to become involved. The most commonly uttered phrase at the bedside of a dying patient is ''if only I could do something!'' Too often the professional caregiver is misled into thinking that these words are always a shortened form of ''if only I could do something to prevent his death!''

In our society few people have seen death. Many have never even seen a lifeless body. It should not be surprising that the image frequently held of death is the theatrical view of a person sitting upright crying for help or mercy, then strangling and falling lifeless to the bed. It is almost always necessary to discuss with the family how death will occur. This is especially important when a single family member keeps the night vigil or when the patient goes home to die. It is necessary to explain what one can expect death to be like for this person—those things which may occur that require some action (for example, consistent difficulty swallowing or choking requires cessation of oral feedings), and those symptoms which may occur for which there is no action (for instance, Cheyne-Stokes respirations, cyanosis, or even convulsion or hemorrhage if these are likely). Every effort needs to be made to prepare the family for what they will encounter without unduly increasing their innate fears. Next to being alone with the patient at the moment of death, most people express the fear that something will happen to hasten the loved one's death and that the family member will be responsible. Many also fear that they will desert the loved one in his time of suffering. When families include medical personnel, it is often assumed that this giving of information and correcting of misconceptions is superfluous. In most cases one can assume that their fears and misconceptions are as great as those of the less medically sophisticated.

What of the bereaved after the patient dies? Should these clients be forgotten, as so often they are? How much better it would be if the bereaved felt free to return to the nurse who helped them with their anticipatory grief to receive additional aid in working out their bereavement. Again the task sounds insurmountable until the component tasks are analyzed. The nurse can assure the bereaved of the normalcy and necessity of grief and the other strange feelings experienced. She can serve as a resource for those times after the initial period of grieving when others have returned to normal life and the bereaved is supposedly doing well. She can help the bereaved recognize that anniversaries and certain special days pose a problem of reactivated grieving, and she can help plan for these periods. She can assess when grief is becoming a threat to the emotional health of the individual and refer him to a self-help group (such as Theos*) a family counseling agency, the appropriate clergy, or a mental health center. In summation, as she did before, she can listen and she can care.

The Nurse

What of the nurse? How does she cope with her dying patients? Who assesses and helps her meet her needs? How does she deal with her grief? For years nurses have been cautioned not to get "too involved." Efforts have been made to differentiate between empathy and sympathy. Lists of therapeutic responses and behaviors have been distributed and are constantly being requested by nurses in threatening situations. The problem with each of these ways of coping is that it consists of building walls to avoid potential problems. To help dying patients, the walls which isolate nurse from patient must be removed. Nurse Johns can give Mr. P a bath, get his pain pill, and change his soiled colostomy bag. Mary Johns, R.N., a human being, can care about Mr. P as a person, assess his needs, support his worth and individuality, counsel his family, and mourn his death. How much Mr. P requires emotionally and physically of Mary Johns depends on his needs. How much Mary can give depends on her as a person and on her needs at the moment. Arbitrary standards are very difficult to set.

Not every nurse is capable of caring for terminal patients. To expect this of every nurse is to relegate person-to-person interactions to the level of technical skills. The complexities of human development prepare individuals who have a variety of capabilities. Each is worthy for his own area of expertise. It is impossible to say that for a nurse to be able to care for dying patients she must possess characteristics A, B, X, and Z. Possibly all that can be said is that a nurse who can succeed in the care of the terminally ill is one who is comfortable being a person caring about another person in a nursing situation. She is capable of receiving satisfaction from helping that person deal with a very difficult problem, not in herself achieving any predetermined goal.

Some nurses cry with almost every patient. Some rarely cry. Crying itself is neither unprofessional and improper nor a measure of the value of a relationship. Caring and giving are the essential behaviors. The appropriateness of the behaviors which manifest this caring can be measured only within the context of a given relationship based on the norms and the personalities of the persons involved. Grief is the response to the loss of someone or something which is valuable or worthwhile, someone or something about which one cares. When one has known and cared about a patient, grief is inevitable when he dies. Acceptance of

*Theos is a group of young widows and widowers who help one another with the process of grieving. Headquarters is Penn Hills, Pennsylvania.

this feeling of loss as part of the cost of knowing and caring for another human being is the first step in dealing with these feelings. Group support and evaluation is the next valuable component. Whether this group support is provided as structured therapy or unstructured meetings in response to need is not important. That it occurs and is accepted and promoted is vitally important. Nurses involved in the day-to-day care of dying patients can be tremendously supportive to one another. However, in this high stress environment, it is also essential that administrative and supervisory personnel recognize the emotional and physical demands made upon these nurses and give them the recognition and support they deserve. This support needs to consist of more than a passing ''keep up the good work, girls!'' Duty time set aside for professional development, staff input into management decisions, regular rotation to a less stressful environment, and professional counseling are methods suggested by various experts in the field of cancer nursing. Basic to all of these methods is the acceptance of the nurse's feelings as a human being.

Being able to leave death and dying and go on to living is also important to the nurse's emotional health and continued value in working with dying patients. This does not mean that when a particular patient with whom one has been working suddenly worsens, a family member has not been to visit, or a problem develops, one goes off duty without a thought to the patient. Such is not possible. Often a phone call to see if the problem has been resolved, asking the help of another nurse on duty, a talk with an in-tune friend, or a good cry are the order of the day. One of the gifts the dying patient gives his nurse, if she can accept it, is a new respect and love for life and living.

As comfort and expertise in caring for dying patients develop, certain problems can arise for the nurse. First, one tends to abbreviate the assessment process based on generalizations formulated through experience. One must constantly remind oneself that only by validating one's assumptions with each and every patient can their validity be assured. (Possibly 99 percent of the time a patient wants to be relieved of pain. What of the one patient who cherishes the pain as a sign that he is still alive!) Second, self-confidence comes with experience, and certainly the comfort it brings is beneficial. Too much self-confidence can lock one into a set pattern of response. Too much confidence in a list, a pattern, stages, or a particular technique breeds habit and routine. When something becomes too habitual it loses its individuality, its person-to-person quality. Third, meeting one's own needs must always be considered. Only through adequate self-gratification is one able to give to another. So often one acts without sufficient thought to one's own needs. Without forethought, these unmet needs can interfere with the perception, interpretation, or fulfillment of the patient's needs. As one becomes comfortable with dying patients, the need for self-evaluation and insight is less urgently felt. It is when one cares the most about a patient that one must be most careful about a thorough assessment, individualized care, and self-evaluation.

Basically all of these problems for the nurse are part of the overall problem of patient care—setting realistic goals and implementing acceptable interventions within the operational limits. In working with dying patients, initially the crucial issue is accepting the inevitability of death and the value of realistic goals of living within this limit. Later the problem becomes one of accepting the restriction imposed by the abilities, wishes, and resources of the patient and his family, the acceptable alternatives, and the day-to-day weaknesses and limits of oneself as a nurse and as a person.

References

1. Michaelson M: The love that lights the last days of a brave young mother. Todays Health, December 1971, p 49–53; "The Lyn Helton Story." Film. New York, American Cancer Society, 1972
2. Glaser BG, Strauss AL: Awareness of Dying. Chicago, Aldine, 1965
3. Brim O, Freeman HE, Levine S, Scotch NA: The Dying Patient. New York, Russell Sage Foundation, 1970
4. Quint J: The Nurse and the Dying Patient. New York, Macmillan, 1967
5. Weisman AD: On Dying and Denying. New York, Behavioral Publications, 1972
6. Schoenberg B, Carr A, Peretz H, Kutscher AH (eds). Psychological Aspects of Terminal Care. New York, Columbia University, 1972
7. Ross EK: On Death and Dying. New York, Macmillan, 1969
8. Engel GL: Grief and grieving. Am J Nurs 64:94, September 1964
9. Parkes CM: Bereavement. New York, International Universities Press, 1972
10. Abrams R: Not alone with Cancer. Springfield, Ill, Thomas, 1974
11. Benoliel JQ: Care and cure: problems and priorities. Paper presented as part of program, Quality of Survival and the Cancer Patient. University of Pittsburgh School of Nursing–Western Pennsylvania Regional Medical Program, Pittsburgh, June 13, 1973
12. Baskerville MT: Another Dimension of Care: Spiritual Consolation. Proceedings of the National Conference on Cancer Nursing. Sponsored by the American Cancer Society, Sept 10–11, 1973. Chicago, American Cancer Society, 1974, p 49

Bibliography

Abrams R: Not Alone with Cancer. Springfield, Ill, Thomas, 1974
Aquilera DC: Crises: Death and dying. ANA Clinical Sessions 1968. New York, Appleton, 1968
Avorn J: Beyond dying. Harper's, March 1973, pp 56–64
Barclay V: Professional Education Audio Tapes for Nurses, No. 3100–3103, American Cancer Society, 1973
Benoliel JQ: Talking to patients about death. Nurs Forum 9:255–268, 1970

Bowlby J: Grief and mourning in infancy and early childhood. Psychoanal Study Child 15:9–52, 1960

Carlozzi CG: Death and Contemporary Man: The Crisis of Terminal Illness. Grand Rapids, Mich, Fermans, 1968

Cassette Program on Death, Grief and Bereavement. Univ Minnesota, Center for Death Education and Research, 1971

Domning JJ, Stackman J, O'Neill P, et al: Experiences with dying patients. Am J Nurs 73:1058–1064, June 1973

Epstein C: Nursing, the Dying Patient. Reston, Va., Reston Publishing Co., 1975

Fiefel H (ed): The Meaning of Death. New York, McGraw-Hill, 1959

Fond KI: Dealing with death and dying through family-centered care. Nurs Clin North Am 7:53–64, 1972

Friedman, SB, Chodoff P, Mason JW, Hamburg DA: Behavioral observations on parents anticipating the death of a child. Pediatrics 32:610–625, October, 1963

Fulton R (ed): A Bibliography on Death, Grief, and Bereavement 1845–1972. Univ Minnesota, Center for Death Education and Research, 1973

————: Death and Identity. New York, Wiley, 1966

Glaser BG, Strauss AL: Time for Dying. Chicago, Aldine, 1968

Goldfogel L: Working with the parent of a dying child. Am J Nurs 70:1675–1679, August, 1970

Gray VR: Grief. Nursing 74 4:25–27, Jan 1974

————: Dealing with dying. Nursing 73 3:26–31, June 1973

Griffin JJ: Family decision: a crucial factor in terminating life. Am J Nurs 75:795–796, May 1975

Hiscoe S: The awesome decision. Am J Nurs 73:291–293, February, 1973

Jackson EN: Telling a Child About Death. New York, Channel Press, 1967

Kavanaugh RE: Facing Death. Los Angeles, Nash, 1972

Krant MJ: The organized care of the dying patient. Hosp Prac. 7:101–108, January 1972

Maguire D: Death by Choice. New York, Doubleday, 1974

Marino EB: Vinnie was dying. Nursing 74 4:46–47, Feb 1974

May R: Love and Will. New York, Norton, 1969

McNulty B: Care of the Dying. Nurs Times 68:1505–1506, 1972

Mervyn F: The plight of dying patients in hospitals. Am J Nurs 71:1988–1990, October 1971

Mitford J: The American Way of Death. New York, Simon and Schuster, 1963

Parad HJ: Crisis Intervention: Selected Readings. New York, Family Service Association of America, 1971

Perspectives on Dying. Costa Mesa, California, Concept Media, 1972

Prattes OR: Helping the family face an impending death. Nurs 73 3:17–20, February 1973

Quint J: The dying patient: A difficult nursing problem. Nurs Clin North Am 2:763–773, 1967

Reed E: Helping Children with the Mystery of Death. New York, Abingdon, 1970

Rinear EE: Helping patients die. Pa Nurs 26:2–8, 1974

Rinear EE: Helping survivors of expected death. Nursing 75 5:60–65, March 1975

Ross EK: Letter to a nurse about death and dying. Nurs 73 3:11–13, October 1973

————: What is it like to be dying? Am J Nurs 71:54–61, January 1971

Saunders C: Care of the Dying. London, Macmillan, 1959

Schwartz LH, Schwartz JL: The Psychodynamics of Patient Care. Englewood Cliffs, NJ, Prentice-Hall, 1972

Ujhely GB: What is realistic emotional support? Am J Nurs 68:758–762, April, 1968

Vernon GM: Sociology of Death. New York, Ronald Press, 1970

Verwoerdt A: Communications with fatally ill patients: Tacit or explicit? Am J Nurs 67:2307–2309, November 1967

Waechter EH: Children's awareness of fatal illness. Am J Nurs 71:1168–1172, June 1971

Whitman HM, Lukes SJ: Behavior modification for terminally ill patients. Am J Nurs 75:98–101, January 1975

4
Pain

Pain. Emotional pain—Physical pain. Psychogenic pain—Somatogenic pain. Acute pain—Chronic pain. Epicritic pain—Protopathic pain. Sharp pain, stabbing pain, cutting pain, burning pain, aching pain, gnawing pain, nagging pain, debilitating pain, demoralizing pain, agonizing pain, excruciating pain. You are a nurse. You have come across a lot of pain in your experiences. You have sensed it, heard it, seen it, touched it, held it in your arms, cried out because of it, and cried inside because of it. How does it grab you in your gut? What does it do to the inside of your head? You have despised it, hated it. You have attacked it, struggled with it. You have a certain respect for its awesome power, for it has defeated you and others many times. It is often the enemy of your patients and thus your enemy, too. Many times the fight against it has been successful or the battle has been brief, and you have been able to help patients to endure and to conquer the pain during this transient time. Then you have felt victorious, useful, strong, competent. At times, however, the battle has been protracted or the pain has withstood the combined power of everyone's seemingly best defenses and weapons. Then it has frustrated you, made you feel inadequate, useless, weak, incompetent, helpless, impotent. Perhaps then you have recoiled from it, withdrawn from it because you could not cope with it any longer. You avoid it in order to escape your own pain. It can be heartrending to be a powerless witness to suffering and agony, when the desperate, pleading eyes, the taut, contorted faces, the silent or audible cries of anguish call out to you, the helper, for help. But you have no more help to offer. You have exhausted your own endurance and ability to do anything more. But have you exhausted your abilities? Knowledge can be power, and power can be control. Are you sure you understand pain well enough to fight the enemy most effectively? Is it possible that some additional information, some other approach, plan, or ploy, some forgotten or new strategy might be successful in reducing the scale of the battle before it has worn on so long as to deplete and devastate?

The purpose of this chapter is to explore the facts, fiction, and facets of pain with the possibility in mind that better-armed and better-educated, we, the helpers, will be equipped more adequately to help patients in their struggles against pain in cancer and that we can perhaps help to change some of the attitudes toward cancer and to correct some of the misconceptions regarding the relationship between pain and cancer.

THE SIGNIFICANCE OF PAIN IN CANCER

The fact that some pain is usually experienced at least some time during the course of a cancer patient's illness is significant in many respects. Probably the most general and widespread importance of this association is that the concept of cancer becomes locked to the notion of pain. The only other concept which may be more universally linked with cancer is death. Most people do not make sophisticated distinctions between types of pain. Their perception of pain in cancer is that of a gruesome, horrible, uncontrollable pain which results in the worst imaginable kind of suffering. The paralyzing fear which results from this presumption adds to all the other fears people have regarding cancer and exacerbates the common emotional reactions to cancer which make efforts to conquer and control the disease so difficult. This universal linkage in the minds of people between cancer and horrendous pain is fallacious, and since it is so detrimental, we must attempt to dispel the illusion.

The pain that people associate with cancer is usually a sequela only of uncontrolled cancer, and even in far-advanced cancer, pain is often neither as prevalent nor as severe as is believed. Some cancer patients have little or no pain even in terminal stages, and there are many disorders which are commonly much more painful than most cases of cancer. Even when pain does become a severe problem in cancer patients, avenues of treatment are numerous and should be sufficient to control it. The health professions may have been at fault in the past for making less than the most vigorous attempts to completely alleviate severe pain in cancer patients. Thus they may have contributed a sizable share to present misconceptions. But this form of neglect has been and is changing and, hopefully, so is public understanding of the nature of pain in cancer.

People should understand that there is nothing inherent in a neoplasm itself which causes pain. That is why pain is usually only a late symptom of cancer. This message now seems to have been conveyed to the public, but it serves to create anxiety about pain itself. Pain, if related to or believed to be related to cancer, may be heralded as an indication of a late stage of disease and thus a sign of incurability or hopelessness. This is not necessarily so, either. Whether or not cancer ever causes pain and the point in the person's illness when cancer does cause pain depend on the location of the tumor, the stimulation of pain-sensitive fibers by a variety of processes, and other physiologic, pathologic, psychologic, and sociologic phenomena. Not all of these things relate entirely to the stage of the person's disease or the degree of curability. Discussion of the terminology of pain, the physiology of pain, and the mechanisms of pain in cancer should help clarify some of these statements.

TERMINOLOGY OF PAIN

Pain is an elusive term to define. It is a sensory and a perceptual phenomenon and, as with all such phenomena, is very subjective. Pain is relevant to a wide variety of disciplines which define it according to their own particular viewpoints and interests. Theologians, philosophers, behaviorists, physiologists, neurologists, and many others would all add different facets to the meaning of pain. There is not sufficient time to consider all of these here, so, for the purposes of this chapter, a basic, primarily physiologic definition of pain is used to delineate the kind of pain most often dealt with. Accordingly, Sternbach defines pain as

> An abstract concept which refers to (1) a personal, private sensation of hurt; (2) a harmful stimulus which signals current or impending tissue damage; (3) a pattern of responses which operate to protect the organism from harm.[1]

This definition of pain serves for the academic discussion of pain in this chapter, but for purposes of an operational definition of pain in the clinical setting, Margo McCaffery proposes one which allows clinicians to rise above all the disputes and come to grips with pain on the level where it really belongs in these situations, with the people who are suffering. Thus the authors are grateful to Ms. McCaffery for defining pain so workably, so simply, and so succinctly by stating that "Pain is whatever the experiencing person says it is and exists whenever he says it does."[2] It should become obvious later in this chapter why this definition works so well with cancer patients and how it avoids unnecessary hassles, particularly in far-advanced or terminal illness, where a need to assess the motives of patients claiming to experience pain is absurd. Although these two definitions of pain will serve as a basis for most of the content of this chapter, it is helpful to understand certain distinctions between types of pain.

Physical versus Emotional Pain

One of the most general distinctions between terms used to describe pain is that of physical versus emotional pain. Emotional pain arises solely from emotional bases. Probably the clearest example is seen in grief. The overriding sensations and feelings in emotional pain are different from those in physical pain, and patients know that the source of their pain is emotional. Emotional pain can, however, be as severe and incapacitating as, if not more incapacitating than, physical pain. The whole huge realm of problems related to cancer is fraught with instances and types of emotional pain, from feelings experienced by the cancer patient himself to those which families, friends, and even whole communities incur. The subject of emotional pain in cancer is, however, covered in other chapters, primarily in Chapters 2 and 3. It is recognized that emotional pain can often be manifested in some somatic symptoms, including physical pain, and the reverse is true: physical pain always has at least some emotional components. This chapter is concerned with physical pain, but some influences of emotions on physical pain are discussed.

Psychogenic versus Somatogenic Pain

Another distinction made between types of pain is psychogenic or functional pain versus somatogenic or organic pain. Psychogenic pain originates in the psyche, the seat of our emotions. Somatogenic pain originates in the soma, the body. The actual physical sensation is the same, however, in both types of pain. Psychogenic pain differs from emotional pain in that the emotional origin of the pain is unrecognized in psychogenic pain, and the painful sensation itself is believed to be the same as physical pain originating from a somatic or organic cause. Actually, the distinction between functional and organic pain is relevant only in terms of how the patient can best be helped, not in terms of whether or not the pain is real, and there are probably few situations in which pure organic pain or pure functional pain can be identified. There are usually elements of both in patients experiencing pain. The classic forms of psychogenic pain, where emotional conflict is clearly the basis for physical pain, are the conversion hysterias. Most other situations are less clear-cut. People with hysterical personalities (hysterics), for example, tend to react more intensely to organic pain, and there are other emotional processes, such as depression or close introspection, which tend to exaggerate or even initiate somatic pain.[3] Therefore, for the purposes of this chapter, it is assumed that most persons who are diagnosed and treated as cancer patients have primarily somatogenic pain.

Acute versus Chronic Pain

One other significant dichotomy in types of pain is that of acute and chronic pain. Acute pain is intense and usually occurs suddenly but subsides within a relatively short time, either spontaneously or after treatment. Chronic pain is continuous or regularly recurs for an indefinite period of time. Chronic pain which has been present over a long period of time and which has been resistant to attempted therapies is referred to as intractable pain. The sources of acute and chronic pain are often different, and the actual sensations may differ. Chronic pain is often a duller pain or ache and is more often visceral in origin. Acute pain is usually sharper, more localized, and generates from either cutaneous or visceral sources. It is important, however, to note that chronic pain can often be quite intense and fairly well localized.

Both acute and chronic pain are encountered in cancer patients. Acute pain may occur as a symptom of cancer but is most often experienced during diagnostic procedures and after surgical treatment. Chronic pain may also be symptomatic of cancer but is present most often in patients with far-advanced or terminal illness. Occasionally it occurs as an adverse effect of treatment, usually surgery or radiotherapy, which has otherwise been successful in treating the disease process. This discussion is meant to include both types of pain, although, as it will be pointed out more clearly, chronic pain is far more taxing and devastating to both patients and personnel.

When considering the nature of acute and chronic pain, the function and meaning of pain are often pondered. The common view of the merit of pain is that some types are essential and beneficial, while others are not. Acute pain does usually serve the purpose of warning the victim of existing or impending harm or damage, and few seriously challenge the benefit of this. In many instances, though, pain continues even after the danger has been removed, and in chronic diseases particularly, the alarm function seems redundant, superfluous, excessive. The pain in these situations seems to take on a purely destructive quality.

There are those who go beyond the usually accepted benefit of acute pain as a warning of harm and give even chronic pain value in a philosophic context. Some religious teachings have tended toward this higher meaning of pain in viewing it as punishment for sin or as an ordeal through which one is able to strengthen his will and his character, perhaps even find his way to God. Buytendijk gives voice to somewhat similar beliefs in his writing. He says:

> Modern man regards pain merely as an unpleasant fact, which, like every other evil, he must do his best to get rid of. To do this, it is generally held, there is no need for any reflection on the phenomenon itself.[4]

He feels that:

> A person who through his sympathy conjures up the suffering of the whole world, who is sensible to the cry of creation for release from pain, becomes aware in this *cri de coeur* that the problem of pain cannot be waived, any more than can the problem of sickness, death, evil, and sin. In each of these phenomena we sense a sinister disharmony, a conflict with the fundamental reasonableness of life. But in pain alone we actually experience a cleavage in the most natural of all organic unions—that of our personal and physical being.[5]

The shattering experience of disharmony described above "abandons us to utter senselessness; this elemental senselessness of pain drives us not only to protest, but also to seek the active cause outside the boundaries of experience."[6] Thus, "pain teaches us how unfree, transitory, and helpless we really are, and how life is essentially capable of becoming an enemy to itself."[6]

He summarizes some of his thoughts as follows:

> The nature of pain contains its significance. "Vitally" speaking, it is without sense, nor has it any bearing on psychic functions. Its meaning is existential, therefore ontological and metaphysical. . . . Its purpose is fulfilled in the attitude which the man who is afflicted by it adopts to his own bodily existence, to himself and to the ground of his being in the world, to God.[7]

Whether or not the realizations which Buytendijk describes are indeed basic aspects of the human condition or just certain perceptions which result from unique or special circumstances shall not be debated here, nor shall the implications that pain is the only pathway to the awareness Buytendijk discusses. Whether or not one sees these consequences of pain as either necessary or beneficial is a matter of opinion, but it cannot be denied that chronic pain does often have some of the effects described above, and nurses should be fully aware of them. These and other effects of chronic pain will be elaborated further in a later section. It is important for health professionals to be in touch with their own beliefs and feelings about pain, for these influence the way they react to patients in pain. It is equally important to be aware of the variable and personal meanings pain has for the persons experiencing it. Conflicts arise when the helpers and the afflicted hold opposing or mutually exclusive views. Ideally, it would seem that medical people should strive to help patients attain their own goals within the context of their own needs and beliefs. Some patients might consciously choose to endure pain for a variety of reasons, while others would strive to eliminate it at any cost. It seems unfortunate to these writers that we so often impose our own values upon patients without attempting to determine how well they coincide with those of the patient. Or even when we do abide by the patient's values, we tend to judge them. The stoic may be seen as stubborn or stupid, or he may be highly respected and revered. The person who wishes to avoid pain at any price may be seen as cowardly or unmanly, or he may be seen as manipulative, cunning, and smart. It is difficult to avoid judging patients on the basis of our own values, for we are human, too, and we have our needs and beliefs, but we are in a helping profession, and few of our patients are grateful for the help which is imposed against their wishes or for the feelings they get when it is offered with negative judgments.

PHYSIOLOGY OF PAIN

Nurses who have a basic understanding of the prevailing theories regarding the origin, transmission, and recognition of pain can anticipate patients' pain in certain circumstances and can offer, at times, explanations to patients or sound information which may assist them in coping with pain. Knowledge of the basic physiologic aspects of pain may also equip nurses to alter some of the variables affecting the pain experience, perhaps to the extent of alleviating the pain. And, of course, nurses cannot grasp the basis for treatment nor explain as much to patients without this background. In the interest of time and space, only that material related to the physiology of pain which is considered essential for the implementation of the above-stated functions and goals is presented.

Several theories which explain various aspects of the physiology of pain have been proposed, but points of all these current theories are still disputed, and none seems fully adequate in incorporating all the presently available data regarding pain. Three categories of pain theories will be explored in this section: specificity theory, based on concepts proposed by von Frey, pattern theory, based on Goldscheider's work, and Melzack and Wall's recently expounded gate control theory, which attempts to reconcile the inadequacies of the older theories as well as elucidate additional evidence regarding the mechanisms of pain.

Somatogenic pain begins with a physical or chemical stimulus capable of exciting sensory receptors and of sufficient intensity to initiate an impulse which will ultimately be consciously recognized as pain. The source of these noxious stimuli may be external or internal. Heat, pressure, and other types of trauma may be observable external physical causes of stimulation, while pressure, anoxia, or inflammation may be inobservable, internal sources of stimuli for pain. These sources of stimuli seem to result in pain when the integrity of cells or tissues is threatened. When cellular damage is impending, certain chemicals are released. These chemicals in turn are believed to stimulate sensory receptors, which initiate an impulse which is transmitted directly via sensory somatic afferent neurons or indirectly through visceral afferent fibers in sympathetic nerve trunks to the posterior root ganglion, as illustrated in Figure 4.1 The cell bodies of all sensory nerve fibers are in the posterior (dorsal) root ganglion. Fibers conducting pain impulses then leave the posterior root ganglion by way of the posterior root, which carries both motor efferents and sensory afferents, and enter the spinal cord, where they are transmitted to the brain by mechanisms and tracts to be discussed in the following sections.

Various substances have been implicated as the chemical mediators responsible for exciting pain receptors, including histamine, plasma kinins, lactic acid, acetylcholine, 5-hydroxytryptamine (serotonin), and potassium and hydrogen ions. It is likely that several of these substances are involved in the production of most pain.

Specificity Theory

In the specificity theory, pain is explained as a primary sensation, such as sight or hearing, with special peripheral receptors, neuronal transmitters, and receivers in the central nervous system. The pain pathway is seen as a straight-through

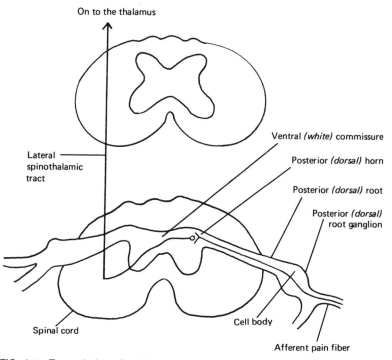

On to the thalamus

Ventral *(white)* commissure

Posterior *(dorsal)* horn

Posterior *(dorsal)* root

Posterior *(dorsal)* root ganglion

Lateral
spinothalamic
tract

Cell body

Spinal cord

Afferent pain fiber

FIG. 4.1   Transmission of pain from peripheral fibers to the lateral spinothalamic tract.

transmission system, where the intensity of pain perceived is directly related to the intensity of the stimulus applied. Peripheral pain receptors are believed to be specific nociceptors which are distinct from other main groups of sensory receptors (mechanoreceptors and thermoreceptors). This theory maintains that free nerve endings are the nociceptors. These nerve endings generate impulses carried by specific nerve fibers (pain fibers), which are the A-delta and C fibers in peripheral nerves. These fibers carry the impulse of pain primarily to the lateral spinothalamic tract in the anterolateral part of the spinal cord, although some impulses do seem to travel via the ventral or anterior spinothalamic tracts. The spinothalamic tract then transmits the impulse to a pain center in the thalamus.

This theory obviously does not account for the vast discrepancies which exist between the intensity of stimuli present and the perceptions of pain which result. Although it is commonly believed that the receptors excited by intense, noxious stimulation are specialized to respond to these particular kinds of stimuli, it is debated whether or not stimulation of the receptor must always elicit pain and only the sensation of pain.[8] In regard to the supposed specialized fibers which conduct the impulse, it is also possible that a small number of fibers may exist that respond only to intense stimulation, but, again, this does not necessarily mean that they produce pain and only pain when stimulated. There is unquestionable evidence that certain spinal cord tracts and other central nervous system pathways carry most impulses related to pain. This does not necessarily mean that they therefore comprise a specific pain system. Melzack and Wall place the specificity theory in the following perspective:

> Physiologic specialization is a fact that can be recognized without acceptance of the psychologic assumption that pain is determined entirely by impulses in a straight-through transmission system from the skin to a pain center in the brain.

Pattern Theory

Pattern theories of pain arose as a reaction against the deficiencies of the specificity theory. These theories stress stimulus intensity and central summation as the critical determinants of pain. Melzack and Wall relate the history of these theories, as described below:

> Goldscheider proposed that the large cutaneous fibers comprise a specific touch system, while the smaller fibers converge on dorsal horn cells which summate their input and transmit the pattern to the brain where it is perceived as pain. Other theories have been proposed, within the framework of Goldscheider's concepts, which stress central summation mechanisms. Livingston was the first to suggest specific neural mechanisms to account for the remarkable summation phenomena in clinical pain syndromes. He proposed that intense, pathological stimulation of the body sets up reverberating circuits . . . in spinal internuncial pools that can then be triggered by normally non-noxious inputs and generate abnormal volleys that are interpreted centrally as pain.[10]

Melzack and Wall also describe a theory related to theories of central summation which proposes that:

> A specialized input-controlling system normally prevents summation from occurring, and that destruction of this system leads to pathologic pain states. Basically, this theory proposes the existence of a rapidly conducting fiber system which inhibits synaptic transmission in a more slowly conducting system that carries the signal for pain. These two systems are identified as epicritic and protopathic, fast and slow, phylogenetically new and old, and myelinated and unmyelinated fiber systems. Under pathologic conditions, the slow system establishes dominance over the fast, and the result is protopathic sensation, slow pain, diffuse burning pain, or hyperalgesia.[10]

Although the above concepts of pattern theories do help to explain many clinical aspects of pain, the association of fiber type and size with a particular pain modality is not well supported. The smaller, unmyelinated nerve fibers (C fibers) are known to conduct impulses at a much slower velocity and seem to have a higher threshold for excitation than the larger, myelinated fibers (A-delta fibers), but beyond this their relationship to specific types of pain is unclear. It is, however, now commonly accepted that "temporal and spatial patterns of nerve impulses provide the basis of our sensory perceptions. The coding of information in the form of nerve impulse patterns is a fundamental concept in contemporary neurophysiology and psychology."[11]

Gate Control Theory

Psychologist Ronald Melzack and physiologist Patrick Wall were the originators of a theory which incorporates substantiated portions of both groups of older theories into one which purports to better account for presently available evidence regarding pain mechanisms. Their gate control theory has had a valuable heuristic effect, even though many have received it with careful skepticism, and some have offered strong points of refutation.

The gate control theory proposes that the perception of and reaction to a pain-producing stimulus applied to the skin are the result of interplay between three systems within the spinal cord: (1) cells within the substantia gelatinosa (SG) in the dorsal horn of the spinal cord, (2) central transmission cells (T cells) in the dorsal horn, and (3) afferent fibers in the dorsal column of the cord (Fig. 4.2).

The SG cells act as a gating mechanism which controls the transmission of afferent signals to the T cells. The impulses which are the output from the T cells

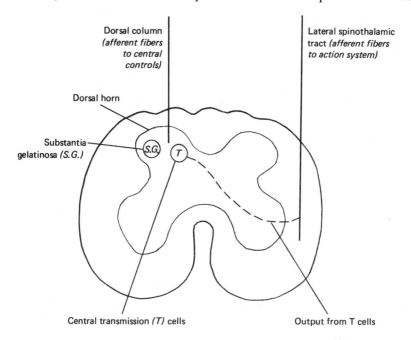

FIG. 4.2. Anatomic location of gate control mechanisms in the spinal cord.

cross the spinal cord to the side contralateral to the side innervated and ascend, mainly via the spinothalamic tract in the anterolaterel part of the cord, to the brain centers comprising the action system, which is responsible for pain perception and response. The crossing of the pain fibers to the contralateral side of the cord does not occur entirely at the level of the entrance of the impulse into the spinal cord but over a large area which may extend two to four segments superior to the entry point. Some pain-carrying fibers may ascend or descend in the ipsilateral side for several centimeters before crossing to the contralateral side.

There are two major brain systems which seem to receive output from the dorsal horn T cells. As illustrated in Figure 4.3, anterolateral fibers project impulses by way of the spinothalamic tract into the somatosensory thalamus and by way of the paramedial ascending system to the limbic midbrain area and medial thalamus. In

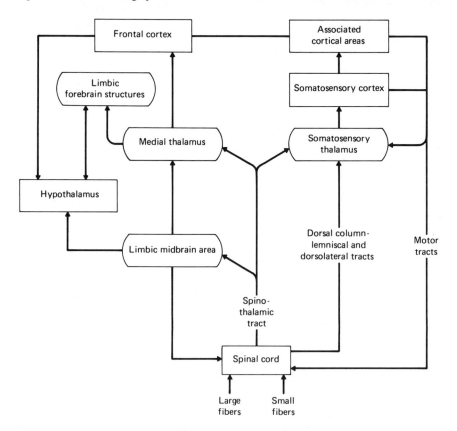

FIG. 4.3.   Schematic diagram of the transmission of output from T cells to the various areas of the brain and the interrelationships of ascending and descending fibers. (Adapted from Melzack and Casey: In Kenshalo (ed): The Senses: Proceedings of the First International Symposium on the Skin Senses, 1968, p 430. Courtesy of Charles C Thomas, Publisher, Springfield, Illinois.)

addition to these areas affected by output from the T cells, fibers in the dorsal column project impulses by way of lemniscal and dorsolateral tracts into the somatosensory thalamus and cortex.[12] The paramedial system leads to reticular and limbic structures which affect the powerful motivational drive and unpleasant effects that trigger the organism into action. Neospinothalamic and lemniscal paths lead to the somatosensory thalamus, where the location and dimension of the painful area are registered and consciously recognized, and on to the cerebral cortex, which affects evaluation of the input in terms of past experience and exerts control over activities in both the discriminative and motivational systems. These three categories of activity are presumed to interact with one another to provide perceptual and cognitive information regarding the pain and the motivational tendency toward it.

The third system involved in the interplay within the spinal cord involves afferent fibers in the dorsal column of the cord. Signals which reach the spinal cord are apparently transmitted to both the SG cells and to these fibers. Afferent signals which reach these fibers bypass the gating mechanism (the SG cells) and are transmitted directly to central controls. There they activate selective brain processes which result in transmission of descending signals to the spinal gate (SG cells). These return impulses then influence the modulating properties of the spinal gate (SG cells) and may have either an excitatory or an inhibitory effect. These descending messages account for the influence of numerous variables which seem to affect the pain experience. These variables, discussed more fully in a later section, include such things as attention, memory, conditioning, the meaning of the pain, and other emotional factors. The gate control theory thus accounts for their effect on the reaction to pain by incorporating them into the sensory perception of pain. To summarize, the two factors affecting the gating mechanism (and thus the transmission of pain impulses to higher centers) are the above-described signals descending from the brain and the afferent impulses reaching the spinal gate from the periphery.

The postulated effect of afferent impulses on the spinal gate has thus far proved to be the most therapeutically useful aspect of the gate control theory. Afferent impulses reach the gate by way of large-diameter and small-diameter fibers, illustrated in Figure 4.4. It seems that large-diameter fibers can be selectively stimulated by electrical impulses (also touch, vibration, message, and other stimuli) because they have a lower threshold for excitation than do small-diameter fibers. Small-diameter fibers are believed to conduct at least some cutaneous pain signals. The gate control theory proposes that impulses traveling over large-diameter fibers excite SG cells, which in turn exert effects which serve to inhibit further transmission of impulses from other fibers. Impulses from small-diameter fibers interfere with the above inhibitory effects and thus serve to enhance transmission of signals to the T cells; they open the gate. Furthermore, efferent impulses descending from the brain add another effect on the gate, which may be either excitatory or inhibitory, as previously described. Thus, as can be seen,

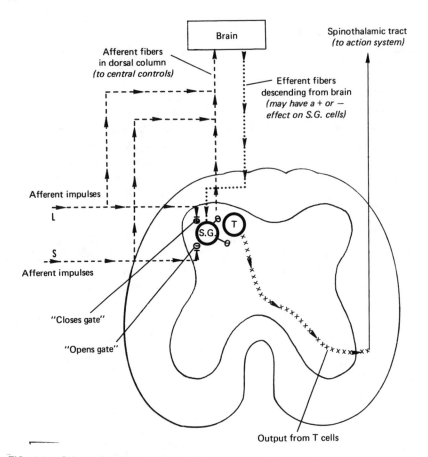

FIG. 4.4. Schematic representation of the gate control theory. (L large-diameter fibers; S small-diameter fibers; + excitatory; − inhibitory)

output from the T cells depends on a very complex combination and interaction of effects based on the number of active afferent fibers and their rate of firing, the ratio of input from large-diameter and small-diameter fibers carrying afferent impulses, and the activity of brain centers. The signal which ultimately triggers the action system in the brain occurs when the output from the T cells reaches a critical level.

The gate control theory provides a rationale for the ability of nonpain-producing stimuli to decrease the perception of pain-producing stimuli.[12] Several clinical applications of this concept will be discussed in the section on treatment of pain.

Pain Threshold

One sensory concept of pain which seems to be generally misunderstood has to do with pain threshold. Under normal circumstances, pain threshold follows the usual pattern of other senses: pain will be perceived in response to a noxious stimulus only when that stimulus reaches a critical intensity which is strong enough to elicit pain. The level of intensity of a stimulus which is required to cause pain is called the pain threshold. Contrary to widespread belief, the pain threshold seems to be quite similar for most people, other variables being constant. What does vary among persons is their pain tolerance, defined under experimental conditions as "the duration of time or the intensity at which a subject accepts a stimulus above the pain threshold before making a verbal or overt escape response."[13] As generally used, it alludes to a person's ability or disposition to endure pain. Thus, it seems that most persons feel pain at the same level of intensity of a stimulus (under controlled conditions), but their reaction to it shows a wide range of differences. These concepts seem to fulfill the requirements of the gate control theory.

MECHANISMS OF PAIN IN CANCER

With some understanding of the physiologic and sensory aspects of pain, one should be able to comprehend some of the mechanisms whereby cancer causes pain. The need for understanding the bases of pain in cancer has already been mentioned. One very basic fact must be firmly grasped if one is to approach pain in cancer with a realistic attitude: there is nothing inherent in a neoplasm itself, benign or malignant, which causes pain. Cancer often does cause pain, however, as a result of its characteristic properties of uncontrolled growth, invasiveness, and ability to metastasize. Whether or not pain is present in cancer, the nature of pain in cancer, and the methods of managing pain in cancer thus depend on the histologic type and the virulence of the malignancy itself, its location, and the manner in which it is affecting the tissues in which it is growing. One way a tumor may result in pain is to compress adjacent tissues and cause ischemia, obstruction, or distention. Invasion of surrounding tissues by tumor may involve actual nervous tissue itself. Pressure on and destruction of nerves, nerve roots, nerve trunks, and even the spinal cord itself may cause severe pain. Pain may also be caused by bone involvement and by the pathologic fractures which may result. Although bone itself is relatively insensitive to pain, the periosteum is very pain sensitive. Involvement of vertebrae may cause vertebral collapse with compression of nerves, roots, and the spinal cord. Involvement of lymphatics and obstruction of blood flow may cause pain from vessel distention or compression, ischemia, or stretching of pain-sensitive tissues from edema. Intestinal obstruction, which characteristically causes cramping abdominal pain, occurs frequently with intraabdominal malignancies. Extreme overfilling of hollow viscera, such as the esophagus, stomach, ureters, and bile ducts, also causes pain, presumably because of overstretching of the tissues themselves. Other causes of pain resulting from malignant growth are infection, inflammation, ulceration, and necrosis.

One must remember that tissues vary greatly in their sensitivity to pain. For instance, the lung parenchyma is almost entirely insensitive to pain, but the pleura and bronchi are quite sensitive. Other tissues which have a rich supply of nerve endings are skin and mucous membranes, subcutaneous tissue, tendons, muscles, arteries, veins, the parietal layer of the peritoneum, the ureters, the bladder, and the urethra. Tissues which are relatively insensitive to pain are the spleen, the kidneys, the visceral layer of the peritoneum, and the parenchyma of the liver. Some tissues elicit pain only in response to certain stimuli, eg, the intestines are insensitive to clamping and cautery but register pain with stretching or spasmic contraction.

EFFECTS OF PAIN

Knowledge of the effects of pain is an invaluable aid in the assessment of pain and in the overall evaluation of the patient's condition and of the actions to be taken. Pain effects can be thought of as physiologic and nonphysiologic.

Physiologic Effects

The physiologic effects of pain may be divided into short-term and long-term effects. Immediate physiologic effects of acute cutaneous pain serve to prepare the organism for a fight-or-flight reaction and include elevation of pulse rate, blood pressure, and rate of respiration, pupil dilatation, increased perspiration and muscle tension, and arousal of psychic reactions. These effects and their protective functions are shown in Figure 4.5.

Severe visceral pain may, on the other hand, slow the pulse and cause a drop in the blood pressure. Digestion and emptying of the stomach may be delayed, contributing perhaps to the nausea and vomiting often seen with intense visceral pain. Abdominal pain may result in a more costal type of respiration, while chest pain causes respirations to be more abdominal.

Chronic, intense pain may result in various debilitating physical disorders. The patient's emotional state is often a strong factor in the initiation and progression of many of these. Immobility may result from an effort not to move parts which feel pain with motion. Pressure sores, muscle weakness, inadequate circulation, constipation, and even contractures may ensue. Lack of motivation, extreme fatigue from lack of sleep, and weakness often contribute to immobility. Later sequelae of prolonged immobility may include decalcification of bones, with osteoporosis and formation of renal calculi. Nausea, fatigue, inactivity, and depression may all be factors in the extreme nutritional depletion which is often seen in patients with protracted pain. Poor hygienic practices, again often resulting from summations of weakness, apathy, and inactivity, may combine with poor nutrition in causing unhealthy conditions of the mouth, skin, and perineum. The

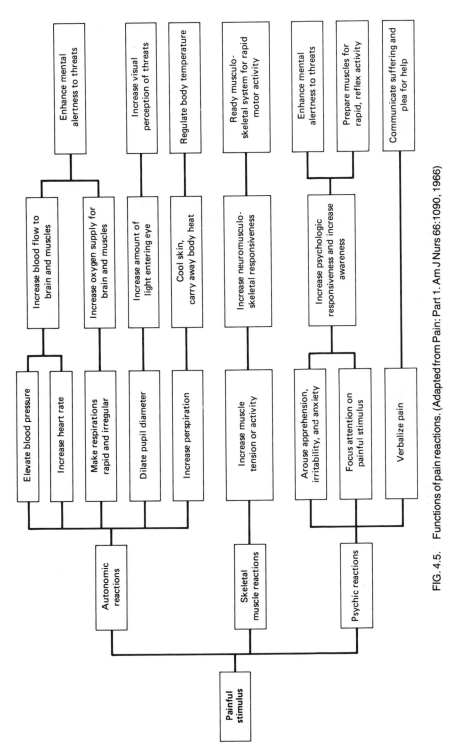

FIG. 4.5. Functions of pain reactions. (Adapted from Pain: Part 1. Am J Nurs 66::1090, 1966)

patient's general appearance may be very unappealing. This often serves to further reduce morale, unless, of course, despair has already reached such depths that the patient does not care about his appearance or hygiene any longer.

Nonphysiologic Effects

It is obviously impossible to separate physiologic effects of pain from the emotional effects, but alterations in patterns of living and in ways of perceiving existence which invariably occur in patients who suffer long-standing pain can be discussed separately. Chronic pain may drain financial resources if it requires costly treatment, as it usually does. It may greatly disrupt personal and family relationships for various reasons—financial strain, inability to function in roles previously played, and changes in emotional outlook. Values, too, may change for people who experience chronic pain. The changes are often somewhat similar to those seen in grief. People who have suffered greatly in one form or another may come closest to what is elemental in their life, and they may have no concern with what they see as trivial, superficial aspects of human existence. They may see through the complexities of their being, their life, into what is most meaningful to them. Once the suffering and memories of it have receded, they may revert back to their older perspectives, or they may be permanently changed by their experiences. At times these effects may be interpreted as good, at other times as bad. If the pain can be tempered in time, a state of inner peace and calm may have been achieved through the realization and retention of what is actually important in life. If, however, the anguish wears on too long, the person may be embittered, defeated, and destroyed by it.

The person's focus of attention is another sphere which nearly inevitably changes in chronic pain. Sternbach describes the narrowing which takes place:

> We cannot place a psychologic distance between ourselves and the hurt, and we are not merely threatened, but invaded and occupied. It is not any longer a matter of *having* a body that has a hurt member, but we *are* a body that is almost entirely pain. The pain is insistent, and crowds out all other feelings, ideas, and perceptions. It persists, exhausts us as though we had fought, and lost, a strenuous battle.[13]

The patient with this type of pain may have no other interest; the pain may become a consuming problem which completely dominates his life. The poem quoted below is a firsthand, bitterly agonizing expression of this invasion and occupation of the whole person by pain.

It's pain I want to talk about—
Not the searing of chicken-frying spatter
Or cold stab of knife in stale dishwater.

Or when the child within you smashes
   and tears for release.
Even that ends.

I mean the kind you eat with, walk with, lie with—
That sits, vulture-hunched on your shoulder.
And won't go, won't go, won't go away.

He lives in your room and eats at your place
And steals your soft cool pillow and your sleep—
What sleep there is.
He talks on in that agonizing flat voice
   long after lights are out.
And you die for sleep.

Turn away, shut your eyes, ignore him if you can.
He'll shout in your ear and drum on your nerves
   with steel-tipped shoes.

To live with pain is to ask release from other loves.
The cheerful lie, "Yes, better—better—"
Is stopped at your lips
And the shrew within you screams
   "Alone—Leave me Alone."
Alone with my jealous lover.

He'll desert some day—but only when oblivion
   seduces me.
Or I can leave him—but only to go on to nothingness,
With black moist earth on my lids
And soft green mold in my ear.
Not yet will I submit, but when I do *you'll* never know
For death does not cry in pain or bloodless lips scream
Pity.
And stiff hands write no poems.[14]

Le Shan also writes in absorbing detail of the "*universe* of the patient in chronic pain."[15] He compares it quite convincingly with the universe of the nightmare. He sees these similarities as:

> (1) Terrible things are being done to the person and worse are threatened; (2) others, or outside forces, are in control and the will is helpless; (3) there is no time-limit set, one cannot predict when it will be over.[15]

Thus, "the patient lives during the waking state in the cosmos of the nightmare."[15] Le Shan notes, as does Buytendijk, that chronic pain seems utterly senseless to most patients in our culture, and he feels that this weakens the ego. This lack of perceived meaning of pain in our antimetaphysical culture may cause us to see a senselessness in the universe, which "weakens our belief that our efforts have validity and point."[15] Pain further weakens the ego, Le Shan feels, because it reduces our connection to and our interaction with the environment. He explains this as follows:

> Time and space are the basic framework for our exchanging energy with the cosmos and thus replenishing the strength of our psychic coherence. Pain weakens our relationship with this framework. There is a pulling to the center, a centripetal force that brings our energies and our consciousness into ourselves and away from all else and all others. . . . There is a real loss of time perspective in pain—we are pulled to the immediate. The intensity and duration of the stimulus bind us to it. Our libidinal energy is pulled back from its objects and used as a defensive wall against the pain. However, this shift of the libido increases our focusing of attention on the pain and thereby makes it fill our life-space to a greater degree and reduces our ability to deal with it. The lost objects can no longer sustain us and help us maintain our inner integrity and sense of being, purpose and meaning. Pain permits personal existence to continue with little assistance from our usual orientation, defenses, safeguards, and associations. . . . In the loud loneliness of pain, only our existence is real. We float alone in space, conscious only of the suffering.[16]

Le Shan states that these reactions press us strongly toward a psychic regression, and we return to the body image, the feelings, helplessness, and dependency of childhood. A similar belief by Sternbach is noted later in this chapter in the section dealing with personality as a variable in the total pain experience (p. 64). Other problems in cancer, such as depression, malnutrition, fatigue, and general debility, may enhance this deterioration of self. Physiologic and emotional depletions and alterations caused by protracted pain will, however, vary from person to person, probably depending on personality differences, life styles, and the beliefs and other support systems unique to the person.

Patients in pain need support and encouragement. The first step in alleviation of pain is to instill confidence in the patient that every effort will be made to help him realize his goals for pain relief. One must then assume responsibility for fulfilling this commitment. *Staying,* combined with a demonstrated ability to manage the pain effectively, are requisites in this commitment. Benoliel and Crowley present these concepts in their paper on pain and discuss what this requires from the work setting. They note that:

> To stay requires a deep conviction of the worth of what one is doing and an awareness of the help one can bring. The maintenance of such an approach is almost impossible in settings which are organized around cure as the prime goal. Providing person-centered care in such situations involves both recog-

nition of the strains involved and a strong support system for the staff. The capacity for staying means being able to give with no guarantee of return. The patient who is in pain and the patient who is terminally ill are in a limited position to provide feedback that makes one feel good about what one is doing. A strong support system can help to make up for this.[17]

VARIABLES IN THE TOTAL PAIN EXPERIENCE

Now that some of the basic biologic aspects of pain have been discussed, it is necessary to consider some other variables in the total pain experience. Many writers separate the pain experience into two components: a sensory or perception component and a reaction component. The reaction component consists of all those variables other than noxious stimuli which influence the overall pain experience of an individual. These influences are responsible for the divergent responses to pain which are seen.

Ethnic Factors

Many studies have verified that cultural and ethnic factors affect the pain experience. The classic study in this area is Zborowski's work on responses to pain in Jewish, Italian, Irish, and "Old American" groups of patients. In the Jewish and Italian patients, he concluded that:

> As both cultures allow for free expression of feelings and emotions by words, sounds, and gestures, both the Italians and Jews feel free to talk about their pain, complain about it, and manifest their sufferings by groaning, moaning, crying, etc. They are not ashamed of this expression. . . . This behavior, which is expected, accepted, and approved by the Italian and Jewish cultures, often conflicts with the patterns of behavior expected from a patient by American or Americanized medical people. Thus they tend to describe the behavior of the Italian and Jewish patient as exaggerated and overemotional. The material suggests that they do tend to minimize the actual pain experiences of the Italian and Jewish patients regardless of whether they have the objective criteria for evaluating the actual amount of pain which the patient experiences. . . . Uninhibited display of reaction to pain as manifested by the Jewish and Italian patient provokes distrust in American culture instead of provoking sympathy.[18]

In the "Old American" patients, Zborowski found little emphasis on emotional complaining. Even though possibly reacting strongly, these patients tend to do it alone. To them, "emotionality is seen as a purposeless and hindering factor in a situation which calls for knowledge, skill, training, and efficiency."[19] This is the type of behavior expected by American health professionals. Patients who do not follow this pattern are seen as deviants, hypochondriacs, and neurotics.

It is interesting to note that the similar responses manifested by the Jewish and Italian patients do not reflect the same underlying attitude toward pain. The Italian attitude is characterized by a "present-oriented apprehension with regard to the actual sensation of pain," while the Jewish patients tend to manifest "a future-oriented anxiety as to the symptomatic and general meaning of the pain experience."[18] Thus it can be seen that ethnic factors can be significant in a patient's total response to pain. While awareness of these factors is helpful in evaluating, accepting, and understanding patients' responses to pain, it must be remembered that there is a great deal of intragroup variation among ethnic groups, and there are many other influences which affect the patient's response to pain.

Personality

Personality is a complex concept which plays a leading part in the pain experience. It has been rather convincingly argued that pain, especially chronic pain, is associated with early childhood experiences and punishment. Sternbach describes the fantasies which result from this association and feels that the following are modal for our society, even though they are not always consciously perceived:

> We examine ourselves to discover the wrongdoing which brought on the punishment, pain, and promise to do right in order to end the punishment. We act as though we are dealing with a parental figure who will harm us if we are bad. . . . There is threat of bodily harm by the punitive parent. . . . We fantasize destruction by an angry, punishing parent—a terrifying fantasy most of us in our culture have had as children. . . . As we fall back on our childhood responses and attitudes, we call for help, for the good parent to take away the hurt. We are sorry, we promise to be good, and the punishment should stop. But the hurt stays with us. It seems as though we are unloved and abandoned—the good parent does not help us.[20]

Sternbach also notes that early experiences with pain are frequently associated with separation anxiety. This results from the combination of an angry parent, punishment, and pain. The child in this situation fears the loss of the parent's love and even the potential loss of the parent. For this reason, for some persons pain may signal impending loss.

Another facet of the pain response related to personality is the way in which pain is involved in interpersonal relationships and the degree of reward associated with pain and particular responses to it. In this respect, pain may be a means of relating to and communicating with others who are important, and it may reflect a person's needs. Pain may be used to get attention or sympathy. It may be used to manipulate. Even though not consciously trying to influence others, the patient has needs, and his expression of pain often serves to satisfy these needs. Sternbach says, "The best clue to what the patient wants, and how he wants it, is to observe our own or others' responses to him."[21] Experiencing pain can, then, be rewarding, especially if it leads to sympathy, interest, affection, or other desired responses from others. Likewise, particular ways of reacting to pain may be more or less reinforced. Sternbach provides an example which illustrates how responses to pain can be rooted in interpersonal relationships with significant others:

> Consider the "nonresponder," the patient who, despite clear physiologic evidence of experiencing pain, voices no complaint. He has recently had radical surgery, and as we see him on the ward there are beads of sweat on his face, his eyes are dilated, pulse and respirations rapid, face drawn, body tense. He has not asked for any medication, and when we ask how he feels, he says, "Pretty good." "Do you hurt?" "Yes." "Badly?" "Yes." "How bad is it?" "Well, I wouldn't want it any worse." When he is given his analgesics, it is easy to see respect and admiration on the faces of the ward personnel, and deference in their behavior. It takes little imagination to see this patient as a child being reinforced for not being a "crybaby," for being somebody's "brave little man." Clearly he has little choice in his behavior; love and support, in his experience and personal phenomenology, are gifts that come wrapped as respectful admiration, and must be earned by silent suffering.[22]

Anxiety

In numerous studies it has been amply demonstrated that anxiety greatly magnifies the response to pain. In fact, many persons feel that anxiety is the major factor related to pain behavior and that the two seem to be correlates of each other. It is thus exceedingly beneficial to try to reduce the patient's anxiety as one method of altering his response to pain. There are many ways in which nurses can assist in this. Some of these are discussed or implied in the discussion of methods of treating pain (pp. 68–90).

Significance of the Pain Itself

There are several variations in response to pain that reflect the significance of the pain itself. Some types of pain are less socially acceptable than others. A headache is less of a stigma than rectal pain and is thus much more likely to be expressed. Some types of pain represent a severe threat. If the pain interferes with a person's occupation or his usual life patterns, this will be reflected in the way he reacts to it. Some types of pain are more frightening than others because of their relationship to harmful diseases.

The general relationship of pain to cancer has been discussed in the introduction to this chapter, but more should be said about the way pain is perceived in a patient already diagnosed or previously treated for cancer. The malignancy and the potential real or imagined consequences of it totally preoccupy many cancer patients at various stages of their illness. During these times, they focus intensely on their bodies and tend to attribute any physiologic alterations to effects of the tumor. Pain, or other untoward symptoms, may thus mean to them that they are getting worse, that their tumor has recurred or metastasized, or that they are approaching death. Sometimes pain does accompany these developments; other times it does not. Health professionals also tend to lean to this myopic view of pain in patients who have or have had cancer. Patients and personnel alike need, at times, to be reminded that cancer patients are prone to all the noncancer-related illnesses and pains that affect mankind, and many of these other ailments can be alleviated if they are correctly diagnosed and treated. Cancer patients get headaches, toothaches, stomachaches, muscle aches, backaches, chest pains, and a variety of other aches and pains from causes entirely unrelated to their tumors. If this is recognized, there are many situations in which fear can justifiably be reduced, and treatment may more rightfully be aimed at the appropriate cause of the pain.

In conclusion, it can be seen that a myriad of phenomena can affect a person's overall pain experience and his reaction to it. Even the same patient will not react to the same pain the same way all the time. To be optimally effective in assisting the patient in pain, the nurse must be aware of these factors. Only by combining knowledge of the sensory and reaction components of pain and the great variability in pain experiences can the nurse hope to find the best methods of understanding and handling pain in each individual patient.

ASSESSMENT OF PAIN

All the areas discussed so far play a part in the assessment of pain—a difficult and inexact task which is requisite in any attempt to alleviate pain. Nurses, who are often responsible for initiating certain forms of treatment, must, if they are humane and truly concerned, learn to be more effective in this regard. There is much incriminating evidence that they do not make full use of their skills in this area. It is difficult to arrive at a fairly realistic estimate of the type and severity of a subjective, personal, private, unique sensation in an individual who will react to pain in a manner different from all other persons. One can try, however, by observing, communicating, and correlating basic knowledge with the individual's particular needs, traits, and circumstances in mind.

Observation

There are several physical parameters which are usually indicative of pain. This is where observation comes in—observation for facial expression, body position, resistance to movement, tension in a part or parts of the body, respirations, perspiration, evidence of anxiety, restlessness, and lassitude. Checking the blood pressure and pulse may be helpful.

Communication

Although recognition of physical indicators of pain is important, verbal communication is the most essential aspect of pain assessment. If the patient does not volunteer information, he should be questioned about pain. Although it is always desirable to avoid putting words into a patient's mouth, it may be necessary to help the patient pinpoint and describe in better detail the pain he is experiencing. It seems beneficial to avoid as much as possible use of the word "pain" in talking with patients. A word such as "discomfort" is a good substitute—it does not have the same connotations that the word "pain" has, and its use prevents the association of feelings often attached to the word "pain." It also seems likely that patients might be more accepting of treatment other than pain medication if they perceive their unpleasant sensations as discomfort rather than pain. Avoidance of the word "pain" should not be carried to extremes, though. In instances where there is no doubt that the patient is experiencing excruciating pain, use of euphemisms may be inappropriate and may even alienate patients.

Recently a number of forms have been devised to enable patients to more accurately describe and quantify the pain they are experiencing. An example of one such questionnaire is shown in Figure 4.6. This form was prepared on the basis of much preliminary research.[23] It is currently being used as an experimental tool and will probably be revised, but as it now stands it is a valuable tool in assessing the patient's pain, in planning treatment, and in evaluating the results of measures instituted to control pain. Nurses could easily use this type of questionnaire with patients. Its merits are apparent.

Knowledge

The other aspect of pain assessment is knowledge—knowledge of the part of the body causing pain, how pain is transmitted, what factors contribute to it, and in what situations pain may be expected to occur. In the final analysis, though, the authors subscribe to McCaffery's definition of pain and believe that the patient's verbal report is the only reliable information about the existence of, the nature of, and the severity of pain. This does not, however, exclude other aspects of

Patients name _____   Age _____
File No. _____   Date _____
Clinical category (eg, cardiac, neurologic, etc.):   _____

Diagnosis: _____

            _____

            _____

Analgesic (if already administered):
    1. Type _____
    2. Dosage _____
    3. Time given in relation to this test _____
Patient's intelligence: circle number that represents best estimate
    1 (low)   2   3   4   5 (high)

****

This questionnaire has been designed to tell us more about your pain. Four major questions we ask are:
    1. Where is your pain?
    2. What does it feel like?
    3. How does it change with time?
    4. How strong is it?

    It is important that you tell us how your pain feels *now*. Please follow the instructions at the beginning of each part.

FIG. 4.6.A.   McGill-Melzack Pain Questionnaire, p 1.

assessment mentioned above, which may be very helpful in managing pain in cancer patients. All these factors, then, can be taken into account and related to other variables of the individual patient. Accurate pain assessment is essential in the diagnosis of pathology, in the determination of treatment, and in the evaluation of the effectiveness of measures used to alleviate pain.

TREATMENT OF PAIN

No discussion of pain would be complete without some attention to methods of treatment. In many situations, major decisions regarding treatment are made by the physician, but there are some effective measures which nurses can initiate, and patient-nurse-physician collaboration in many decisions regarding patient care seems to be gaining ever wider acceptance among health-care personnel. However, even treatment which is determined only by the physician should be understood by the nurse so that she can assist in interpreting it to the patient and in evaluating its effects on the patient.

In any type of pain, determination of the procedures to alleviate it should take into consideration (1) the immediate cause of the pain, (2) the intensity, site, mechanism, type, and probable duration of the pain, (3) the nature of the underlying disease, (4) the patient's age, physical and mental status, life expectancy, and responsibilities to his family and community, (5) the availability and practicality

Where Is Your Pain?

Please mark, on the drawings below, the areas where you feel pain. Put E if external, or I if internal, near the areas which you mark. Put EI if both external and internal.

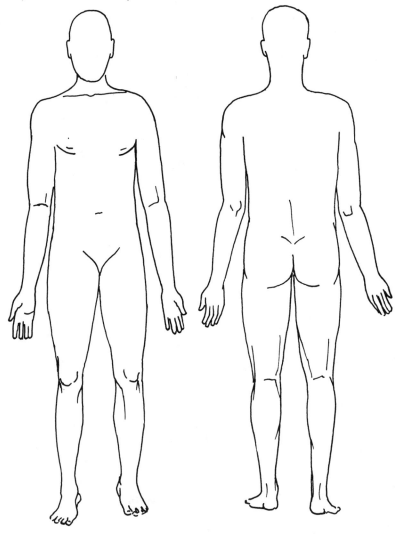

FIG. 4.6.B.   McGill-Melzack Pain Questionnaire, p 2.

of treatment methods, (6) the side effects or complications of each method of treatment, and (7) the patient's and family's values, beliefs, and preferences.

Analgesics are the most frequent type of treatment for pain in cancer, but there are many other forms of treatment which may be helpful and perhaps even more desirable in treating pain in cancer patients. As will be noted in more detail later,

What Does Your Pain Feel Like?

Some of the words below describe your present pain. Circle *ONLY* those words that best describe it. Leave out any category that is not suitable. Use only a single word in each appropriate category—the one the applies best.

1	2	3	4
Flickering	Jumping	Pricking	Sharp
Quivering	Flashing	Boring	Cutting
Pulsing	Shooting	Drilling	Lacerating
Throbbing		Stabbing	
Beating		Lancinating	
Pounding			

5	6	7	8
Pinching	Tugging	Hot	Tingling
Pressing	Pulling	Burning	Itchy
Gnawing	Wrenching	Scalding	Smarting
Cramping		Searing	Stinging
Crushing			

9	10	11	12
Dull	Tender	Tiring	Sickening
Sore	Taut	Exhausting	Suffocating
Hurting	Rasping		
Aching	Splitting		
Heavy			

13	14	15	16
Fearful	Punishing	Wretched	Annoying
Frightful	Gruelling	Blinding	Troublesome
Terrifying	Cruel		Miserable
	Vicious		Intense
	Killing		Unbearable

17	18	19	20
Spreading	Tight	Cool	Nagging
Radiating	Numb	Cold	Nauseating
Penetrating	Drawing	Freezing	Agonizing
Piercing	Squeezing		Dreadful
	Tearing		Torturing

FIG. 4.6.C.   McGill-Melzack Pain Questionnaire, p 3.

responses to treatment for pain seem to show much susceptibility to suggestion. It seems that the more confidence the patient has in the success of a particular method, the more likely it is that the method will be effective for him. Such suggestibility is claimed to be particularly operative in certain methods for pain relief which do not fit well with present Western scientific thought—acupuncture, faith healing, relief from administration of a placebo, and hypnosis.

How Does Your Pain Change With Time?

1. Which word or words would you use to describe the *pattern* of your pain?

1	2	3
Continuous	Rhythmic	Brief
Steady	Periodic	Momentary
Constant	Intermittent	Transient

2. What kind of things *relieve* your pain?

3. What kind of things *increase* your pain?

How Strong Is Your Pain?

People agree that the following 5 words represent pain of increasing intensity. They are:

1	2	3	4	5
Mild	Discomforting	Distressing	Horrible	Excruciating

To answer each question below, write the number of the most appropriate word in the space beside the question.

1. Which word describes your pain right now? _____

2. Which word describes it at its worst? _____

3. Which word describes it when it is least? _____

4. Which word describes the worst toothache you ever had? _____

5. Which word describes the worst headache you ever had? _____

6. Which word describes the worst stomachache you ever had? _____

FIG. 4.6.D.   McGill-Melzack Pain Questionnaire, p 4. (Courtesy of R. Melzack. Copyright R. Melzack, Oct 1970.)

Certain types of radiotherapy, chemotherapy, and surgery may help to relieve pain by exerting an effect on the tumor itself or on areas adjacent to the tumor. Other methods of pain relief may alter the sensation of pain, the transmission of painful impulses, or the patient's reaction to the pain.

Radiotherapy

Radiotherapy is very effective in palliating pain caused by a variety of types of localized malignancies. In certain types of malignancies, only a relatively small dose of radiation is required to dramatically relieve the most severe pain. In patients who fall into this category, undesirable side effects are seldom seen. In other types of tumors, the dosage of radiation required to successfully palliate pain may approach levels required for curative therapy. These patients will thus experience the same side effects as patients being treated for cure, and they often feel quite ill from the treatments before pain is controlled. The nurse must be aware of the intent of radiotherapy (cure of palliation) in order to help the patient maintain realistic goals. The nurse should also be aware of the total dosage and area to be irradiated in order to know whether or not to anticipate, observe for, and help prepare the patient for untoward effects. Since radiotherapy is usually effective for pain only from localized areas of disease, systemic therapy (chemotherapy) or more indirect methods of pain control (eg, analgesics, neurosurgery) must be employed for widespread pain from widely disseminated disease (carcinomatosis).

In head and neck cancers, large lesions not amenable to curative irradiation or surgery often cause pain which will respond adequately to moderate doses of radiotherapy. When a large tumor mass involves the oral cavity, patients often have either trismus or severe pain behind the mouth and ear. With these far-advanced, localized lesions, a small number of previously unirradiated patients may benefit from high dosages of radiotherapy (approaching those of attempt at cure—around 5,000 rads total dose fractionated over a period of five to seven weeks). Split-dosage radiotherapy, allowing one or two rest periods of two to four weeks during the total course of therapy, is being used more often, especially for patients who cannot tolerate the side effects inherent in the single series of daily treatments.[24]

Severe headache associated with intracranial tumors, either primary or metastatic, can occasionally be relieved by cautious, steady irradiation of the whole brain. The pounding headache occurring with the superior vena cava syndrome (superior vena cava obstruction) seen sometimes in lung cancer or lymphoma usually subsides dramatically with mediastinal irradiation.

Pain from lung lesions which involve the brachial plexus, such as Pancoast tumors (tumors extending from the lung apex), can become excruciating. Radiation therapy may be worth trying, although it is seldom significantly effective, as other measures are also rarely effective. Radiotherapy may be effective for pain from rib or chest wall involvement from lung tumors. Pain in the bony thorax caused by metastatic lesions (usually from primaries in the lung or breast) can be palliated by moderate doses of radiation, since these metastases seem to respond well to much smaller doses than do the primary tumors.

Pain due to soft-tissue involvement of the breast with ulceration and bleeding can be lessened with a rapid course of radiotherapy in moderate doses. Pain due to osteolytic breast cancer metastases to pelvic bones can be markedly alleviated in a high percentage of cases (around 80 percent) with radiotherapy delivered to the involved area in doses of 2,500 to 4,000 rads in two to four weeks. Pain due to breast cancer metastases to bones of the extremities may be relieved in over 50 percent of patients treated with radiotherapy.[24]

Radiotherapy may be helpful in the management of pain in cancer patients with abdominal involvement. When diversionary bowel surgery is definitely contraindicated in patients with gastrointestinal obstruction, radiotherapy may, under well-defined circumstances, be used in hopes of attaining some relief of the obstruction. Most patients with genitourinary obstruction from primary kidney or ureteral tumors or from lymph node or retroperitoneal cancer may obtain pain relief from radiotherapy when radiation beams can be properly focused on involved areas. Preferably, exploratory laparotomy, to assess tumor extent, and urinary diversion (skin ureterostomy or ileal pouch) are carried out before initiating radiotherapy. When splenomegaly or splenic infarctions in chronic leukemia cause acute pain, rapid relief can be obtained with rather small doses of radiation (700 to 2,000 rads in ten days to three weeks).[24]

Pain from several pelvic sources may be reduced by radiotherapy. Multiple sites of pelvic intestinal obstruction are only rarely helped by radiotherapy, but it may be worthwhile to try, since surgery is contraindicated. Rectal tenesmus in unresectable rectal carcinoma may be palliated with high doses of radiation, as may perineal recurrence of rectal cancer, where even small lesions cause great discomfort in the sitting position. Extensive bladder cancer may cause urinary tenesmus, in which case interstitial implantation of any of a number of radioactive isotopes or external supervoltage irradiation may afford relief, although urinary diversion may be required if the patient has a chronically contracted bladder and infected urine.

Pain from many types of primary bone tumors may be alleviated with radiotherapy. Painful lesions in Ewing's sarcoma and multiple myeloma can generally be relieved if selected sites can be identified. A therapeutic trial of irradiation may be worthwhile, too, in osteosarcomas or chondrosarcomas, although the chance of pain relief is not great in these lesions.

Painful lesions in other types of malignancies which may respond to radiation therapy include osteoblastic metastases to the pelvis from prostatic cancer and metastatic lesions in bones of the extremities from bronchogenic, prostatic, thyroid, or kidney cancers, and lymphomas. The dysphagia which often accompanies esophageal cancer can usually be attenuated with a palliative course of radiotherapy when cure is not possible, although, as in many situations, the treatment intensifies the symptom before relieving it.

Chemotherapy

Chemotherapy with cytotoxic drugs is less often effective than either radiotherapy or surgery as a means of treating the source of pain in malignant diseases. However, it is the only direct method available for treating generalized pain in widely disseminated diseases, and drugs given by infusion or perfusion may even be helpful for pain from some types of localized lesions. Generally the dosage of drugs required to palliate pain in cancer must be so high as to cause whatever side effects the drugs used are known to exhibit.

Pain in certain head and neck tumors may respond to infusion of chemotherapeutic drugs via branches of the external carotid artery. Combination therapy, using oral methotrexate and external irradiation, has been used in the management of pain in certain far-advanced head and neck tumors.[24]

Painful widespread osseous metastases from breast cancer may often be controlled successfully by either chemotherapy or surgery which alters sex hormones. In premenopausal patients, androgens may be administered for recurrences which appear after a well-defined sequence of surgery to remove sources of estrogen has been successfully employed. Estrogen therapy may be used for patients who are more than five years past menopause. When hormone therapy becomes ineffective for either of these groups of patients, alkylating agents, such as 5-fluorouracil (5-FU) and cyclophosphamide (Cytoxan), may be effective. More recently, other types of chemotherapeutic drugs have been used, such as some of the antibiotics, and protocols of several drugs in combination are being used often. Painful bony lesions from prostatic cancer may be reduced by the administration of estrogen in the form of stilbestrol.

In most other malignancies where chemotherapy is employed, the drugs are given to control various aspects of the disease process and not specifically to alleviate pain, although they may certainly have that specific effect if they are successful in controlling the disease. For example, severe bone pain in acute leukemia may be alleviated by chemotherapy, but the drugs are not given primarily for that purpose.

Surgery

A number of surgical techniques may be quite beneficial in relieving pain arising from the effects of various malignancies. These may be procedures aimed at the source of the pain or neurosurgical methods devised to interrupt the transmission of painful impulses.

GENERAL SURGERY.   Surgical procedures aimed at the source of pain in malignancies may include removal of the neoplasm itself (with no intent to cure) to alleviate pain due to compression, obstruction, pressure, ulceration, or necrosis. Thus, a simple mastectomy may be performed to afford pain relief from a fungating breast malignancy which is incurable. Some surgical procedures may be aimed at relief of the terribly uncomfortable effects of obstruction, such as a purely palliative colostomy in bowel cancer or a urinary diversion in cases of upper genitourinary obstruction. Surgical drainage of abscesses relieves pain. Pain caused by vertebral involvement which impinges upon the spinal nerves or cord can be relieved by decompressive surgery.

Pain from osseous metastases in patients with breast or prostatic cancer can often be controlled with a well-defined sequence of surgery and chemotherapy. The aim of such therapy is to alter the hormonal milieu in which the cancerous tissue is growing. Since the breast and prostate are both comprised of hormone-dependent tissues, this therapy can be effective in causing a regression of symptoms. In premenopausal females, removal of the ovaries to decrease estrogen production is the initial surgery. If the patient responds well to this hormonal ablation, either adrenalectomy or hypophysectomy may be performed when symptoms recur. Either of these procedures eliminates the adrenal glands as a source of estrogen production. In men with painful osseous metastases from prostatic cancer, bilateral orchiectomy may be performed to decrease symptoms by removing the source of testosterone. As mentioned earlier, once these ablative procedures have been successfully employed, further recurrences may be managed with hormone therapy and, as a last resort, nonhormone chemotherapy.

NEUROSURGICAL AND NEUROLOGIC TECHNIQUES.   A wide variety of neurosurgical and neurologic techniques have been employed in the management of pain in cancer patients. Cancer is the most common cause of pain which requires neurosurgical intervention, although neurosurgery is used for cancer patients only when the cause of pain cannot be treated directly and when the intensity and chronicity of the pain justify this form of treatment.

Much of the argument for use of neurosurgical procedures stems from the disadvantages of using medications to control pain, especially when the drugs are poorly considered and excessively prescribed, as they often are. This sentiment is expressed quite well in the following excerpt:

> Hypnotics, whilst in effect giving blessed relief, bite away a little more of the time left and many patients prefer to endure the pain rather than submit to such curtailment. It is terrible to die of pain and nowadays rarely necessary. By the term, "dying through pain," we must include patients who require such high doses of hypnotics that they spend their days in confusion and intermittent pain. Early pain relief and preservation of consciousness are the right of all dying from cancer.[25]

The neurosurgical and neurologic techniques used to relieve chronic pain are discussed in the following sections.

Interruption of Peripheral Nerves.   Peripheral nerve interruption involves destruction of somatic and autonomic sensory (afferent) and motor (efferent) fibers. There are several drawbacks to the procedure. It results in complete lack of sensation, which includes pain, temperature, deep touch, position, and vibratory senses, in the portion of the body served by the nerve. Also, some degree of paralysis and trophic changes occur with the interruption of motor and sympathetic fibers, and the pain may recur in time. This procedure is helpful only for pain localized in a small area, such as part of an extremity. Cranial nerve section may occasionally afford considerable pain relief in cancers of the head and neck.

In patients suffering from visceral pain alone, separation of a portion of the sympathetic chain, the splanchnic nerves, or both has been attempted in hopes of affording some pain relief. Sympathectomies have not, however, achieved any outstanding significance in the treatment of chronic pain.

Interruption of Sensory Roots.   Posterior rhizotomy involves division of the sensory root of the spinal nerve. It destroys transmission of all sensory modalities from the part of the body supplied by the nerve. Since severed nerve roots do not regenerate, sensory loss is permanent. The production of complete anesthesia negates the use of this procedure in treating pain in an extremity and pain in sacral segments carrying sensation from the bladder and rectum. Because of sensory overlap, one or two roots above and below the roots serving the affected body area must also be resected. This requires an extensive laminectomy.

Section of Pain Tracts.   There are a number of methods now being used to interrupt spinal and cerebral tracts carrying painful impulses in patients with diffuse, severe, intractable pain. These are usually patients with far-advanced disease. Chordotomy, or cordotomy, is a general term referring to destruction of a portion of the spinothalamic tract. Thalamotomies are procedures done to destroy certain thalamic nuclei. Other procedures include leukotomies or lobotomies, surgeries performed in the area of the cerebral cortex. The mortality rate is high for many of these procedures, and another major problem in all the chordotomies and thalamotomies is the tendency for the pain to recur. Not all procedures are even initially successful, but when they are, a large percentage of patients begin to lose initial analgesia within months after completion of the successful procedure. Loss of analgesia may proceed over a year or more to the point where the pain is equal in intensity to that which was present before surgery.

Chordotomy.   There are a number of types of chordotomy which may be performed on cancer patients who are experiencing intractable pain. These include unilateral, bilateral, surgical, and percutaneous procedures. The effectiveness of many of these procedures has been amply documented, providing that patients are carefully selected according to established criteria for the most appropriate procedure. Surgery is performed in the side contralateral to the pain, since pain fibers cross at the level of the spinal cord.

The level at which the anterolateral portion of the spinal cord (the spinothalamic tract) must be destroyed depends on the location of the pain. For higher levels of pain, higher lesions must be created. Since the level of analgesia obtained usually drops several segments postoperatively, surgery must be performed at least five to six spinal segments above the highest level of pain. For relief of pain in the lower half of the body, high thoracic tractotomy is adequate. For pain originating in the thorax, upper extremities, or shoulders, high cervical or medullary tractotomy is indicated. Since pain and temperature are the only sensations transmitted by the spinothalamic tract, other sensations remain intact after spinothalamic tractotomy. Frequent complications occur, however. They may be transient symptoms due to cord edema or permanent residuals due to cord damage. Hemiparesis on the same side as the surgical lesion may occur from effects of fibers of the corticospinal (pyramidal) tract. Involvement of the spinocerebellar tracts may cause ataxia. Bladder function and sexual function are commonly impaired, although the effects are usually transient in unilateral procedures. In bilateral procedures, most patients suffer some type of permanent impairment, which may be bladder retention or incontinence. Sexual function in males is lost following bilateral chordotomy.

Unilateral chordotomy is preferred to bilateral when the pain can be well lateralized, since there is less risk of complications with a one-sided procedure. When bilateral chordotomy is necessary, it can be performed in one stage at the thoracic level. At higher levels, two separate procedures at least several days apart are recommended, as there is a serious risk of respiratory failure in one-stage procedures performed at high levels. Sleep apnea, where respiration is normal when the patient is awake but gradually fails when he is asleep, is a dreaded complication.

The classic chordotomy is a surgical chordotomy or an open chordotomy, as it has come to be called. It is a major surgical procedure, usually performed under general anesthesia, in which a laminectomy is carried out to expose the cord. The spinothalamic tract is then surgically incised. This procedure has now largely been replaced by a nonsurgical technique known as "percutaneous chordotomy," although some neurosurgeons maintain that there are advantages to an open procedure in certain patients if the patients are good surgical risks.

Percutaneous chordotomy is the transcutaneous insertion, into the spinal cord, of a needle through which an electrode is passed to coagulate and destroy spinothalamic fibers. It is usually performed in the radiology department. A spinal needle is inserted on the appropriate side of the patient's neck just medial to the carotid pulsation until the anterior surface of the vertebral body is encountered.[26] Once the needle is believed to be in its proper place in the cord, verification of its position is obtained by air myelogram. After the target is selected, the stylet of the spinal needle is replaced by the electrode. A radiofrequency lesion generator is then used to create the lesion. A small current is given for a short period as a test stimulus. Response to this stimulus is used to confirm the proper position of the electrode. A higher current is then used to enlarge the lesion until satisfactory analgesia is obtained. The patient is conscious during the entire procedure and may experience a great deal of pain at various points in the process, especially when the dura is penetrated and when the current is delivered. The main advantages of a percutaneous rather than an open chordotomy are obviation of the need for general anesthesia and for spinal surgery. Recovery after percutaneous chordotomy is rapid, although patients must be closely observed for at least 24 hours for complications mentioned above. All necessary precautions related to a loss of pain and temperature sensation in the areas of analgesia must be explained to any patient undergoing a procedure to ablate transmission of pain impulses over the spinothalamic tract.

Destruction of Thalamic Nuclei. Lesions in various portions of the thalamus stereotactically produced by implanted electrodes have provided pain relief in some patients with widespread malignancies. However, there is controversy over the most appropriate target areas, and few centers provide enough experience in the procedure to enable stereotactic surgeons to gain the necessary skill for the detailed localization required.[27] In addition, significant sensory deficits and dysesthesias can occur, and there is a very high relapse rate (up to 50 percent or more). For these reasons, thalamotomies have rather limited application for cancer patients with chronic pain.

Ablation of Cortical Areas.   In very special circumstances, surgery may be performed on cortical areas in an attempt to manage pain. In this type of surgery, the reaction of the patient to his pain and to his overall condition seems to be altered, while his perception of the pain may remain intact. When questioned, patients upon whom this surgery has been performed may verbalize or acknowledge the presence of pain, but the pain no longer seems to trouble them.

After its initial use in psychiatric patients, frontal lobotomy or leukotomy, severance of frontothalamic projection fibers, was tried as a method of pain relief in some patients. The unilateral procedure produces fewer alterations in the patient's emotional outlook and behavior than do bilateral procedures, but both procedures cause very disturbing psychosocial changes which are ethically and aesthetically repugnant to most people. Lobotomy may still be performed, however, in very exceptional cases where life expectancy is very short, suffering and fear are paramount in the patient's existence, and all lesser procedures have been unsuccessful.

Cingulumotomy (cingulotomy) is another sensory cortical ablative procedure which may be performed in unusual cases of intractable pain in cancer patients. In this procedure, fibers transmitting messages related to pain are interrupted bilaterally in the area of the cingulate gyrus. The area to be destroyed is localized with x-ray techniques, and the lesions are completed with a stereotactic frame and a radiofrequency probe. Since there is reportedly less intellectual impairment and less interruption in affect and social response with this procedure than with a frontal lobotomy, it may have a broader range of application than lobotomy, although cases where it is the most appropriate and acceptable procedure are still relatively rare.

Regional Nerve Blocks.   Regional nerve blocks are a very effective form of neurologic intervention for treatment of pain which can be localized to a specific area of innervation. They are less effective once the patient has become addicted to narcotics. Procedures used may include unilateral or bilateral blockage of sensory segments of specific peripheral spinal nerves, intercostal nerves, or the celiac plexus. The procedure for regional nerve block is relatively simple, although it can be quite painful, but it carries some risk of complications. When spinal nerves are injected, there is some possibility of lower extremity muscle weakness and bladder or bowel dysfunction. Hypesthesia of the skin over the dermatomes or other areas blocked is expected. Local anesthetics are usually injected first to determine response. If response is good, neurolytic agents such as phenol or alcohol may be used to obtain long-lasting results. The duration of pain relief with injection of neurolytic agents is variable, averaging several months. If the block is unsuccessful, it can be repeated within a few days.

Cervical spinal blocks may be used for patients with head and neck cancers. Thoracic spinal nerve blocks or intercostal nerve blocks may be effective for patients with thoracic pain. Lumbar or sacral roots may be injected for lower abdominal or lower extremity pain. These procedures may enable control of pain arising from breast, lung, uterine, bladder, prostatic, or rectal malignancies. Management of intractable intraabdominal pain in patients with nonresectable cancers of the stomach, pancreas, liver, or gallbladder can often be achieved with a celiac plexus block.

Barbotage.   Another neurologic technique which has been successful in treating some patients with abdominal or thoracic pain due to metastatic cancer is barbotage. Through a needle inserted into the spine in the subarachnoid space at T_1 to T_6, cerebrospinal fluid is withdrawn into a syringe in 10 ml amounts, then reinjected into the subarachnoid space. This sequence is repeated 15 to 20 times. In a series of 40 cancer patients treated in this manner, 28 had good relief from pain, 6 had partial relief, and 6 were unchanged; the longest period of pain relief lasted four months.[27] When the pain recurs, the procedure can be repeated as many times as necessary, and no adverse effects have been noted. The mechanism by which barbotage relieves pain is unclear.

Peripheral Fiber and Dorsal Column Stimulation.   Application of the gate control theory to clinical relief of chronic pain has created several techniques which employ selective stimulation of large-diameter fibers in an effort to close the spinal gating mechanism and inhibit transmission of painful impulses carried via small-diameter fibers. From traditionally well known maneuvers to diminish pain, such as touch, massage, pressure, light scratching, and application of heat or cold, the gate control theory has enabled progress to more sophisticated and more effective techniques of selectively stimulating large-diameter fibers. Large-diameter fibers are more excitable than small-diameter fibers, and thus they can be selectively stimulated. Initially, mechanical vibrators were applied over painful parts. Then needle electrodes were used to apply electrical current to areas around the nerve supplying the painful part. More recently, electrodes have been implanted in the posterior columns of the spinal cord in an effort to activate many more large fibers of primary afferent neurons. Small, battery-operated stimulators and receivers are attached to the electrodes. Patients can regulate the frequency, pulse duration, and current intensities of the impulses delivered.[28] Electrical stimulation is now also applied with transcutaneous electrodes. Because roughly half of the patients treated with peripheral fiber stimulation do not receive significant pain relief, percutaneous stimulation is now used to test response before electrodes are implanted.

Electrical stimulation presently is being used in three different ways. (1) Stimulation is provided to the surface of the skin over the painful area by the transcutaneous method. (2) A peripheral nerve implant is used to apply stimulation to peripheral nerves. (3) Electrodes implanted in the dorsal column are used to stimulate fibers in the spinal column. The transcutaneous method, in which a charge is delivered through electrodes applied to the skin, is the simplest. For peripheral nerve implants, an electrode is attached to the nerve and connected to a subcutaneously implanted radio receiver. A transmitter is worn externally. The dorsal column stimulator works on the same principle, except that a major, painful surgical procedure (laminectomy) must be carried out under general anesthesia in order to place the electrodes in the dorsal column of the spinal cord, usually in the thoracic area. The location and nature of the pain determine which of these procedures might be most effective for individual patients. Not everyone with chronic pain is considered a candidate for large-fiber stimulation. A number of criteria, including an emotional profile of the patient, are used in most centers to select prospective patients.[29]

The success rate in different series of patients treated by peripheral fiber stimulation varies greatly. In one series of patients who were screened before treatment, most patients experienced a 75 to 85 percent relief of their chronic pain.[29] Stimulation causes a buzzing or tingling sensation in the area stimulated. With the dorsal column stimulator, this sensation radiates from the site of the stimulator down the spinal cord to the feet.[27] Some patients, although experiencing relief of pain, find the alternative sensations unpleasant or intolerable. Whereas the effects of one application of current to a peripheral nerve may be prolonged (up to 10 hours in one patient), the effects of dorsal column stimulation may cease with termination of the stimulus, although the requirements for control of pain by stimulation vary from patient to patient.[27] It is reported that electrical stimulation is not as effective when patients have had previous neurosurgical treatment of the pain, such as chordotomy. Drug dependence is not a contraindication for use of electrical stimulation to relieve pain. Patients who are dependent on medications are gradually weaned from the drugs as they gain confidence that their pain can be controlled by electrical stimulation.[30]

Acupuncture. Analgesia as a result of acupuncture is a mystery to Western scientists, but some persons attempt to explain its effectiveness on the basis of the gate control theory. It has not been used very much in this country to date, although American physicians are beginning to take some interest in it. Little more can be said unless and until more experience with acupuncture in relief of pain is available.

Hypnosis, Wake-imagined Analgesia, and Distraction

Hypnosis and wake-imagined analgesia (WIA) are two methods of pain control that have much in common. Both are presumed to be effective at least partly on the basis of distraction and reduction of anxiety. Hypnosis is an old technique which has been shown to attenuate pain responses in many cases. WIA is a new term for an ancient practice which has also been successful in reducing pain in many situations. In WIA the patient uses his imagination to try to recreate a previously experienced pleasant sensation in place of pain. In the strictest sense of WIA, the patient imagines the specific painful sensation as being a sensation other than painful.[2] For example, if a patient is suffering low back pain, he may imagine that someone is giving him a back rub. In a broader sense, WIA may be used to evoke pleasant or relaxing sensations of a more general nature which are not a specific substitute for the particular pain sensation or area of pain. For example, the patient may imagine that he is floating in a cool lake on a hot summer day. In both hypnosis and WIA, patients must be susceptible to suggestion. Some persons believe that WIA is essentially the same as hypnotic analgesia except for the absence of hypnotic induction and trance, and some experiments have found that hypnotically suggested analgesia appears to be no more effective than WIA in reducing pain reactivity.[31] Neither of these methods are very effective for severe, intractable pain, partly because of the intensity of the pain and the state of fatigue seen in this kind of pain. Patients must be able to concentrate with both these methods. Patients who are debilitated or physically exhausted cannot concentrate very well. However, both of these techniques may be very helpful for severe spasmodic pain, which, because of its timing and unpredictability, is difficult to manage with other methods of pain control.

Although distraction is believed to be a common element in both hypnosis and WIA, it can be used for pain control in a broader range of patients, as it does not necessarily require the patient's cooperation; it can be imposed by external stimuli. Distraction can be quite effective in reducing the patient's awareness of a painful sensation, and there are innumerable ways in which it can be used. It seems that distraction is more effective when patients are actively involved in the distraction and when as many sensory modalities as possible are utilized (sight, touch, smell, hearing). As with hypnosis and WIA, distraction is much more useful in patients experiencing pain which has a fairly well defined time limit, such as those undergoing painful diagnostic or treatment measures. It is of less value in chronic or severe pain. The more severe the pain, the more powerful the distraction must be, and not all patients are distracted by the same sets of stimuli. To maximally involve the patient in distraction, one must be aware of activities or situations that are the most exciting, interesting, or absorbing to individual patients. Watching television, reading books, or knitting are not potently distracting activities for many people! Even effective distractions need to be varied or altered after a period of time, as they lose their effectiveness if they become monotonous, boring, or tiresome.

Audioanalgesia, the use of intense auditory stimulation to reduce awareness of pain, is probably a form of distraction. Pleasing music or simply loud noises or cacophony may be used to increase tolerance to pain. This technique has been used mainly in dental practice, but it would seem to have implications for environmental aspects of patients in chronic pain.

Other aspects of the environment which capture the senses and the imagination are conducive to distraction, and pleasing surroundings may also do much to improve morale and to promote relaxation. The use of colors, objects, sights, and sounds which are interesting and soothing is recommended for patients in chronic pain. It is assumed by many that pain is often more severe at night because of the absence of any forms of distraction.

Medications

Medications in our drug-oriented culture are by far the most widely and frequently used treatment for pain in cancer patients. This seems unfortunate, for as already noted, there are numerous other treatment methods available, many of which are more direct and less harmful for long-standing pain. However, it must be emphasized that it is essential that patients have confidence in the method of pain relief employed, and many patients have confidence only in drugs to relieve pain. If it is decided, for whatever reasons, that pain should be controlled by medications, then drugs should be used wisely, intelligently, and humanely to attain the level of effects desired by the patient.

Medications may relieve pain by specifically counteracting the cause of pain, such as steroids for inflammation or antibiotics for infections, or by modifying the perception of and reaction to the sensation of pain. The pharmacology of these medications is much too involved to fully include here, but since administration of medications has largely been delegated to nurses, some general principles and some details particularly relevant to the use of analgesics are included.

Medications given primarily for the purpose of altering the sensation of pain or the patient's response to it are called "analgesics." A few analgesics are specific for certain types of pain, eg, Pyridium, which is a urinary tract analgesic, but most are nonspecific and can be used interchangeably for various types of pain. Analgesics which are opiates or opiatelike drugs are called "narcotics," and, in general, they are stronger and more effective for intense pain than are nonnarcotic analgesics. They also result in drug dependence when given over a prolonged period of time. With the present concern in American society over drug abuse, it may be helpful to clarify some terms that are loosely bandied about before considering the applicability of certain drugs in treating cancer patients in pain.

Drug abuse and drug dependence are different. Each implies a certain set of physiologic and behavioral components. Drug abuse implies the use of drugs in such a way that the effects of usage are more destructive than constructive either for society or for the individual.[32] Drug dependence, having largely replaced the older term "drug addiction," may be either physical or emotional, although some authorities prefer not to categorize the psychologic need for drugs as drug dependence.[33] As most commonly used, it refers to a state in which a person will manifest physical withdrawal symptoms when deprived of an addicting drug which has been taken over a period of time. The withdrawal symptoms are also called an "abstinence syndrome," and the exact symptoms will vary with the drugs being used. Those most commonly seen include nervousness, restlessness, fever, rhinorrhea, nausea, vomiting, muscle cramps, and increased blood pressure and respiratory rate. Psychologic dependence is defined as a craving for the drug, based on a need to alter mood or emotional outlook. It is clearly recognized that various drugs have different abuse liabilities and different potentials for either physical or emotional dependence. Drug abuse may occur without drug dependence, and drug dependence may be present without drug abuse, although the two often coexist. Rarely does one need to be concerned with drug abuse in cancer patients experiencing pain. However, the old term "drug addiction" carries associations of drug abuse, and we are plagued today in many situations with persons who assume that "drug addiction" is bad in all persons under all circumstances and is to be avoided at any cost. At present, the search for a drug that will effectively relieve intense pain with no risk of dependence has been unsuccessful, and adequate relief of severe pain with medications necessarily induces some risk of drug dependence. A general rule in using analgesics to control chronic pain is to give the smallest dose of the weakest analgesic which will effectively control the pain and to give the drug by mouth if at all possible. The patient's pathology must also be considered when prescribing the dosage and route of administration. Drugs which are detoxified in the liver, for example, may rapidly build up to dangerous levels in cancer patients with liver involvement.

A number of different chemicals are employed in pain relief. Aspirin, a salicylate, is still one of the most effective drugs available for mild to moderate pain, and it is one of the few analgesics which seems to have an additive effect when given with other analgesics, especially the narcotics. Although it is contraindicated in patients with bleeding tendencies, aspirin can safely be given in fairly large doses to many other patients. Gastrointestinal bleeding is problematic in some patients with long-term use of this drug, however. All analgesics presently classified as narcotics have similar positive and negative effects, which will be discussed later. Many narcotic antagonists are also potent analgesics and have a lower addiction liability than do narcotics, but there are other hazards associated with their use. Pentazocine (Talwin), a drug chemically related to potent opiate antagonists, has been widely used in recent years, but it occasionally causes the distressing psychotomimetic effects which occur so frequently with the other narcotic antagonists, and addiction to Talwin has not conclusively been ruled out. As with other narcotic antagonists, it cannot be administered to a patient dependent on narcotics, as it will precipitate an abstinence syndrome.

SIDE EFFECTS OF ANALGESICS. Nonnarcotic analgesics, in general, have few problematic side effects other than the bleeding tendencies noted with aspirin. When such potent narcotics as Demerol and morphine must be given, side effects begin to appear. All narcotics have similar side effects which are dose-related, and all have comparable addiction liability at equianalgesic dosages. Different individuals, however, may respond better to certain of these drugs and may show fewer side effects.

Hypotension and sometimes even cardiovascular collapse can follow administration of narcotics. Narcotics also depress respirations and the cough reflex, and they increase the possibility of lung complications, especially in older patients and postoperative patients. They do, though, allow for better respiratory exchange and effective coughing by permitting less painful breathing and coughing, especially in patients who have had major thoracic or abdominal surgery. Respiratory and circulatory depressant effects can be specifically counteracted by narcotic antagonists.

The side effect of increasing intracranial pressure contraindicates the use of narcotics in patients in whom this may be a problem. Dizziness, postural hypotension, sedation, malaise, anorexia, and constipation are other side effects which must be anticipated.

One of the most problematic side effects of narcotics is tolerance, an inevitable sequel of treating a patient's chronic pain with narcotics. Tolerance occurs when the patient requires higher and higher dosages of a drug to get the same effects. It is heralded by a shortened duration of the effect of the drug. Tolerance occurs quite rapidly with some drugs, such as morphine and morphine-related drugs. With administration of these drugs two times a day, tolerance can begin to develop in one to two weeks. The duration of tolerance, however, is also short. Following abstinence of one to two weeks, tolerance may be completely eliminated.[34]

An unfortunate fact is that there is considerable cross-tolerance among narcotics, so that switching from one to another may not solve the problem of tolerance. If the usual therapuetic dose of another narcotic is substituted for a drug the patient has been receiving in high doses, the patient actually experiences less pain relief. Even more discouraging is the fact that cross-tolerance also occurs between some nonnarcotics and narcotics. For this reason, chronic users of tranquilizers, hypnotics, and alcohol are resistant to potent analgesics.

Since tolerance to the most serious side effects, such as respiratory depression, develops simultaneously with tolerance to analgesic effects, patients who are tolerant to a drug can safely be given fairly high dosages. There is, however, a peak dosage beyond which higher dosages yield little more return in terms of pain relief. Some physicians suggest alternate administration of several different drugs to retard the development of tolerance.

Drug dependence or addiction is a risk in the long-term administration of narcotics. It is a factor which the physician, the nurse, and the patient often concern themselves with excessively. In any patient with uncontrolled or advanced cancer, the only reasonable concern should be that tolerance will develop to the point where the effectiveness of potent drugs is exhausted before the patient's life is over. Patients may needlessly suffer by refusing to take medication because of their lack of understanding about drug addiction, and in many instances nurses greatly contribute to this misunderstanding. Nurses may tell patients not to take too much medication or they will become addicted, or they may be reluctant to give drugs and may even withhold them for fear that the patient is becoming addicted. In cases of pain medications used for transient illness or surgery, drug habituation is extremely rare, and in cases of incurable cancer, the problem should be nonexistent, for the patient carries his drug dependence with him to the grave.[35] Intelligent use of narcotics at the appropriate time should obviate the need for the overzealous concern about addiction shown by many nurses.

PLACEBO PHENOMENON.   A myth about analgesics that must be dispelled has to do with the placebo phenomenon. A placebo is defined as a pharmacologically inert substance. Not infrequently, placebos may be administered to patients who do not obtain adequate pain relief from potent analgesics in order to determine whether the patient has real pain. This error is a great disservice to the patient. It is estimated that one-third of the entire patient population would respond favorably to a placebo at certain times and under certain circumstances. The degree of pain relief will vary, and a person who responds once to a placebo may not respond consistently. Patients who react to placebos often experience the same effects that they receive from drugs being given for pain, including time of onset, peak effect, duration of action, and side effects. It has been shown that placebos may actually cause changes in laboratory data. Generally speaking, patients tend to respond more to placebos given with great stimulus impact. For example, intravenous placebos are more effective than intramuscular ones, while intramuscular ones are more effective than oral placebos.[2] Researchers have been unable to observe any superficial characteristics which distinguish patients who receive relief from placebos from those who do not.

Apparently the decisive factor in obtaining relief from a placebo is confidence in the ability of the substance administered to relieve the pain. This involves the patient's rapport with his caretakers (trust), the enthusiasm with which the substance is given (suggestion), and the prior relief obtained from use of medications (classical conditioning). This certainly means that the manner in which nurses attend to pain needs to be given some thought. A positive, confident approach implying that a particular method of treatment will relieve pain may do much to insure that that method actually will work. It also seems to imply that pain medication is not the only method capable of relieving pain. Other measures tried, however, will probably be ineffective unless the patient is convinced that they will help him. McCaffery's statement aptly summarizes what conclusions can be drawn from a positive placebo response.

> Clearly it is a gross injustice to the patient to believe that his positive placebo response means he is a neurotic who has no cause to feel pain in the first place. *A much more accurate conclusion about the placebo reactor is that he very much wants to be relieved of his pain and that he trusts something or someone, perhaps the nurse, to help him obtain pain relief.*[36]

Use of placebos for pain in cancer patients is not generally recommended for several reasons. For one thing, the faith of the patient is an essential element in the success of any kind of treatment. If a placebo is given and fails to relieve pain, the patient has justification to distrust the caretakers and may suspect that they do not believe he is having pain. Once the patient's suspicion is aroused, he may begin to have doubts about other aspects of his care. Also, placebos do not solve any nursing problems, with the possible exception of tolerance and addiction. Administration of a placebo takes as much time and effort as administration of a pharmacologically active drug. There are those who advocate alternating placebos with narcotic analgesics for patients who have chronic pain to cut down on the risks of tolerance and dependence. Perhaps this is reasonable, but the authors feel that the risk of betraying trust generally outweighs any advantages of placebo administration. Nurses who cannot in good conscience administer placebos should decline to do so.

ROUTE OF ADMINISTRATION.   The route of administration of an analgesic is an important consideration. There is a definite difference in the effect achieved by various routes. Switching from one route to another without changing dosages may mean that the patient is either receiving an inadequate dose or an overdose. For example, oral Talwin is only about one-third as effective as intramuscular Talwin.[37] Oral Demerol is only about one-fourth as potent as parenteral Demerol, and oral morphine is only about one-sixth as effective as the parenteral form.[35]

Many patients seem to prefer an injection rather than oral medication for pain. This is true because often the oral dose is the same as the parenteral dose prescribed, and the patient soon learns that the oral form does not provide adequate relief. Also, the peak effect of parenteral medications usually occurs within an hour, while oral medications may not peak for several hours. However, if an appropriate dose of oral analgesic is ordered, patients may be controlled quite well orally, and there are many advantages over the parenteral route. Methadone (Dolophine), for example, is absorbed very well orally and has a long duration of effect. Several oral doses per day can be substituted in many patients for frequent injections of even very potent narcotics. Oral medications are much easier to take at home, are less costly, require less equipment, are less time-consuming to prepare, are less painful to take, and entail fewer complications. In severely thrombocytopenic patients, oral medications are mandated to avoid unneccessary hematoma formation which may result from injections administered with needles of even the smallest gauge. Oral medications are also highly desirable for severely leukopenic patients, for whom unnecessary breaks in the integrity of the skin present a major threat of infection. Most drugs, even narcotics, can be effective orally if given in high enough dosages. Table 4.1 lists commonly used analgesics and shows equianalgesic doses by the intramuscular and oral routes of administration.

One route of administration seldom used is the intravenous route, although there are instances where intravenous analgesics could be used very effectively. Patients who need to be observed closely for side effects and patients with severe pain are good candidates for this method. Side effects can be observed almost immediately after injection, with the person giving the drug still in attendance to treat the effects. Severe pain can be relieved almost immediately with intravenous analgesia, and the dosage can be titrated much more accurately to suit the patient's need. For patients who cannot absorb oral medications and who have circulatory problems which impede intramuscular absorption, intravenous administration of drugs may be a satisfactory solution. For patients who require continuous intravenous infusions, intravenous analgesics present few additional hazards and can bypass risks incurred with parenteral injections in thrombocytopenic, leukopenic, or debilitated patients.

TIMING.   Timing is one of the most essential aspects of successful pain relief with medications. It is a well-documented observation that analgesics are more effective when given before the pain becomes severe. Once pain becomes unbearable, the patient becomes more anxious and more difficult to treat. Therefore, early, adequate relief is an important principle in analgesic therapy. This knowledge could be used in many situations where pain can be anticipated, such as in painful dressing changes, so that analgesics could be given before these procedures are initiated.

PRN ORDERS.   Timing is dependent upon the protocol for administration of analgesics, and this usually involves PRN orders. The main reason for use of PRN orders is that they avoid unnecessary doses of medication. After acknowledging some value in PRN orders, one must also recognize the problems they create.

The processes involved in the use of PRN orders put the patient in a very dependent position. In almost all instances, the patient must request the medication before he receives it. This implies that the patient is in possession of sufficient faculties to do this and to make a sound decision regarding the advisability of his receiving a medication at a particular time. When a patient does request medication, he has no assurance that he will receive it promptly or even at all. He has no control over the situation; he is at the mercy of the nurse. Obviously, this must make patients feel that they must not alienate nurses or cause them displeasure, for there is always the possibility, hopefully remote, that the administration of pain medications could be used consciously or subconsciously in a punitive manner by the nurse. Then, too, the request for medication often comes when the nurse is busy and must interrupt her work to tend to it. This may foster a feeling of resentment on the part of the nurse, especially if the patient makes frequent requests. The distress of a nurse hearing frequent requests for PRN pain medications may not seem so callous if it is seen in light of the fact that she may have spent a good part of her day checking medication orders, searching for narcotics keys, and making frequent trips back and forth to the medication room for single doses of medication, each time having been taken away from some other activity.

And one must not overlook the communication problems in the use of PRN orders. The nurse often learns of a patient's request for medication from another person, usually the person providing direct care. There may have been considerable delay in the relay of this message from this person to the nurse. The nurse may herself be busy and may further add to the delay by not attending to the request

TABLE 4.1.
Equianalgesic Doses of Commonly Used Analgesics by Intramuscular and Oral Routes of Administration*

POTENCIES OF ANALGESICS EMPLOYED FOR SEVERE PAIN, EXPRESSED IN INTRAMUSCULAR (IM) AND ORAL (PO) DOSES APPROXIMATELY EQUIVALENT TO A 10 mg IM DOSE OF MORPHINE

	IM (mg)	PO (mg)	Major Differences from Morphine
Oxymorphone (Numorphan)	1	6	None
Hydromorphone (Dilaudid)	1.5	—	Shorter acting
Levorphanol (Levo-Dromoran)	2	4	Relatively high PO to IM potency
Phenazocine (Prinadol)	3	15	None
Metopon	3	18	None
Heroin	4	—	Shorter acting
Dextromoramide (Palfium)	7.5		High PO to IM potency
Piminodine (Alvodine)	7.5	—	None
Methadone (Dolophine)	10	20	Relatively high PO to IM potency
Morphine	10	60	—
Oxycodone	15	30	Shorter acting Relatively high PO to IM potency
Dipipanone (Pipadone)	20	—	None
Methotrimeprazine	20	—	Phenothiazine—unlike morphine
Anileridine (Leritine)	30	50	Relatively high PO to IM potency
Alpharprodine (Nisentil)	45	—	Very short acting
Pentazocine (Talwin)	60	180	Narcotic antagonist analgesic
Meperidine (Pethidine, Demerol)	75	300	None
Codeine	130	200	Relatively high PO to IM potency Relatively more toxic in higher doses
Dextropropoxyphene (Darvon)	240		Similar to codeine but more toxic in high doses

TABLE 4.1 (Cont.)

POTENCIES OF ORAL ANALGESICS FOR LESS SEVERE PAIN, EXPRESSED IN TERMS OF DOSES APPROXIMATELY EQUIVALENT TO 650 MG OF ASPIRIN

	PO (mg)	Salient Features
Pentazocine (Talwin)	30	Weak narcotic, narcotic antagonist, high analgesic potential, low addiction liability
Codeine	32	Weak narcotic, high analgesic potential, relatively low addiction liability
Meperidine (Demerol)	50	Narcotic, high analgesic potential, high addiction liability
Propoxyphene (Darvon)	65	Weak narcotic, low analgesic potential, low addiction liability
Aminopyrine (Pyramidon)	600	Nonnarcotic, low analgesic potential, no addiction liability, risk of agranulocytosis
Aspirin (ASA)	650	Nonnarcotic, antiinflammatory, low analgesic potential, no addiction liability or tolerance
Phenacetin (Acetophenetidin)	650	Similar to aspirin but with limited antiinflammatory properties
Acetaminophen (Paracetamol)	650	Similar to phenacetin, less potential renal toxicity
Sodium salicylate	1000	Similar to aspirin

From Houde: In Clark, Cumley, McCay, Copeland (eds): Oncology, 1970, Vol 3. Courtesy of Yearbook Medical Publishers.

immediately. The principle of early relief does not fit into this system. Solutions to these problems are not easy, but innovations should be tried in hopes of removing some of these obstacles. One solution which seems eminently reasonable is the administration of pain medications in adequate doses at specified intervals. Another hope might lie in allowing patients to administer their own medications.

One of the shortcomings of nurses in using pain medications is that they fail to use therapeutic and supportive measures along with the medication. There are many measures available to the nurse in promoting comfort and alleviating pain. Meaningful interaction alone has been convincingly shown to be effective in helping to relieve pain.[38] Improving the patient's understanding of his pain may serve to decrease anxiety and allow for more self-control. Helping the patient to find some meaning in his pain or supporting the meaning pain has for the patient may make the pain more tolerable. The meaning, however, must come from the patient; we cannot impose our own, but we can assist patients in exploring avenues by which they can arrive at their own meaning. Any measures which improve the patient's general physical and mental health will enable him to better cope with pain. Proper nutrition, adequate rest and relaxation, recognition of the need to deal with depression, and many other basic and general observations and concerns will contribute greatly to the patient's ability to respond to any measures instituted to manage pain. No attempt is made here to include all the measures the nurse might use to help relieve pain. The heart of the matter lies in adequately evaluating the pain and then using the most direct, the most effective, and the least harmful measures to obtain the level of pain relief desired by the patient.

If the concepts and facts of this chapter are kept in mind, the humane, concerned, and inventive nurse should be able to suggest and devise numerous measures to promote the comfort of cancer patients in pain. Virginia Jarratt provided the words which seem an excellent summary to this entire discourse.

> In no area of nursing practice is there more opportunity for independent action based on sound application of knowledge than in discovering the patient's particular needs for pain relief, in revealing the measures that work best for him, and in solving the problem of pain. And I submit that in no area have we overlooked our responsibilities more.[39]

References

1. Sternbach RA: Pain: A Psychophysiological Analysis. New York, Academic Press, 1968, p 12
2. McCaffery M: Nursing Management of the Patient with Pain. Philadelphia, Lippincott, 1972, p 8
3. Mastrovito RC: Psychogenic pain. Am J Nurs 74:514–59, March 1974
4. Buytendijk FJJ: Pain: Its Modes and Functions. Trans by O'Shiele E. Chicago, University of Chicago Press, 1962, p 15
5. *Ibid:* p 26
6. *Ibid:* p 27
7. *Ibid:* p 132
8. Melzack R, Wall PD: Psychophysiology of pain. In Yamamura H (ed): Anesthesia and neurophysiology. Int Anesthesiol Clin 8:3–34, 1970
9. *Ibid:* p 7
10. *Ibid:* p 9
11. *Ibid:* p 11
12. *Ibid:* p 19
13. Sternbach: *op cit,* p 63
14. McNamer PJ: Pain: terminal. Am J Nurs 70:1483, July 1970
15. Le Shan L: The world of the patient in severe pain of long duration. J Chronic Dis 17:120, 1964
16. *Ibid:* p 121
17. Benoliel JQ, Crowley DM: The Patient in Pain: New concepts. Proceedings of the National Conference on Cancer Nursing. Sponsored by the American Cancer Society, September 10–11, 1973, Chicago, American Cancer Society, 1974, p 74
18. Zborowski M: Cultural components in responses to pain. In Folta JR, Deck ES (eds): A Sociological Framework for Patient Care. New York, Wiley, 1966, p 264
19. *Ibid:* p 266

20. Sternbach: *op cit*, pp 83–84
21. *Ibid:* p 88
22. *Ibid:* pp 88–89.
23. Melzack R, Torgerson WS: On the language of pain. Anesthesiology 34:50–59, 1971
24. Gunn WG, Posnikoff J: Palliation of pain in cancer patients. GP 40:125–132, 1969
25. Hitchcock E: The surgical relief of pain. Practitioner 198:781, 1967
26. Therrien B, Salmon J: Percutaneous cordotomy for relief of intractable pain. Am J Nurs 68:2594–2597, December, 1968
27. Janetta PJ, Selker RG, Albin MS, et al: The neurosurgical approach to the relief from pain. Curr Probl Surg Feb 73
28. Sweet WH, Wepsic JG: Treatment of chronic pain by stimulation of fibers of primary afferent neuron. In Yahr MD (ed): Trans Am Neurol Assoc 93:103–107, 1968
29. Gaumer WR: Electrical stimulation in chronic pain. Am J Nurs 74:504–505, March 1974
30. Goloskov J, Le Roy P: Use of the dorsal column stimulator. Am J Nurs 74:506–507, March 1974
31. Barber TX, Hahn KW: Physiological and subjective responses to pain-producing stimuli under hypnotically suggested and waking-imagined "analgesia." J Abnorm Psychol 65:411–418, 1962
32. Dimijian G: Contemporary drug abuse. In Goth A (ed): Medical Pharmacology, 6th ed. St. Louis, Mosby, 1972
33. Eddy NB: Drug dependence. In Payne JP, Burt RAP (eds): Pain: Basic Principles—Pharmacology—Therapy. International Symposium on Pain, Rottach-Egern, Germany, October, 1969. London, Churchill-Livingstone, 1972
34. Goth A: Medical Pharmacology, 6th ed. St. Louis, Mosby, 1972
35. Rogers A: Pain and the cancer patient. Nurs Clin North Am 2:671–682, 1967
36. McCaffery: *op cit*, p 165
37. Beaver WT, Wallenstein SL, Houde RW, Rogers A: A clinical comparison of the effects of oral and intramuscular administration of analgesics: Pentazocine and phenazocine. Clin Pharmacol Ther 9:582–597, 1968
38. McCaffery M, Moss F: Nursing intervention for bodily pain. Am J Nurs 67:1224–1227, June, 1967.
39. Jarratt V: The keeper of the keys. Am J Nurs 65:69, July 1965

Bibliography

Aagaard GH: Use of drugs in control of chronic pain. Northwest Med 69:689–692, 1970
Barber TX: The effects of "hypnosis" on pain. Psychosom Med 25:303–333, 1963
Batterman RC: Pain relief with analgesic agents. DM, August, 1968.
Batzdorf U, Weingarten SM: Percutaneous cordotomy: A simplified approach to the management of intractable pain. Calif Med 112:21–26, 1970
Beecher HK: The use of chemical agents in the control of pain. In Knighton RS, Dumke PR (eds): Pain. Boston, Little, Brown, 1964
Bonica JJ: Current concepts of the pain process. Northwest Med 69:661–664, 1970
Botton JE: Neurosurgical procedures for the management of intractable pain. Clin Orthop 73:101–108, 1970
Casey KL, Melzack R: Neural mechanisms of pain: A conceptual model. In Way EL (ed): New Concepts in Pain and Its Clinical Management. Philadelphia, Davis, 1966
Copp LA: The spectrum of suffering. Am J Nurs 74:491–495, March 1974
Crue BL (ed): Pain and Suffering. Springfield, Il, Thomas, 1970

Derrick WS: The management of chronic pain. CA 23:269–274, 1973

Dickey R, Minton, J: Levadopa—Relief of bone pain from breast cancer. N Engl J Med 286:843, 1972

Drakontides AB: Drugs to treat pain. Am J Nurs 74:508–513, March, 1974

Ewing G: Pain. Can Nurs 61:443–445, 1965

Gorbitz C, Leavens M: Alcohol block of the celiac plexus for control of upper abdominal pain caused by cancer and pancreatitis. J Neurosurg 34:575–579, 1971

Hackett TP: Pain and prejudice: Why do we doubt that the patient is in pain? Med Times 99:130–141, 1971

Kolodny AL, McLoughlin PT: Comprehensive Approach to Therapy of Pain. Springfield, Il, Thomas, 1966

Lim RKS: Pain. Annual Review of Physiology. Palo Alto, Calif, Annual Reviews, 1970, Vol 32, pp 269–285

Loan WB, Dundee JW: The clinical assessment of pain. Practitioner 198:759–768, 1967

McLachlan E: Recognizing pain. Am J Nurs 74:496–497, March, 1974

Melzack R, Wall PD: Pain mechanisms: A new theory. Science 150:971–979, 1965

Merskey H, Spear FG: Pain: Psychological and Psychiatric Aspects. London, Bailliere, Tindall, Cassell, 1967

Moss FT, Meyer B: The effects of nursing interaction upon pain relief in patients. Nurs Res 15:303–306, 1966

Murray JB: Psychology of the pain experience. J Psychol 78:193–206, 1971

Pain: Part 1, Basic concepts and assessment. Am J Nurs 66:1085–1108, May, 1966

Parker RG: Pain relief for the cancer patient through selective radiation therapy. Northwest Med 69:665–668, 1970

Perret G: Management of pain in the patient with cancer. In Hickey RC (ed): Palliative Care of the Cancer Patient. Boston, Little, Brown, 1967

Pilowsky I, Bond MR: Pain and its management in malignant disease. Psychosom Med 31:400–404, 1969

Raney JO: Pain, emotion and a rationale for therapy. Northwest Med 69:659–661, 1970

Shealy NC, Mortimer JT, Reswick JB: Electrical inhibition of pain by stimulation of the dorsal columns. Anesth Analg 46:489–491, 1967

Siegele DS: The gate control theory. Am J Nurs 74:498–502, 1974

Stravino VD: The nature of pain. Arch Phys Med Rehabil 51:37–44, 1970

Uihlein A, Weerasooriya LA, Holman CB: Percutaneous electric cervical cordotomy for the relief of intractable pain. Mayo Clin Proc 44:176–183, 1969

Wall PD, Sweet WH: Temporary abolition of pain in man. Science 155:108–109, 1967

Wang RIH: Pain and principles for its relief. Mod Treat 5:1083–1093, 1968

Wilson CB: Surgical control of pain in the cancer patient. Oncology 23:44–48, 1969

5
Infection

Infection is probably the most significant cause of morbidity and mortality in cancer patients, yet it is an area sparsely represented in nursing literature. Although a complex and frequently perplexing field, it is one with many major implications for nursing practice.

The severity of an infection depends on the number and virulence of the etiologic organism and the resistance of the host. Cancer patients, as a whole, are very vulnerable to infection because of a wide range of possible impairments in resistance. Many of the common malignancies occur mainly in older persons, at a time when immunologic functions of the body gradually begin to decline. The general debility often seen in the aged and in the patient with far-advanced cancer also seems to reduce resistance to infection. The uncontrolled growth, invasion, and obstruction characteristic of malignancies create sites and situations very favorable to the growth of microorganisms.

All three major forms of treatment for cancer—surgery, radiotherapy, and chemotherapy—confer significant risks of infection. Most types of radiotherapy and chemotherapy are immunosuppressive in themselves. Radical surgery always induces a considerable liability of infection, and lymph node dissection, either alone or in combination with major surgery, may impose additional risks. Malignancies of the reticuloendothelial and hematopoietic systems cause immunologic derangements due to the basic pathology of the diseases. Inadequate granulocyte production, seen in acute leukemias and chronic myelogenous leukemia and with the use of intensive chemotherapy and radiotherapy, may enable opportunistic, possibly endogenous, organisms to become pathogenic. When infections do occur in cancer patients, treatment with antibiotics may disturb the balance of normal microbial flora and result in further infections by opportunistic organisms. All of these factors combine to make many cancer patients exceptionally prone to infection. After a brief review of some of the rudiments of infection and host resistance, causes of infection in cancer patients and preventive care will be explored. Treatment of infections in cancer patients will then be considered.

GENERAL CONSIDERATIONS

In order to understand the mechanisms that cause infections in cancer patients and the rationale behind prevention and treatment of infection in these patients, some basic information about infection and host resistance must be grasped. Infections are caused by microorganisms and result when a microbe which is not part of the normal flora in a particular body site enters a receptive site, becomes established, and multiplies.[1] Infections may also occur when microbes normally found in a particular area of the body cause disease. Many organisms which are normal, harmless residents in one area of the body can cause severe infections when introduced into areas where they are not normally found. *Escherichia coli (E. coli)* is, for example, a normal intestinal organism which can and frequently does cause infections in nearly any other body site. Organisms which are normal microbial flora of the body are called "endogenous" or "resident" organisms. Infections caused by these organisms are called "autoinfections." Organisms not normally found in the body are called "exogenous" organisms.

Various distinctions are made between types of infections. Acute infections are those which develop rapidly and usually result in a high fever and severe illness, while chronic infections develop more slowly with milder but longer-lasting symptoms. Local infections are those which are confined to specific localities, while systemic infections are those which spread throughout the body. Local infections may, however, cause systemic symptoms. Usually these systemic symptoms are caused by the toxic substances (toxins) elaborated by certain microorganisms. Sometimes a local infection will seed organisms into the bloodstream which cause infections, often abscesses, at other sites. A primary infection is the initial infection causing illness. This is usually an acute infection caused by an invasive organism. A secondary infection or superinfection is another infection which occurs during or after a primary infection. Secondary infections are often caused by organisms which are not very virulent but which can establish an infection once the body's defenses have been weakened by the primary infection. These normally nonpathogenic or noninvasive organisms are called "opportunists," and the infections they cause are called "opportunistic" infections. These organisms may be endogenous or exogenous. Antibiotic therapy often causes superinfections from opportunistic resident organisms. Bacteremia is a term used to denote the presence of nonmultiplying bacteria in the blood. Septicemia denotes the presence of organisms which are actively multiplying in the blood.[2]

Endogenous organisms reside in the body. In order to cause infection, they require a change in their balance or in their environment which is favorable to their excessive proliferation or transport to a susceptible site where they are not normally found.

Exogenous organisms must somehow get to receptive sites in order to cause infections. The areas through which microorganisms enter the body are called "portals of entry." Some organisms enter almost exclusively through one portal of entry. Others may enter through any of the ports. Portals of entry include the respiratory tract (via the nose and mouth), the gastrointestinal tract (via the mouth), the genitourinary tract (via the urethra), the skin and mucous membranes (via breaks in their integrity), and blood (via insect bites, injections with contaminated needles, or blood transfusions). The portals of exit for a disease-causing organism are usually the same as the portals of entry for the particular agent.

Exogenous Pathogenic Microbes

All exogenous pathogenic microbes can be categorized as either bacteria, viruses, protozoa, or fungi.

BACTERIA.   Bacteria cause the majority of infections occurring in human beings. Bacteria are subdivided according to their morphology into cocci (spherical), bacilli (cylindrical or rod-shaped), or spiral forms (curved rods or spirals). A further distinction between bacteria is made on the basis of the gram stain. Organisms which do not stain with the gram stain are called "gram-negative" organisms (cocci or rods). Those which do stain are called "gram-positive" organisms. Gram-negative bacteria are chemically more complex than are gram-positive organisms and contain endotoxins in their cell walls. These endotoxins are very toxic and are responsible for the severe systemic symptoms often seen with infections caused by gram-negative organisms.

VIRUSES.   Viruses, which are perhaps the simplest form of life known, are also common pathogens. They consist of only a strand of nucleic acid surrounded by a protein coat. Since virions (virus particles) lack some components essential to their replication, they can exist only as obligate intracellular parasites. Viruses enter cells and use the cellular organelles to reproduce themselves. Some viruses cause cellular death; others seem to exist in a commensal relationship, causing no obvious harm or benefit. Since all viruses contain only one type of nucleic acid, the broadest classification of viruses is based on whether the virus contains deoxyribonucleic acid (DNA) or ribonucleic acid (RNA). Included in the DNA viruses are parvoviruses, adenoviruses, papovaviruses, adeno-associated viruses, herpesviruses, and poxviruses. Included in the RNA viruses are picornaviruses, tagoviruses, myxoviruses, paramyxoviruses, coronaviruses, leukoviruses, rhabdoviruses, and reoviruses. In addition to causing many of the common ills known to mankind (warts, cold sores, the common cold, pneumonias, chickenpox, shingles, mononucleosis, smallpox, encephalitis, influenza, rabies, polio, measles, and others), various viruses in the above group are capable of producing cancer in animals. Such viruses are called "oncogenic" viruses.

Some human malignancies have been linked with certain viruses. Viral etiology has been implicated in leukemias, lymphomas, breast cancer, cervical cancer, and other malignancies. In fact, the oncogene theory proposes that all cells of vertebrate species contain viral oncogenes in their chromosomes. These oncogenes are transmitted from parent to offspring as part of the normal genetic material. Normally these oncogenes are repressed, but sometimes agents de-repress them (carcinogens—radiation, chemicals, viral infections) and cause cell transformation and growth of a malignancy. The possible viral etiology of human tumors is a complex, exciting field which is presently being intensely investigated. Of all areas of tumor research, breakthroughs in this area and in the area of tumor immunology seem to hold the most promise of ultimate control of human malignancies.

PROTOZOANS.   A few protozoans are capable of causing disease in man. Protozoa, the only pathogenic microorganisms classified in the animal kingdom, are single-celled organisms, the lowest forms of animal life. Amebic dysentery (amebiasis), trichomonas vaginitis, malaria (caused by species of *Plasmodium*), various types of sleeping sickness (caused by species of *Trypanosoma*), and a few other infections uncommon in this country are caused by protozoans.

FUNGI.   A number of types of fungi, yeasts and molds, are pathogenic in man. Some of them infect only integumentary tissue (skin, hair, and nails). These are called "dermatophytes," and they cause various types of infections, many of which are a form of ringworm. Other fungi cause deep infections or systemic diseases which are often extremely difficult to treat. These include species of *Aspergillus* (aspergillosis), *Blastomyces* (blastomycosis), *Candida* (moniliasis, candidiasis, thrush), *Coccidioides* (coccidioidomycosis), *Cryptococcus* (cryptococcosis), *Histoplasma* (histoplasmosis), and *Sporotrichum* (sporotrichosis). *Candida albicans*, it should be noted, is an endogenous organism of the mouth, intestinal tract, and sometimes the vagina.

Endogenous Microbes

Most of the endogenous microflora of the body are bacteria, although some fungi and viruses may exist in certain parts of the body without evidence of disease. Many resident microorganisms never or only very rarely cause diseases. Others are potential pathogens, opportunists. Some microorganisms which are normally pathogenic can be harbored in certain persons without causing disease. Such persons are called "carriers." Body sites which commonly harbor either commensal and/or opportunistic organisms are the skin, the gastrointestinal tract, the genitourinary tract, the vagina, the upper respiratory tract (nose and nasopharynx only), the eye, and the bloodstream. Table 5.1 lists the common endogenous organisms in these areas.

TABLE 5.1
Common Endogenous Organisms of the Human Body*

BODY AREA	MICROBIAL FLORA	OPPORTUNISTIC
Skin		
(General)	Staphylococcus species	X[†]
	Cryptococcus, Candida	X
	Sarcina species	
	Gram-negative bacilli	X
	Gram-positive sporeformers	
External ear	Staphylococcus species	
	Diphtheroid bacilli	
	Mycobacterium species (nonpathogenic)	
Axilla and groin	Mycobacterium smegmatis	
	Staphylococcus albus	X
	Diphtheroids	X
Eye		
Conjunctiva	Corynebacterium xerosis	
	Neisseria species	
	Small gram-negative bacilli	
Respiratory tract		
Nose and Naso-		
pharynx	Neisseria species (nonpathogens)	
	Staphylococcus species	X
	Streptococcus species	X
	Corynebacterium pseudodiphtheriae	
	Diplococcus pneumoniae	X
	Haemophilus influenzae	X
	Neisseria meningitidis	X
	Klebsiella pneumoniae	X
Larynx, trachea, bron-		
chi and lungs, and		
accessory nasal		
sinuses	No normal flora recognized	
Gastrointestinal		
tract		
Mouth and		
oropharynx	Micrococcus species	
	Staphylococcus species	X
	Streptococcus species	X
	Gram-positive bacilli including lactobacillus and aerobic sporeformers	
	Veillonella (gram-negative cocci)	
	Gram-negative bacilli	X
	Spirochetes—Treponema species (nonpathogens)	
	Vibrios	X
	Vincent's spirillum	
	Fusiform bacillus	
Stomach	No normal flora recognized	

TABLE 5.1 (Cont.)

BODY AREA	MICROBIAL FLORA	OPPORTUNISTIC
Intestine		
Small intestine		
Duodenum	Usually none	
Jejunum and upper ileum	Usually few	
Lower ileum	α-streptococci	
	Streptococcus faecalis	X
	Staphylococcus species	X
	Sarcinae	
	Lactobacillus species	
	Clostridium perfringens	X
	Veillonella	
	Escherichia coli	X
	Yeasts	X
Large intestine	Coliform bacilli, including E. coli, C. freundii, and Enterobacter aerogenes	X
	Salmonella species Proteus species	X
	Enterococci	X
	Staphylococcus species	X
	Clostridium species including Cl. tetani and Cl. perfringens	X
	Bacteroides	X
	Lactobacillus species	
	Thermophilic bacteria	
	Spirochetes	
	Pseudomonas aeruginosa	X
	Friedländer bacillus	
	Aerobic sporeformers, including Bacillus subtilis	
	β-streptococci	X
	Certain fungi	X
	ECHO viruses	
Genitourinary tract		
Bladder	None	
Urethra		
-Female	Usually none, or few cocci (nonpathogenic)	
	Mycoplasma	
Male	Diphtheroids	
	Staphylococcus species	
	Gram-negative bacilli	
	Mycoplasma	
Preputial secretions (male and female)	Mycobacterium smegmatis	
Vagina		
Prior to puberty and after menopause	Coliforms	
	Diphtheroid bacilli	
	Micrococcus species	
	Streptococcus species	

TABLE 5.1 (Cont.)

BODY AREA	MICROBIAL FLORA	OPPORTUNISTIC
Between puberty and menopause	Lactobacillus species Diphtheroid bacilli E. coli Staphylococcus species Streptococcus species	X
	Anaerobic cocci and bacilli Yeasts	X

*Adapted from Volk and Wheeler: Basic Microbiology, 3rd ed. 1973. Courtesy of Lippincott
†Potential pathogens are indicated by X.

HOST RESISTANCE

The body has several lines of defense against invasion by microorganisms. In general, these are called "immunologic defense mechanisms" or "host resistance." One type of resistance is nonspecific. The second line of resistance is specific for the organism and is thus called "specific resistance" or "specific immunity."

Nonspecific Resistance

Nonspecific defenses include both mechanical and chemical barriers. The skin itself prevents entry of microbes, while certain glands in the skin secrete substances which are lethal for many bacteria and fungi. Additional examples of nonspecific resistance include the mechanical action of cilia on the mucous membranes of the respiratory tract and the washing and chemical effects of tears in the eyes.

The above deterrents are often ineffective in preventing the entrance of microorganisms into the body. Therefore, other types of nonspecific mechanisms are activated when organisms get by these first lines of defense. Phagocytosis is a major process in combating organisms which have entered a part of the body where they are capable of causing infection. The tissue destruction that occurs when an organism initiates an infection causes the release of certain chemicals which attract to the affected area cells capable of phagocytizing the etiologic organisms. This process is called "chemotaxis." The cells attracted to the infected area must be capable of migrating into the area and engulfing, digesting, and removing the offending organisms, dead cells, and other debris. Two types of cells are primarily responsible for this very important action, leukocytes and macrophages. Leukocytes are white blood cells produced by the bone marrow and lymphatic tissues that circulate in the blood. Macrophages are found mainly in tissues, where some of them are capable of wandering from one place to another (wandering macrophages). Leukocytes active in phagocytosis are polymorphonuclear cells, also called granulocytes, polys, or PMNs. They are produced in the bone marrow. There are three types of granulocytes: neutrophils, basophils, and eosinophils. The neutrophils constitute over 60 percent of the white cells circulating in a healthy person's blood, and they are the granulocytes which carry out phagocytosis. An abnormally low total white blood cell count is called "leukopenia." Since it is the granulocytes in general and the neutrophils specifically that are usually reduced in leukopenia, the terms "granulocytopenia" and "neutropenia" are used to describe more specifically the same condition. A drastic reduction in the number of circulating leukocytes severely jeopardizes a person's resistance to infection.

There are also macrophages and other cells capable of phagocytizing substances in the organs and tissues of the reticuloendothelial system (eg, the liver, spleen, and lungs). These fixed macrophages are not mobile, but they will destroy organisms that reach them by way of the blood or lymphatic circulation. Lymph nodes are believed to play a major role in confining infections to local areas. Organisms which reach lymph nodes in the area are filtered out, phagocytized, and prevented from spreading to other areas by way of lymphatic channels or blood.

Specific Resistance

The lymphatic tissues are primarily responsible for producing the cells involved in specific immunity. Specific immunity, or acquired immunity, is an immune response to a specific microorganism based on the body's recognition of some portion of the microorganism as an antigen. An antigen is a substance which the body recognizes as foreign and which thus causes the production of certain elements that initiate processes that ultimately inactivate the antigenic material. Certain microorganisms, notably many viruses and bacteria, carry antigens on their cell surface which activate specific immune responses. Obviously, specific immunity develops only after the person has been exposed to the specific antigen. With a second exposure to the same antigen the body is able to react quickly and destroy the antigen before much harm is done.

The cells circulating in the blood which are produced primarily by lymphatic tissue are called "lymphocytes," and they are the second most numerous white cell found in normal blood. They usually constitute around 20 percent of the circulating white cell population. Lymphocytes produced in the peripheral cortical areas of lymph nodes are called thymic-dependent lymphocytes (T cells). They are small, long-lived lymphocytes and are believed to be responsible for a type of specific immunity called "cellular" immunity. Lymphocytes produced in the more cortical areas of lymph nodes are called B cells, and they are also believed to play a role in specific immunity.

The two different types of specific immunity identified are humoral immunity and cellular immunity. Humoral immunity depends on the production of antibodies by plasma cells. It is believed that plasma cells themselves are derived from lymphocytes seeded throughout lymphatic tissue. These B cells (lymphocytes) are believed to originate at some time from the lymphoid tissue in the gut. Cellular immunity depends on the production of small lymphocytes by lymphocyte precursors in lymphatic tissue. Certain antigenic substances will precipitate only one of these responses. Most, however, seem to initiate both responses to some degree. Factors which seem to determine whether a humoral or a cellular response to antigens occurs include the size of the antigenic particle and the route of entry. The size of antigens required to initiate antibody synthesis is much smaller than the antigen size necessary to induce a cellular immune response. Injections of antigens into the skin tend to cause strong cellular immune responses, while intravenous antigens cause strong humoral immune responses.

There is reason to believe that all lymphocyte precursors originate at some time in the bone marrow. From the bone marrow, it is postulated that some pass through the thymus and on to more peripheral areas of lymphoid tissues, where they colonize and cause more differentiated lymphocytes (T cells) to be released into blood, lymph, and other tissues. Some pass from the bone marrow through lymphoid tissue in the gut into more cortical areas of lymphoid tissue, where they further differentiate. It is believed that plasma cells, responsible for immunoglobulin production, are derived from these lymphocytes (B cells) (Fig 5.1).

HUMORAL IMMUNITY.   The antibodies which circulate in the bloodstream as products of the humoral immune response are classified into five types, called "immunoglobulins"—IgG (Immune globulin gamma, or gamma globulin) IgA, IgM, IgD, and IgE. Of these, IgG is quantitatively the most important class, as it accounts for more than 80 percent of the immunoglobulins (antibodies) found in serum. Persons who have an impairment in antibody synthesis are greatly handicapped in their resistance to infections caused by certain antigenic microorganisms.

CELLULAR IMMUNITY.   The cellular immune response involves the reaction of the whole lymphocyte with the antigenic substance, rather than just a compound elaborated by the cell. From this derives the term "cellular" immunity. "Delayed hypersensitivity" is an older term sometimes used synonymously with cellular immunity. A defective cellular immune response also subjects a person to risk of infection, especially from those organisms which cause strong cellular immune responses.

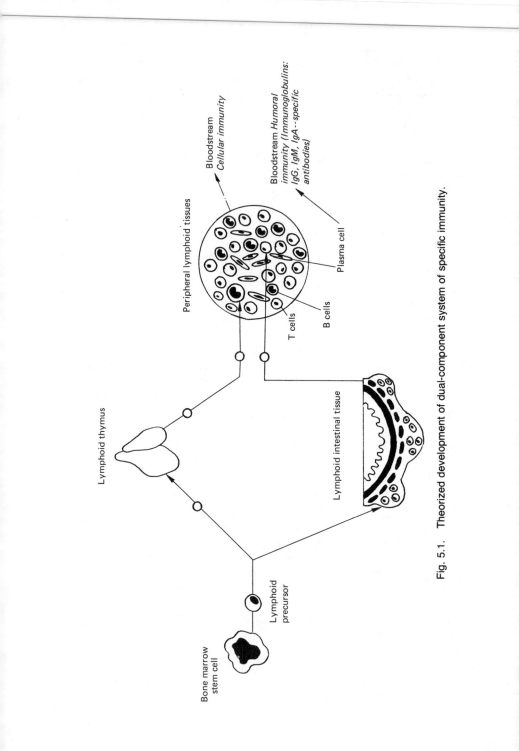

Fig. 5.1. Theorized development of dual-component system of specific immunity.

Bone marrow stem cell

Lymphoid precursor

Lymphoid thymus

Lymphoid intestinal tissue

Peripheral lymphoid tissues

T cells

B cells

Plasma cell

Bloodstream *Cellular immunity*

Bloodstream *Humoral immunity (Immunoglobulins: IgG, IgM, IgA - specific antibodies)*

102

Other Immunologic Terms

Several other terms often used to distinguish between types of immunity are "active" versus "passive" and "artificial" versus "natural." Active immunity is acquired by an exposure to antigens and the production of antibodies in response to them. Natural active immunity is immunity acquired as a result of infection by the etiologic antigenic microorganism. Artificial active immunity is acquired by vaccination with the killed or attenuated organism or its toxoid. Passive immunity is acquired by the transfer of preformed antibodies or cells from one person to another. In artificial passive immunity the antibodies formed by one person are injected into another person. Natural passive immunity is the transfer across the placenta of antibodies from the mother to the fetus. Passive immunity lasts only a short time. Active immunity lasts much longer, from years to a lifetime.

IMMUNITY AND CANCER

Although tumor etiology is not included in the scope of this text, it should be noted that specific immune responses are now believed to play a major role in the development of malignancies. Current thinking is that malignancies represent some failure in immunologic surveillance. There is much evidence to support this view, including the phenomenon of spontaneous tumor regression, the positive correlation between older age and the tendency to develop a malignancy (immunologic defenses decline with age), the association between autoimmune diseases and certain malignancies, the increased incidence of malignancies in patients receiving therapy which is immunosuppressive (transplant patients and cancer patients treated with intensive chemotherapy or radiotherapy), the identification of antigens on tumor cells, the presence in the blood of antibodies to tumor antigens, and the well-documented observation that lymphocyte infiltration into tumor-bearing areas is favorable to the patient's prognosis. Treatment of malignancies is now taking immunologic factors into account. It is believed that many tumors can be controlled if the number of their cells is reduced to a level which can be successfully held in check by the body's immunologic mechanisms. The older view of treatment was that every single malignant cell had to be eradicated if control of the disease was to be achieved. Questions as to the advisability of lymph node dissection of clinically negative nodes are being raised, and cancer therapy which results in immunologic suppression is now recognized as a double-edged sword. The specific effects of humoral versus cellular immunity in tumor etiology are unclear. Cellular immunity seems to retard the progression of malignant proliferation in many tumors, while humoral immunity may actually enhance tumor development. Neither of these effects is clear.

Recognition of the role of immunity in tumor growth has resulted in various attempts to bolster immune responses to tumors. Antigenic challenges, stimulation of antibody responses, and attempts to enhance cellular immunity have all been tried in various studies. To date, the only type of this so-called immunotherapy which has achieved any degree of acceptance is the use of BCG (bacilles Calmette-Guerin) vaccine and *Cornyebacterium parvum* to stimulate a general cellular immune response. BCG vaccine has traditionally been used to vaccinate persons who are subject to wide exposure to tuberculosis. It has been injected into various types of tumors in hopes of contributing to control of the malignancy. Although the original studies with BCG were done on leukemic patients in France, it is now being used most often in patients with malignant melanomas. *C. parvum*, another immunostimulant, is presently being used to treat breast cancer patients in some centers.

FACTORS IN INFECTION IN CANCER PATIENTS AND IMPLICATIONS FOR CARE

Age

For the aged cancer patient and the cancer patient who is debilitated, immunologic capacities are diminished, and general preventive measures, applicable to all patients, assume great importance. These patients often acquire severe infections within hospitals. The most common etiologic agents in hospital-acquired, or nosocomial, infections are strains of gram-negative enteric bacilli, fungi, and resistant staphylococci. Therefore, cross-contamination must be avoided. Handwashing before and after each patient contact is probably the most important single step in avoiding cross-contamination. Ideally, each patient unit should have a sink near the door with a dispenser for germicidal soaps to facilitate and act as a reminder for handwashing. Vigorous mechanical friction with handwashing is essential in order to remove transient and resident bacteria from the skin. Nails should be kept clean and short. Good patient hygiene is mandatory, and special attention should be given to body sites which are especially vulnerable to invasion by pathogens (skin, mouth, perineal area).

Adequate nutrition is necessary in patients who are elderly or debilitated to assure the manufacture of serum proteins and an energy level conducive to physical activity. Immobility predisposes to pneumonias, pressure areas which may become necrotic and infected, and other undesired consequences. For the patient who must be bedfast, turning, coughing, and deep breathing must be carried out routinely. Patients who are able to be ambulatory should be as active as their condition permits.

Characteristics of Malignancies

When tumors lower the normal anatomic defense mechanisms, infection is likely to result, but certain measures can often eliminate some of the risk. Local mechanical factors, such as obstructions, which create an environment favorable to proliferation of pathogenic organisms, can often be relieved. Bronchial, gastrointestinal, and genitourinary blockages are infection-enhancing obstructions which can often be treated. Reservoirs favorable to the growth of microorganisms, such as effusions, especially bloody effusions, can be removed. Ulceration may occur with tumor growth or with intensive chemotherapy or radiotherapy, and topical treatment may help to reduce the danger of infection in traumatized tissues. If ulcerated tissue cannot be managed with topical treatments or if the tissue becomes necrotic, excision of the affected tissue may be necessary to control infection. Abscesses must be drained in order to heal.

Immunosuppressive Treatment for Cancer: Leukopenia

High dosages of radiotherapy and certain types of chemotherapy have a toxic effect on the rapidly dividing cells of the bone marrow and may lead to severe leukopenia. For radiotherapy to cause severe bone marrow depression with neutropenia, large portions of the functioning marrow must be irradiated. Certain cancer chemotherapeutic drugs may also depress both humoral and cellular immune responses. Certain alkylating agents, antimetabolites, antibiotics, and vinca alkaloids have been shown to cause all of these impairments.[3] Corticosteroids, used mostly for patients with leukemia or a lymphoma, also seem to depress immune defenses. Fungus infections seem to be the most significant infections associated with long-term corticosteroid therapy. Leukemic patients who produce insufficient or inadequate granulocytes also have severe impairments in nonspecific resistance to infection. They may be leukopenic, or they may have an excess of abnormal granulocytes (leukocytosis) which are incapable of carrying out normal phagocytic action.

Of all impairments in host resistance, leukopenia is the most prevalent and the most problematic in cancer patients. In any patient whose bone marrow is prone to dysfunction, frequent white blood cell counts must be taken in order to monitor granulocyte levels. Radiotherapy or chemotherapy may be halted if granulocytes are markedly reduced. With radiotherapy and certain chemotherapeutic drugs, white cell counts may continue to drift downward for days and even weeks after treatment is suspended.

Since pus does not form in the absence of granulocytes, leukopenic patients may have a locus of infection without typical abscess formation, and an infection which would remain localized and less harmful in a patient with a normal granulocyte count can and often does develop into a septicemia in leukopenic patients. Daily careful inspection of body areas which have a high potential for infection in these patients is required. Wounds must be observed, cleaned, and dressed frequently.

In a markedly leukopenic patient with a temperature elevation, an assiduous search for infection is necessary. While suspicious sites are checked and cultured, either broad-spectrum antibiotics or antibiotics effective for the organisms likely to be the offenders should be promptly initiated. If no questionable lesions are found, multiple urine, sputum, and blood specimens should be submitted for culture and antimicrobial sensitivity. If a specific organism is identified, the antibiotic of choice for the organism is then administered. Not infrequently, however, the site of infection cannot be located in these patients. In acute leukemic patients, about two-thirds of the febrile episodes which occur are assumed to be manifestations of the underlying disease process, as no other signs of infection are identifiable. Fever of undetermined origin also occurs, although less frequently, in other hematologic and lymphatic malignancies, including Hodgkin's disease, chronic lymphocytic and myelocytic leukemia, and lymphosarcoma. As these diseases progress, fever becomes more frequent and is more often associated with an infectious process. Pyrexia in patients with solid tumors nearly always represents an infectious process, although a small minority will manifest an unexplained sustained high fever. Occasionally fever heralds the presence of a cryptic carcinoma.[4] The mechanisms by which fevers of undetermined origin occur in cancer patients have not been elucidated. Conversely, severe infections in cancer patients, including septicemias, may occur without fever, so that such clinical signs as unexplained leukocytosis, leukopenia, thrombocytopenia, tachycardia, hyperventilation, hypotension, and subtle mental changes warrant an investigation for an occult infection.[3]

SITES OF INFECTIONS IN LEUKOPENIC PATIENTS. In any severely leukopenic patient, certain preventive measures should be routine. These measures are based on an awareness of the commonest sites of infection in these patients: the skin, the bloodstream, the perineal area, the bladder and kidneys, the respiratory tree and lungs, and the mouth.

Skin. Since granulocytes are required to phagocytize and wall off infectious organisms, neutropenic patients are deprived of one of the most important nonspecific defenses against infection. Every effort must be made with these patients to avoid the introduction of pathogenic organisms into susceptible sites. Every break in the skin, the body's first defense, is a potential site for entry of infectious microbes. Unfortunately, since leukopenia in cancer patients is a consequence of bone marrow depression or malignant infiltration of the bone marrow, thrombocytopenia often appears concurrently. The bone marrow produces platelets as well as granulocytes, and platelet depletion, or thrombocytopenia, is another consequence of inadequate bone marrow function. With thrombocytopenia, the tendency to bleed excessively may cause extensive breaks in the skin and mucosa, allowing microorganisms easy entry. Skin care and protection are, therefore, vital in leukopenic patients. Injections are to be avoided insofar as possible. Bone marrow aspiration and biopsy, frequently ordered blood tests, and spinal taps all present risks of infection. Hair should be shaved over sites where the integrity of a large area of skin must be interrupted. Keeping the patient's fingernails short and well manicured will help alleviate infections around the fingers and skin infections which could be caused by scratching. Toenails should also be carefully cut and cared for.

Bloodstream.   Intravenous infusions, although often necessary, provide microbes direct access to the bloodstream. Such infusions, therefore, must be handled scrupulously. Needles or catheters should be changed every few days, and all intravenous tubing should be dated and changed every 24 hours. Antibiotic ointment and a sterile dressing to the site of entry should be applied at least once a day. A skin defatting agent, such as alcohol, and an antibacterial agent, such as Betadine, should be used to cleanse any skin site subjected to puncture, since many potential pathogens reside as normal microbial flora on the skin, especially around hair follicles.

Perineal Area.   The perineal area is a source of many pathogens and a frequent portal of entry for microorganisms. Proper perineal care should be performed on a regularly scheduled basis, especially in female patients. Normal females easily contract vaginal and bladder infections from improper wiping after bowel movements or from perineal irritation. Obviously, vaginitis, urethritis, and cystitis are even more likely to occur in leukopenic females. Unless treated promptly, these infections can cause serious difficulties. Complaints of perineal itching or urinary burning, frequency, or urgency should be fully explored. Sexual counseling should be routine for sexually active males and females who are severely leukopenic, although females are much more vulnerable to infections resulting from sexual practices.

Sexual hygiene and sexual practices which are contraindicated should be discussed with leukopenic patients. Cleanliness, avoidance of excessive friction, proper lubrication, and prevention of contamination should be reviewed. Both heterosexual and homosexual anal activity should be discouraged, as the anus is highly susceptible to abscess formation in these patients if any breaks or tears in the membrane occur. There is also a risk of transporting rectal bacteria to sites susceptible to infection (open areas on the skin, the vagina, the urethra, the oral area).

Enemas, rectal medications, and rectal temperatures are contraindicated in patients with dangerously low neutrophil counts, since rectal trauma should be avoided as much as possible. In patients receiving intensive cytotoxic chemotherapy or radiation therapy to the pelvis, irritation of the intestinal mucosa can be expected. This creates an even greater need for avoidance of trauma to the area. If anal fissures or abscesses do form, sitz baths, topical anesthetics, and antibacterial ointments to the area are helpful.

Bladder and Kidneys.   Bladder infections may ascend to cause kidney infections. In addition to the above-mentioned causes of cystitis, bladder catheterization contributes significantly to the risks of genitourinary infections. Bladder catheterization results in a high incidence of bacteria in the urine, bacteriuria. In one study, the incidence of bacteriuria after a single catheterization in 100 male and female ambulatory patients was 1 percent. In hospitalized, debilitated patients, it was around 10 percent.[5] Increasingly, the gram-negative bacilli are reported to be causing bacteriuria. The most common causative organisms in bacteriuria are species of *E. coli*, *Klebsiella-Aerobacter*, *Proteus*, *Pseudomonas*, and *Candida*.

In the leukopenic patient, the risk of infection from bladder catheterization is heightened. Bladder catheterization should be performed only when circumstances demand it. When catheterization is necessary, avoidance of common errors, such as contamination during insertion, inadequate lubrication resulting in trauma to the urethra, and use of an unnecessarily large catheter, will help to reduce the risk of infection.

Indwelling bladder catheters should be used only after careful consideration of the risks, as the incidence of bacteriuria rises sharply with the length of time a catheter is left in place. The incidence of bacteriuria is nearly 100 percent in patients with long-term indwelling catheters. There are, however, some measures which seem to decrease the incidence of bacteriuria in patients with indwelling catheters. Sterile drainage systems, in which all sections of tubing and drainage bottles are sterile and remain closed, should be used, and the system should not be interrupted unless absolutely necessary, which means that the catheters should not be irrigated unless occlusion is suspected. Addition of a germicidal solution to the collection containers may be helpful. Triple-lumen bladder catheters, which allow for infusion of an antibacterial solution into the bladder, can be used with a closed drainage system. This seems to reduce the incidence of bacteriuria significantly. Although cleansing of the urethral area around the catheter with antibacterial solutions and use of antibacterial ointments are sometimes recommended, these practices have not proved very useful in significantly diminishing the incidence of bacteriuria in these patients.[6]

Techniques to anchor the catheter securely to prevent inward and outward movement should help to decrease urethral trauma and the transport of organisms into the urethra. The balloon on a Foley catheter will allow the catheter to move outward only as far as the balloon, but inward and then outward motion is possible unless care is taken to secure the catheter. Firmly taping the catheter to the inner aspect of the thigh is a common method of anchoring the catheter.

Some evidence suggests that systemic administration of broad-spectrum bactericidal agents helps to prevent bacteriuria in patients with indwelling catheters,[6] but prophylactic use of antibiotics is contraindicated in most patients (pp. 118–119). Forcing fluids may help to cut down on bacterial proliferation in the urinary tract, and fluids should always be forced for patients receiving sulfa preparations for urinary tract infections. Pyridium, a urinary tract analgesic, may help to control discomfort in patients with indwelling bladder catheters, although the drug has no effect on infectious organisms.

Respiratory Tree and Lungs.   Infections of the middle ear, sinusitis, pharyngitis, and other infections of the upper air passages and lungs are common, serious infections in many cancer patients. Pneumonias and other lung infections are especially frequent in elderly and leukemic patients. Pneumonias are caused by gram-negative bacilli as well as by pneumococci, staphylococci, and streptococci. Interstitial pneumonias occur and may be caused by *Pneumocystis carinii*, *Toxoplasma gondii*, cytomegalovirus, *Aspergillus*, *Candida*, and *Cryptococcus*. Tuberculosis is particularly prevalent in patients with Hodgkin's disease, but it also occurs often in patients with leukemias or other types of lymphomas and in those with cancer of the lung. Tuberculosis spreads with alarming rapidity in many of these patients.[7]

Pneumonia can sometimes be prevented with certain precautions. In addition to mobility, turning, deep breathing, and coughing, careful screening of personnel and visitors who have respiratory infections and aseptic management of any equipment used for respiratory treatments helps to prevent development of pneumonia in these patients. If the patient is on IPPB therapy, he should have his own mouthpiece and nebulizer. A strong pulmonary regimen with pulmonary physiotherapy may be required in some patients. Leukopenic patients should not share a room with another patient who has a respiratory infection. Ideally, they should not be in a room with a patient who has any type of infection.

Tracheostomies, although frequently essential for supportive therapy, especially in cancer patients undergoing thoracic surgery or extensive head and neck surgery, are accompanied by a substantial risk of respiratory infection. Sterile suctioning technique and careful cleansing of the stoma and tracheostomy tube help reduce the risk of infection in these patients, as does humidification of the air the tracheostomy patient inspires.

Meningitis, which occurs mostly in patients with leukemias and lymphomas, is usually caused by organisms entering by way of the upper respiratory tract. *Cryptococcus neoformans* is one of the commonest pathogens causing meningitis. *Listeria monocytogenes* is found often in patients with lymphatic neoplasias. *Pseudomonas aeruginosa*, *E. coli*, and *Diplococcus* are frequent bacterial agents in the etiology of meningitis in cancer patients.[7] Brain abscesses may also occur, many of them caused by these same organisms.

Mouth.   The oral area is another frequent portal of entry for infectious agents in leukopenic patients. Ideally, the teeth and gums should be in good repair before intensive radiotherapy or chemotherapy is begun. Dental caries or periodontal disease can create serious loci of infections. Fastidious oral hygiene is necessary to decrease the opportunity for infection to begin in this area. Mouth care should be given routinely around the clock. Petroleum jelly or some other lubricant should be used to prevent drying and cracking of the lips. The mouth should be inspected daily for ulcers or white patches. White patches usually indicate moniliasis, a common infection in the oral area, in which case Mycostatin (nystatin) mouthwash is used, or Mycostatin tablets, usually used intravaginally, can be sucked in the mouth. Antiseptic sprays, mouthwashes, or oral irrigations may be used to keep the mouth clean, and water picks can be used to clean the mouth and keep the gums healthy. Teeth should be brushed and cleaned as often as necessary. Other aspects of oral hygiene in cancer patients are discussed in Chapter 6.

REVERSE ISOLATION.   Reverse isolation techniques are additional measures often initiated for patients who have few defenses against pathogenic organisms. It has been shown, however, that reverse isolation does not reduce the incidence of infection in leukopenic patients unless life islands or laminar air flow units are used. Both of these units are generally available only in major cancer centers, and they are expensive to use. Cost and the need for a specially trained nursing staff are not the only drawbacks. Patients may undergo psychotic episodes in these environments of isolation, impersonality, and small, enclosed space, although they are less likely to do so in the laminar air flow units than in the life islands. Psychologic interviews and tests help to screen out patients who may find these units intolerable, and adequate patient teaching and preparation can reduce the stress, but most patients still find the confinement of these units emotionally taxing. Some also become very dependent on the protection against infection afforded by these units. They feel very unsafe and vulnerable, perhaps even angry, when removed from the units.

Life Island.   The life island is a large plastic canopy which encloses the patient's bed. All items inside are sterilized, and the air inside is filtered to remove all airborne microorganisms. Items are passed in and out of the unit through two ultraviolet-radiated locks at the foot of the unit, which remove surface contaminants. All contact with the patient is through arm-length gloves built into the side of the unit.

Laminar Air Flow Unit.   Laminar air flow units or rooms are enclosures which have a constant flow of purified air flowing across the width and breadth of the area to avoid exposing the patient to pathogenic organisms. The air is propelled by fans located behind filters which screen out the microorganisms. The continuous flow prevents airborne microorganisms from moving against the air current toward the patient. Anyone or anything entering the patient's room remains downstream of the patient and thus will not infect him. Visitors need not wear caps or gowns if they follow this principle, but anyone touching the patient must wear a sterile gown, cap, mask, gloves, and shoe covers.[8] The laminar air flow unit is larger and permits much more interaction with the environment and more freedom of activity than does the life island.

Radiotherapy

In addition to the severe leukopenia which may occur in cancer patients when large portions of functioning bone marrow are irradiated and the predisposition to infection caused when irradiated tissues become irritated or ulcerated, radiotherapy may also contribute to infectious complications when it leads to fistula formation. This situation is seen most often in patients with malignancies of the cervix who receive high doses of radiation to the pelvic area, although it may also occur in female patients who receive bladder irradiation or in patients whose intestinal tract is in the field of irradiation. Vesicovaginal, rectovaginal, and vesicorectovaginal fistulas may occur in these patients. The continuous cross-contamination occurring with these fistulas makes the resulting infections very difficult to control. Drainage of abscesses, packing, irrigation, and antibiotics may help in controlling these infections, but corrective surgery is often required to eradicate the fistulas. In extreme cases, diverting colostomies and/or urinary diversions may be necessary to eliminate infection and to relieve the patient of troublesome continuous drainage and offensive odors.

Surgery

Although surgery for cancer is not immunosuppressive, it is often of a radical nature and carries considerable morbidity and mortality from infectious complications. Removal of large blocks of tissue in lengthy procedures results in considerable hemorrhage, decreased tissue perfusion, and creation of dead spaces, all of which combine to produce favorable sites for infection. Dead space should be obliterated wherever possible during surgery.

Many other factors which seem to increase the incidence of postoperative wound infections are present in surgery for many cancer patients: bacterial contamination during surgery (dirty surgery), older age, lengthy procedures, long preoperative hospital residence, previous adrenal steroid therapy, and infection remote from the operative incision.[9] The development of postoperative wound infections can be allayed by gentle handling of tissue to minimize trauma, edema, and interstitial fluid pressure. Proper cleansing of dirty and deep wounds and debridement of devitalized tissues will also help to reduce the occurrence of secondary infection. If postoperative wound infection does occur, adequate drainage must be assured. Removal of skin sutures, spreading of wound edges to the underlying surface, draining loculated areas, and perhaps even extension of the original incision may be necessary to ensure adequate drainage.[9]

Although dissection of clinically negative lymph nodes is now being seriously questioned, many types of surgery for cancer still include resection of regional lymph nodes, and node dissections alone are performed on involved nodes. Regional lymph nodes are believed to act as a filter or a trap for organisms in the area. In addition, regional nodes may be active in the production of lymphocytes which help to control infections in the local area. Lymph node dissection may also disrupt the normal return of lymph in the lymphatic channels and cause lymphedema. The net result of regional or radical lymph node dissection is a heightened vulnerability to infection in the area subserved by the removed lymphatic chain. With axillary node dissection, done most often for breast cancer, the upper extremities are at risk. With inguinal or femoral node dissections, the lower extremities are at risk. Not only are infections hard to control once they have developed in these areas, but they also contribute to the precipitation of lymphedema in the involved part. Precautions must be taken to avoid infection in the involved areas, and patients must be taught to care properly for these vulnerable areas. Breaks in the skin should be prevented, which means no injections or venipunctures in the involved extremities. Hands can be protected from trauma in innumerable ways—wearing a thimble when sewing, wearing gloves when gardening, using insulated gloves to handle hot objects. Feet can be protected by wearing properly fitting shoes or slippers at all times. Constrictive clothing or jewelry should not be worn on the involved extremity. Any break in the skin should be promptly treated by cleansing with an antibacterial soap and application of an antibacterial solution or ointment. Any evidence of infection should be brought to medical attention so that it can be eradicated before damage is extensive.

Gynecologic surgery for cancer may result in fistula formation. The problems and treatment for these fistulas have already been mentioned in regard to their occurrence with radiotherapy (p. 110). Lung surgery or chronic lung infections may also lead to fistula formation in the bronchi, and bronchopleural fistulas are difficult to treat. Adequate drainage of the resulting infected areas and antibiotic therapy may control infections which result from these fistulas.

Malignancies of the Reticuloendothelial and Hematopoietic Systems

Patients with carcinomatosis or advanced metastatic nonlymphomatous solid tumors may show specific defects in immunity. Cell-mediated immunity is impaired earlier and more often than humoral immunity in these patients. However, patients with malignancies of the reticuloendothelial and hematopoietic systems undergo such drastic alterations in their body's defenses against infectious agents that they stand in a category of their own in terms of cancer patients who are predisposed to infections.[10] The specific immunologic derangements in these nonsolid and lymphatic malignancies are related to the type of malignancy. The myeloproliferative disorders, acute leukemias and chronic granulocytic leukemia, are characterized by inadequate neutrophil production. The leukopenia which results is then further aggravated by therapy for the basic disease process, intensive chemotherapy. Until the disease process can be controlled, leukopenia in these patients may be of life-threatening proportions. White blood cell counts below 1,000 are dangerous. It is not unusual to see counts of 500, 200, or even lower in these patients. All the usual precautions against infection must be intensified with these patients. If a remission can be attained, the leukopenia resolves, and patients live normally unless or until the disease recurs.

Patients with certain types of lymphomas, notably Hodgkin's disease, often exhibit defects in cell (lymphocyte)-mediated immunity. They show anergy to many common antigens during exacerbations of their disease and are vulnerable to infections which normally cause delayed hypersensitivity reactions (cellular immune responses), such as tuberculosis. They also show a marked vulnerability to yeast and fungus infections, such as candidiasis, cryptococcosis, histoplasmosis, coccidioidomycosis, and aspergillosis, and to certain viral infections, including varicella (herpes zoster), cytomegalic inclusion disease, and vaccinia (chickenpox). Patients with chronic lymphatic leukemia also show a disposition to develop these viral infections. Patients with uncontrolled lymphomatous disease, especially Hodgkin's disease, should be cautioned against exposure to these fungi and viruses. *Cryptococcus* is transmitted in pigeon droppings, and these patients should avoid contact with pigeons and areas where pigeons gather. Patients with either chronic lymphatic leukemia or Hodgkin's disease should avoid exposure to persons with chickenpox or herpes zoster and to those recently vaccinated. Corticosteroid therapy, administered to many of these patients, appears to predispose to fungal infections.[11]

Patients with multiple myeloma show abnormalities in their immunoglobulins. Multiple myeloma and chronic lymphocytic leukemia especially and also some lymphosarcomas, all lymphoproliferative disorders, may be associated with hypogammaglobulinemia, in which case periodic administration of hyperimmune gamma globulin may help to prevent bacterial infection. The altered antibody response in these patients often results in major bacterial infections, and many of these patients die of bacterial sepsis.

In summary, it must be noted that the wide variety and erratic occurrence of infections in patients with hematologic and lymphatic malignancies proves that there are many contributing factors in the development of infections in these patients. Silver makes this point quite well in the following excerpt.

Although the deficiency of cellular, protein, and immune mechanisms against infection in leukemia, lymphoma, and allied diseases has been broadly outlined, it is emphasized that these gross abnormalities offer only a partial explanation for the frequency of infections observed in the clinic. Although decreases in the number of circulating neutrophils and in the granulocyte reserve appear of paramount importance in acute leukemia, not every decrease in neutrophils is followed by infection, and patients may be neutropenic for relatively long periods of time without developing bacterial complications. Whereas qualitative and quantitative abnormalities of gamma globulin and abnormal antibody response appear of most importance in multiple myeloma, chronic lymphocytic leukemia, and disseminated lymphosarcoma, infection may not occur even in the complete absence of normal gamma globulin and diminished antibody response. Conversely, infection can develop in some patients with normal amounts of gamma globulin and normal antibody response. Although patients with Hodgkin's disease have impaired delayed hypersensitivity, its significance remains to be determined. . . .

Clearly the development of infection in the leukemias and lymphomas is a composite of many factors. In groups of patients with each disease, the major abnormality which apparently pre-disposes to infection may be appreciated. In the individual patient, on the other hand, the development of infection is related to some known causes which may involve neutrophils, macrophages, serum proteins, antibodies, anergy, local tissue factors, tumor infiltration, hemorrhage, therapy, and the relation of the infecting organism to the host, and undoubtedly and unfortunately, a myriad of other causes which, at present, are unknown.[12]

Table 5.2 is a summary of immune defects related to these neoplastic diseases.

TABLE 5.2
Immune Defects in Various Neoplastic Diseases*

SPECIFIC IMMUNITY		NONSPECIFIC IMMUNITY
Humoral	Cellular	
Serum Mediated (Immunoglobulins)	Mononuclear Cell Mediated (Lymphocyte and/or Macrophage)	Polymorphonuclear Leukocyte Mediated (Granulocytes or Neutrophils)
Chronic lymphatic leukemia	Hodgkin's disease	Acute lymphoblastic leukemia
Multiple myeloma	Lymphosarcoma	Acute myelogenous leukemia
Lymphosarcoma	To lesser degree, other lymphomas and leukemias	Leukolymphosarcoma
To lesser degree, other lymphomas and leukemias	Altered due to therapy	Altered due to therapy
Altered due to therapy		

*Adapted from Armstrong, Young, Meyer, Blevins: Med Clin North Am 55:731, 1971

OTHER PREVENTIVE MEASURES

Other than the measures mentioned above which are specific for certain conditions, there are several general measures which help to prevent infection in cancer patients.

Tuberculosis Prophylaxis

Prophylaxis against tubercular infection in cancer patients is indicated in patients with leukemia or a lymphoma who have a positive skin test, patients with a positive skin test who are treated with immunosuppressive agents, and any patient who receives adrenocorticosteroids or prolonged immunosuppressive therapy, regardless of skin test reactivity.[7] Isoniazid (INH) should be given prophylactically to any patient in these categories. Since its antibacterial action is limited to *Mycobacterium tuberculosis*, prophylactic use of INH does not predispose to the development of superinfections.

Proper Use of Antiseptics and Disinfectants

Effective, proper use of antiseptics and disinfectants can be very helpful in both the prophylaxis and treatment of infections in cancer patients. They must be used in dilutions which are maximally therapeutic, and specific preparations are not equally effective against all organisms. Antiseptics are more effective when fewer microorganisms and less organic material are in the area. Therefore, wounds should be thoroughly cleaned, irrigated and/or scrubbed, and rinsed before antibacterials are applied. The area should then be dried before the antiseptic is applied so that dilution does not occur.[13] Some commonly used antiseptics and disinfectants and some of their recommended use-dilutions are given in Table 5.3.

TABLE 5.3
Antiseptics and Disinfectants with Recommended Use-dilutions*

CHEMICAL	USE	USE-DILUTION
Phenolic Compounds		
Cen-O-Phen	Disinfectant	0.6% (1:175)
Lysol	Disinfectant	1 % (1:100)
Phenol	Disinfectant	5 % (1:20)
Staphene	Disinfectant	0.5% (1:200)
Pheno-Cen		
Bisphenolic Compounds		
pHisoHex	External antiseptic	Undiluted (3%)
Gamophen		
Iodine Preparations		
Betadine	External antiseptic	Undiluted (1%)
Iodine tincture	External antiseptic	2% (1:50)
Ioprep	External antiseptic	Undiluted (1%)
Wescodyne		
Chlorine Preparation		
Clorox	Disinfectant	5% (1:20)
Cationic Quaternary		
Ammonium Compound		
Zephiran	External antiseptic	0.1-0.13% (1:750-1:1,000)
Roccal		
Ceepyn	Urinary antiseptic	0.01% (1:10,000)
Miscellaneous		
Alcohol	External antiseptic	Undiluted (70%)
Glutaraldehyde	Disinfectant	Undiluted (1:50)

*Copyright 1969 by Medical Economics Company. Adapted with permission from RN 32:51, 1969

TABLE 5.4
Advantages and Disadvantages of Some Antimicrobials*

	CHEMICAL GROUP	ADVANTAGES	DISADVANTAGES
Effective as Antiseptics and Disinfectants	Alcohol	Inexpensive; rapidly effective against vegetative bacteria; effective against tubercle bacillus; evaporates without leaving residual chemical	Volatile, with no residual activity; on prolonged contact, damaging to rubber and plastic
	Chlorine preparations	Economical	Inhibited by extraneous organic matter; in high concentration, corrosive to metal
	Iodine Preparations	Highly active; compatible with soaps and detergents	In high concentration, some leave stains
Effective as Antiseptics only	Bisphenolic compounds	Generally nonirritating to tissue; compatible with soaps	Bacteriostatic only; slow-acting, with repeated and frequent application required; insoluble in water; inactivated by extraneous organic matter
Effective as Disinfectants only	Glutaraldehyde	Broad-spectrum activity	Relatively expensive; unstable; toxic; on prolonged contact, corrosive to metal; weakly sporicidal
	Phenolic compounds	Rapidly effective; compatible with soaps and detergents; not readily inactivated by extraneous organic matter	In high concentration, irritating to human tissue.
Partially effective as Antiseptics and Disinfectants	Cationic quaternary ammonium compounds (quats)	Relatively nontoxic to tissue; nearly odorless	Against some organisms, bacteriostatic only; not effective against tubercle bacillus; neutralized by soap and anionic detergents; absorbed by gauze and fabrics; inhibited by extraneous organic matter
Ineffective as Antiseptics and Disinfectants	Mercurial preparations	None	Bacteriostatic only; inactivated by organic matter

*Copyright 1969 by Medical Economics Company. Adapted with permission from RN, 32:51, 1969

Table 5.4 indicates the advantages and disadvantages of some of these antimicrobials.

Avoidance of Unnecessary Hospitalization

Another means of cutting down on infections in cancer patients is to reduce the length of hospitalization as much as possible. Many infections in these patients are nosocomial and might have been prevented if the patient had not been hospitalized. Provided that adequate and safe outpatient care and home care are available, many patients with impaired immunity may be safer from infection at home. This depends, of course, on the degree and type of deficiency in host resistance, the type of treatment being administered, and the complexity of other types of care required. Major surgery obviously requires inpatient residence, but minor surgery, chemotherapy, and radiotherapy can all be administered to outpatients if provisions are made for close observation and proper precautionary measures. All patients and families should receive as much explanation as they are capable of absorbing in regard to the patient's risk of developing an infection, preventive measures, signs and symptoms of infection, and treatment. Many patients can be taught to observe for signs of infection and to carry out certain aspects of their own care. Outpatients and their families must understand clearly the risks of infection and the necessary precautions, and they must know exactly what to do when it appears that an infection is developing.

OPPORTUNISTIC INFECTIONS

Opportunistic infections often occur in patients whose immune mechanisms are impaired, whose anatomic defenses are lowered, or who are in environments where antibiotic-resistant bacteria are prevalent (hospitals). These infections occur in severly leukopenic patients, in patients with other immunologic deficiencies, and in patients treated with antibiotics. The infections occur because of the underlying abnormalities. Treatment with antimicrobial agents modifies the balance of and the nature of existing organisms and further predisposes to infections by drug-resistant organisms. So far most of this discussion has been concerned with prevention of infection by exogenous organisms. Opportunistic infections are often caused by endogenous organisms, and they are responsible for a large proportion of the infections which occur in patients with immunologic deficiencies. Some infections caused by exogenous organisms which are very rarely pathogenic might be classified as opportunistic, but the vast majority of opportunistic infections are caused by resident microflora which are, in normal persons, nonpathogenic. Not much at present can be done to deter the development of opportunistic infections. However, many of the general measures to prevent infection by exogenous organisms are probably prophylactic for many infections caused by endogenous organisms, and some severely leukopenic patients are put on routines to cut down on the more commonly infectious opportunistic organisms which occur in the mouth, the bowel, and on the skin. Neomycin or some other intestinal antibiotic may be given orally to suppress intestinal flora. Antibacterial solutions are used to scrub the skin. These measures are routinely used for patients in life islands or laminar air flow units.

The majority of opportunistic infections are caused by resident cocci (staphylocci or streptococci) on the skin, in the mouth, or in the colon; *Bacteroides;* enteric bacteria in the colon (gram-negative rods), such as *E. coli, Klebsiella-Aerobacter,* and *Proteus; Candida,* the most frequent type of fungal infection in these patients, which can cause infections in the mouth, vagina, esophagus, stomach, or bladder; *Aspergillus; Mucor;* and *Nocardia. Pseudomonas* is another opportunistic organism causing an increasing incidence of infection in hospitalized patients, being the causative agent in a high percentage of fatal bacteremias.[3] Any one of these organisms can result in septicemia, a grave development in an otherwise healthy person. In debilitated, leukopenic patients, it is not infrequently the direct cause of death. Patients who survive septicemia may suffer later from organisms seeded in various organs which may cause difficulties with abscess formation in the lungs, brain, kidney, liver, heart, or other body areas.

TREATMENT OF INFECTION

When the best preventive measures fail to allay the onset of an infection in cancer patients, the infection and consequences of it must be treated.

Antibiotic Therapy

The mainstay of treatment for infections is antibiotic therapy. Most antibiotics are effective only against bacteria, although a few are effective against fungi and protozoans. Very few agents, and none of the traditionally classified antibiotics, are effective against viral infections. The organisms responsible for the infection should be identified so that the most appropriate antimicrobial therapy can be used. The antimicrobial agents of choice in life-threatening infections in cancer patients are outlined in Table 5.5. Prophylactic administration of antibiotics to infection-prone cancer patients is a pernicious practice. In patients with defects in immunity, use of prophylactic antibiotics only increases the risk of infections by opportunistic or drug-resistant organisms. Unfortunately, even the wisest antibiotic therapy is often ineffective in leukopenic patients. These patients do not respond nearly as favorably to antibacterial therapy as do patients with normal immune mechanisms, and the mortality rate is high for patients with infections complicating neoplastic disease. Although prophylactic antibiotics may be ordered postoperatively for patients who have undergone extensive surgery, clean surgery in areas where no normal microbial flora exist does not require prophylactic administration of antibiotics.[7] With surgery in which contamination due to organisms in the area is likely (eg, major bowel surgery), it is probably helpful to use prophylactic antibiotics aimed at specific organisms usually found in that area, but they should be given for only one to three days postoperatively, as longer periods of administration are not helpful and may result in superinfections.[7] The incidence of postoperative wound infections may actually be higher in patients who receive prophylactic antibiotics postoperatively.[9]

Injudicious or excessive use of antibiotics can do more harm than good.

TABLE 5.5
Antimicrobial Agents of Choice for Life-threatening Infections*

ORGANISM	FIRST CHOICE†	ALTERNATIVES
Gram-positive Cocci		
Streptococcus pyogenes (Groups A, B, C, and G)	PCN-G	EM, CP, LC
Streptococcus viridans	PCN-G	AP, EM, CP, LC, VC
Enterococcus	PCN-G + STM	AP, CP+STM, EM+STM, VC+STM
Anaerobic streptococcus	PCN-G	TCN
Pneumococcus	PCN-G	EM, CP, LC
Staphylococcus aureus	OX	CP, LC, EM, GM, VC
Gram-positive bacilli		
Clostridium perfringens	PCN-G	TCN, CM, EM
Listeria monocytogenes	EM+TCN	AP, PCN+CM
Gram-negative bacilli		
Salmonella species	CM	AP, CP, PCN-G
Escherichia coli	AP	CI, KN, TCN, GM, PCN-G, GM
Klebsiella enterobacter	GM	KN, CM, CI —
Klebsiella pneumoniae	GM	CP, KN, TCN+STM
Proteus mirabilis	AP	KN, GM, PCN-G, CP
Proteus species	KN	GM, CM, TCN+STM
Pseudomonas aeruginosa	GM	CI, CB, CM
Serratia marcescens	GM	KN
Mima-Herella	TCN	CM, KN, CI
Bacteroides species	TCN	CM, LC, PCN, AP, EM
Higher Bacteria		
Nocardia asteroides	SN	TCN, CS, PCN-G
Mycobacterium tuberculosis	INH+STM	INH+ET, INH+PAS, RF+STM
Fungi		
Aspergillus species	AM-B	—
Mucor species	AM-B	—
Candida species	AM-B	5-FC
Coccidioides immitis	AM-B	—
Cryptococcus neoformans	AM-B	5-FC
Histoplasma capsulatum	AM-B	—
Sporotrichum schenckii	AM-B	—

TABLE 5.5 (Cont.)

ORGANISM	FIRST CHOICE	ALTERNATIVES
Protozoa		
Pneumocystis carinii	PT	SN+PY
Toxoplasma gondii	SN+PY	—
Viruses		
Cytomegalovirus	CA	FUDR
Herpes hominis	IUDR	—
Varicella-zoster	CA	—
Vaccinia	TSC	GG (hyperimmune gamma globulin)

*Adapted from Armstrong: CA 23:148–149, 1973
†Key to Antibiotics:

AM-B	Amphotericin B	GM	Gentamycin
AP	Ampicillin	INH	Isoniazid
CA	Cytosine arabinoside	IUDR	Iododeoxyuridine
CB	Carbenicillin	KN	Kanamycin
CI	Colistin or polymyxin B	LC	Lincomycin
CM	Chloramphenicol	OX	Oxacillin
CP	Cephalothin	PAS	Para-aminosalicylic acid
CS	Cycloserine	PCN-G	Penicillin-G
EM	Erythromycin	PT	Pentamidine
ET	Ethambutal	PY	Pyrimethamine
5-FC	5-fluorocytosine	RF	Rifampin
FUDR	2-deoxy-5-fluororidine	SN	Sulfonamide
		STM	Streptomycin
		TCN	Tetracycline
		TSC	Thiosemicarbazone
		VC	Vancomycin

Identification of the infectious agent should allow prescription of the most effective drug, and the drug should be given in moderation. Superinfections occur when multiple antibiotics, broad-spectrum antibiotics, or inordinately large doses of a single drug are administered. Bactericidal agents, rather than bacteriostatic agents, are preferred for use in patients with altered defense mechanisms.

Initially, antibiotics should be given parenterally in order to avoid the uncertainty of gastrointestinal absorption in seriously ill patients. Some drugs are not absorbed well from the gastrointestinal tract and must be given parenterally in all patients. Intravenous medications must be used for severe systemic infections or for patients in shock or who are thrombocytopenic or have peripheral vascular disease, as intramuscular injections are too risky in these patients.

Certain antibiotics engender a high risk of superinfections. Awareness of the potential of specific drugs for causing superinfections and the type of superinfection likely to occur with their use is helpful in preventing, observing for, and treating the superinfections that occur. Penicillins and semisynthetic penicillins (Ampicillin) tend to cause opportunistic infections with staphylococci and gram-negative enterobacteria. Diarrhea may occur with oral administration of these drugs, possibly due to changes in normal bowel flora. Anogenital *Candida* infections (especially vaginitis) also frequently occur with the use of these drugs. Administration of cephalosporins seems to be followed by a very high risk of superinfection. Cephalothin seems to predispose to *Pseudomonas* infections and should be used cautiously, especially for urinary tract infections.[14] Superinfections also occur with frequency following the use of the tetracyclines. Exogenous strains of *Candida albicans* and *Staphyloccus aureus* are the commonest offenders, causing infections primarily in the respiratory, genitourinary, and gastrointestinal tracts.[14] Severe infections with gram-negative bacilli, *Pseudomonas*, endogenous *E. coli*, and *Klebsiella-Aerobacter*, are also common with tetracycline therapy. A particularly favorable setting for severe opportunistic infections is seen in patients with malignant disease who receive antimetabolite, corticosteroid, and tetracycline therapy.[14] Streptomycin is notorious for its propensity to cause superinfections because of rapid emergence of highly resistant mutants and their subsequent overgrowth. Because of this, streptomycin should probably be reserved for treatment of tuberculosis, where it must always be combined with at least one other antibacterial drug. Kanamycin and neomycin are similar to streptomycin in the causality of superinfections. Polymyxin B and colistin are associated most often with superinfections caused by *Proteus* species. Continued caution and surveillance are required in clinical situations where the risk of superinfections is high.

Aside from superinfections, antibiotics may cause other serious side effects. Some antibiotics are quite toxic, but when an infectious organism is causing a life-threatening infection and is sensitive to only one or two specific drugs, the drugs must be carefully administered in spite of their toxicity. Amphotericin B, for example, is very toxic, but it is the only antifungal agent of proved efficacy in the treatment of systemic mycoses (cryptococcosis, candidiasis, aspergillosis). Renal dysfunction and hypokalemia are the most frequent severe side effects of amphotericin B, but chills, fever, hypotension, and vomiting occur frequently. Phlebitis, anemia, thrombocytopenia, and liver necrosis have also been reported. Blood urea nitrogen and serum potassium levels must be checked every few days while this drug is being administered. Streptomycin causes ototoxicity in many patients when given in high doses over a long period of time. Many other antibiotics are nephrotoxic and ototoxic.

Alteration of Corticosteroid Dosage

For patients with major infections who are on corticosteroid therapy it is suggested that the dosage of steroids be reduced to the effective minimum until the infection is controlled. Corticosteroids suppress and mask many symptoms of severe infection, and there is some evidence that the infection-enhancing effects of steroid therapy are dose related.[15] Paradoxically, corticosteroids are often beneficial in the acute stages of bacterial infection, especially septicemias, where they may reduce fever and enhance well-being in a manner not well understood.[16]

White Blood Cell Infusions

White blood cell (granulocyte) infusions have been used in leukopenic patients in the hope of helping to control infections. Since it is nearly impossible to obtain adequate quantities of granulocytes from normal donors, patients with chronic myelocytic (or granulocytic) leukemia have been used. Blood cell separators allow for retrieval of granulocytes from these patients by leukophoresis. At present, the process is too impractical to be of much value as a general treatment measure, and there is doubt as to its ultimate effectiveness. The infused granulocytes have a very short life span and may not contribute much to the patient's ability to control infection.

Management of Septic Shock

Severe sepsis and bacteremia can result in septic shock. Therefore, treatment of acute infections in cancer patients must sometimes include the management of septic shock. Since patients in septic shock are so ill and their condition is so precarious, they are best handled in an intensive care unit where specially trained nurses are available. A central venous catheter must be used to monitor the central venous pressure (CVP). If the CVP falls below 11 cm of water, plasma expanders are used and fluids are pushed. Urinary output is checked frequently and should be maintained at greater than 50 ml per hour. Blood pressure should be maintained at about 100 mm Hg systolic. If a rising CVP prevents continued use of plasma expanders to maintain urinary output, Isuprel may be given for its inotropic effect and selective vasodilatation. Adrenal corticosteroids may be administered.[3]

Opinions vary regarding some aspects of the management of septic shock. Some clinicians are more likely to use vasopressor therapy than others and might institute Aramine or Levophed therapy early to maintain blood pressure. However, the use of vasopressor therapy seems to increase the risk of acute tubular necrosis. A variety of other therapeutic adjuncts, as yet of controversial value, have been used in the treatment of septic shock.[17]

Regulation of Activity Levels

Septic patients should have a carefully planned activity schedule. If the infection is localized, they may feel well enough to pursue their normal routines. With a systemic infection, however, they often feel weak and tired and cannot tolerate vigorous or lengthy activities. All febrile patients should have their activities limited; most should probably remain in bed, with bathroom privileges. Patients with very high fevers or who are in septic shock should be on absolute bed rest.

Control of Pyrexia

For patients who are very febrile, various measures may be instituted to reduce their fever. Tepid sponge baths, antipyretic drugs, and alcohol baths or cooling mattresses may be used. Since aspirin is contraindicated in patients with bleeding disorders, acetaminophen (Tylenol) is often the preferred antipyretic agent. Chills, which usually precede a spike in temperature, require warm bed covers. When the temperature begins to fall, profuse perspiration may occur. Bedclothes and bed linens may need to be changed frequently to keep diaphoretic patients warm and dry. Unless they are chilling, febrile patients should wear as little clothing as possible to enable the normal heat-regulating processes of evaporation and conduction of heat from skin to air to proceed. A cool room temperature will also facilitate heat conduction from skin to air. Fluids should be forced during febrile episodes to ensure adequate replacement of fluids lost through perspiration and increased excretion. Fluids also help to dilute toxins eliminated by the kidneys and thus help prevent kidney damage. High-calorie, high-protein fluids and those high in sodium and potassium should be offered, as fever increases the metabolic rate, which increases energy requirements, and sodium and potassium are lost with the fluids excreted. Since patients who are febrile are usually also anorexic, adequate fluid and nutrient replacement may be difficult. Approaches to these and other nutritional problems are included in Chapter 6.

Prevention of Cross-contamination

Cross-contamination is an area of concern in the care of cancer patients with infections. All drainage and exudates should be confined as much as possible to infected areas to prevent spread to other body parts. Bulky dressings and frequent dressing changes may be required to provide for proper absorption of drainage. Water-repellent substances may be used to protect uninfected wounds from contaminated drainage. For instance, an abdominal incision can be protected from accidental fecal drainage from a colostomy by taping a piece of plastic between the two wounds. Soiled dressings should be properly disposed of, as should soiled linen and equipment. Principles of medical asepsis are also of paramount importance in preventing spread of infection from patients to other patients and personnel. Personnel can wear gloves to protect their hands from infectious exudate. This is particularly recommended for personnel who have cuts or breaks in the skin on their hands. Patients who are infected with organisms likely to spread should be put in isolation. Hospitals should have an infection control committee to establish infection control policies. A written procedure for isolation should be available.

Control of Odor

Management of infections in cancer patients may also require odor control. Many infectious organisms cause the formation of offensive odors in exudates. *Pseudomonas*, for example, has a very characteristic smell which most people find very objectionable. Changing dressings and/or packing and frequent irrigations will help to control odor. Sprinkling small amounts of deodorizers or spraying atomized deodorizers onto dressings may mask troublesome odors. When local measures are insufficient, various forms of room deodorization may be used. Sprays, liquids, and even machines are available to help control room odors. Distasteful odors interfere with the patient's appetite, his self-image, his willingness to interact with others, his emotional well-being. Odor control may seem insignificant, but it is actually often an essential element in the patient's overall feelings about himself, his illness, and his care.

The hazards of infection in cancer patients are great. Diligent preventive measures and judicious treatment of infections in cancer patients can help to control infection. A summary of measures which may help to prevent infection in cancer patients with immunologic deficiencies is presented in Table 5.6. Table 5.7 is a summary of general measures to prevent infection in cancer patients, and Table 5.8 is a summary of treatment measures for cancer patients with infections.

TABLE 5.6
Measures which May Help Prevent Infection in Cancer Patients with Immunologic Deficiencies*

	LEUKOPENIA	IMPAIRED HUMORIAL IMMUNITY	IMPAIRED CELLULAR IMMUNITY
Provide high-calorie, high-protein diet	XX	XX	X
Consider possible need for vitamin supplementation	XX	XX	X
Plan and implement exercise program appropriate to condition	XX	XX	X
Prevent pressure sores; turn bedfast or very weak patients every hour	XX	XX	X
Wash hands vigorously before and after each patient contact	XX	XX	XX
Monitor white blood count	XX	X	—
Suspend immunosuppressive therapy if granulocytes reduced to dangerously low levels	XX	X	—

TABLE 5.6 (Cont.)

	LEUKOPENIA	IMPAIRED HUMORIAL IMMUNITY	IMPAIRED CELLULAR IMMUNITY
Avoid skin and mucous membrane trauma	XX	XX	XX
Avoid injections if possible	XX	X	—
Avoid intravenous infusions if possible	XX	X	—
If intravenous infusion necessary, date and change all tubing daily;	XX	X	X
apply antibiotic ointment and sterile dressing to insertion site daily	XX	XX	XX
Prepare skin before any puncture or injection with skin-defatting agent (alcohol) and antibacterial solution (Betadine)	XX	XX	XX
Shave hair on skin if sizable areas of skin integrity need to be interrupted	XX	XX	XX
Keep patient's fingernails and toenails short, clean, and well manicured	XX	XX	X
Ensure that proper perineal care is performed for females twice a day	XX	XX	X
Teach females proper wiping technique for bowel movements	XX	XX	XX
Discuss sexual hygiene, techniques, and contraindicated practices in sexually active patients	XX	X	X
Avoid rectal temperatures, rectal medications, and enemas	XX	X	—
Administer stool softeners	XX	X	—
Carefully inspect all body sites with a high potential for infection daily	XX	X	X
Clean and dress wounds as necessary, at least twice daily; use appropriate antiseptics properly	XX	XX	XX
Avoid bladder catheterization unless absolutely necessary	XX	XX	XX
When bladder catheterization is necessary, avoid contamination during catheter insertion, use adequate lubrication, use smallest possible catheter	XX	XX	XX
Use indwelling bladder catheters only after consideration of risks	XX	XX	XX
If indwelling bladder catheter essential, connect to sterile closed drainage system; do not interrupt closed system to irrigate and unless catheter is occluded; anchor catheter securely; force fluids	XX	XX	XX

TABLE 5.6 (Cont.)

	LEUKOPENIA	IMPAIRED HUMORIAL IMMUNITY	IMPAIRED CELLULAR IMMUNITY
Ensure that proper coughing and deep breathing is carried out as often as necessary	XX	XX	XX
Ensure that strong pulmonary regimen is carried out; may include chest physiotherapy	XX	XX	XX
Screen personnel and visitors with contagious infections	XX	XX	XX
Provide patient with individual equipment	XX	XX	XX
Properly clean and disinfect patient's equipment	XX	XX	XX
Avoid placing patient in room with patient with contagious infection; private room desirable when feasible	XX	XX	XX
Repair dental caries and/or periodontal disease	XX	XX	X
Ensure fastidious oral hygiene	XX	XX	X
Ensure that mouth care is performed before and after all meals; antiseptic mouthwashes; sprays; irrigations; water pik	XX	XX	X
Use life island or laminar air flow unit if available	X		
Avoid patient exposure to pigeon droppings	XX	XX	XX
Avoid patient exposure to people with herpes zoster (shingles), chickenpox, measles	XX	XX	XX
Avoid patient exposure to recently vaccinated persons	XX	XX	XX
When appropriate, teach patients and families preventive measures	XX	XX	XX
Provide appropriate explanations, support, and reassurance to patients and families	XX	XX	XX

*XX = Highly recommended
X = Recommended
— = Not relevant or probably not necessary

TABLE 5.7
General Measures to Prevent Infection in Cancer Patients

Relieve obstructions (bronchial, gastrointestinal, genitourinary)

Drain reservoirs of fluid (effusions, hematomas)

Drain abscesses

Excise necrotic or devitalized tissues

Repair fistulas

Preserve lymph nodes if possible

Obliterate dead spaces

Carry out and teach preventive measures to patients who have undergone extensive lymph node dissection in the axilla, groin, or popliteal area (avoid injections, venipunctures, cuts, abrasions, burns, constrictive clothing or jewelry, blood pressures on affected extremities)

Ensure adequate drainage of infected wounds

Minimize length of hospitalization

Teach home care to outpatients and patients being discharged from hospital

TABLE 5.8
Treatment Measures for Cancer Patients with Infections*

	LEUKOPENIA	IMPAIRED HUMORAL IMMUNITY	IMPAIRED CELLULAR IMMUNITY
Administer appropriate antibiotics (antibacterials) judiciously	X	X	X
Reduce dosage of corticosteroid therapy to minimum	X	X	X
Administer hyperimmune gamma globulin	—	X	—
Control fever (antipyretics, alcohol or tepid sponges, cooling mattresses, light clothing, cool room temperature, force fluids, replace sodium and potassium loss)	X	X	X
Manage septic shock (monitor BP, urine output, CVP; administer plasma expanders; vasopressors if necessary to maintain BP and urine output; administer corticosteroids)	X	X	X
Plan activity within limits of tolerance	X	X	X
Avoid cross-contamination	X	X	X
Use medical aseptic techniques	X	X	X
Control odor from drainage	X	X	X
Administer granulocyte infusions (when available; of questionable value)	X	—	—

* X = appropriate
− = inappropriate

References

1. Meyer EA: Microorganisms and Human Disease. New York, Appleton, 1974
2. Volk WA, Wheeler MF: Basic Microbiology, 3rd ed. Philadelphia, Lippincott, 1973
3. Armstrong D, Young LS, Meyer RD, Blevins AH: Infectious complications of neoplastic diseases. Med Clin North Am 55:729–745, 1971
4. Silver RT: Infections, fever, and host resistance in neoplastic disease. J Chronic Dis 16:677–701, 1963
5. Turck M, Petersdorf RG: The role of antibiotics in the prevention of urinary tract infections. J Chronic Dis 15:683–689, 1962
6. Cleland V, Cox F, Berggren H, Mac Innis MF: Prevention of bacteriuria in female patients with indwelling catheters. Nurs Res 20:309–318, July-August 1971
7. Armstrong D: Life threatening infections in cancer patients. CA 23:138–150, 1973
8. The professional nurse and chemotherapy. In Behnke HD (ed): Guidelines for Comprehensive Nursing Care in Cancer. Report of a Series of Continuing Education Seminars in the Care of the Patient with Cancer, held at Memorial-Sloan Kettering Cancer Center. New York, Springer, 1973
9. Andriole VT: Treatment of opportunistic infections complicating surgery. Mod Treat 3:1116–1128, 1966
10. Harris J, Bagai RC: Immune deficiency states associated with malignant disease in man. Med Clin North Am 56:501–514, 1972
11. Louria DB: Treatment of opportunistic fungal infections. Mod Treat 3:1099–1106, July-August, 1966
12. Silver: op cit, p 693
13. Kretzer MP, Engley FB: Effective use of antiseptics and disinfectants. RN 32:48–53, 1969
14. Turck M, Petersdorf RG: Treatment of opportunistic infections complicating antibiotic therapy. Mod Treat 3:1107–1115, July-August, 1966
15. Weinberg AN, Austen KF: Treatment of opportunistic infections secondary to corticosteroid and/or antimetabolite therapy. Mod Treat 3:1147–1161, July-August, 1966
16. Smith H: Antibiotics in Clinical Practice, 2nd ed. London, Pitman, 1972
17. Sanford JP: Treatment and prevention of opportunistic infections of the urinary tract. Mod Treat 3:1162–1170, July-August, 1966

Bibliography

Bodey GP, Watson P, Cooper C, Freireich EJ: Protected environment units for cancer patients. CA 21:214–219, July, August, 1971

Brachman PS: Symposium on infection and the nurse. Nurs Clin North Am 5:85–88, March, 1970

Garrod LP, O'Grady F: Antibiotic and Chemotherapy, 3rd ed. Edinburgh, Livingston, 1971

Louria DB: Treatment of infections arising in patients with neoplasms. Mod Treat 3:1093–1098, July-August, 1966

Mangan HM: Care, coordination and communication in the life island setting. NO 17:40–44, January, 1969

Metcalf D: Initiation of immune responses against cancer cells. CA 22:308–310, September-October, 1972

Mudd S (ed): Infectious Agents and Host Reactions. Philadelphia, Saunders, 1970

Pierce AK, Sanford JP: Treatment and prevention of infections associated with inhalation therapy. Mod Treat 3:1171–1174, July-August, 1966

Rose NR, Milgrom F, van Oss CJ (eds): Principles of Immunology. New York, Macmillan, 1973

Schumann D, Coindreau P: The adult with acute leukemia. Nurs Clin North Am 7:743–761, December, 1972

Scope Monograph on Immunology. Kalamazoo, Michigan, Upjohn Co, 1970

Warner GA: Immunotherapeutic approaches to cancer control. AORN 17:71–74, May, 1973

6
Nutrition

Life cannot be sustained without a continuous supply of energy. Basically, for human beings this requires the intake, absorption, and utilization of substances capable of being metabolized to forms usable for human physiologic functions and the availability of oxygen to complete the chemical reactions which convert these substances into energy. In addition to the minimum energy requirements necessary to support fundamental life processes there are particular nutrients required to support specific processes conducive to the healthy growth, maintenance, and repair of human tissues. With regard to nutrition, sustaining life may differ from promoting optimum health. It may be necessary, at times, to disregard optimum nutrition when it interferes with the implementation of other short or long-term lifesaving measures.

In addition to normal energy requirements, there are certain factors which increase demands for energy. In addition to physical activity, there are many less obvious influences on metabolic needs, such as trauma, which leads to increased energy requirements for healing, and infection, which usually leads to fever and an elevated metabolic rate. The caloric needs, as well as needs for more specific nutrients, such as vitamin C, may escalate in these situations to several times what the patient normally needs. Since infections are a frequent problem in cancer patients, many of whom have impaired immunologic defenses (in association with advanced age, leukemias, lymphomas, or high doses of chemotherapy or radiotherapy), and trauma is encountered often either as a result of the tumor itself or secondary to treatment, many cancer patients have extremely high energy, or caloric, requirements.

The purpose of this chapter is to explore common obstacles to adequate nutrition in cancer patients and to discuss measures to help ameliorate these problems. Since the full scope of this topic is too extensive to be presented here, only selected aspects of certain problems are discussed. It is assumed that the reader has a working comprehension of nutrition and the anatomy and physiology of the digestive tract.

Since the full gamut of nutritional derangements is encountered in different cancer patients, nutrition is a major concern for nurses working with cancer patients, and a great deal of knowledge in this area is required for intelligent nursing practice. Before entering into any specific areas, it is appropriate to discuss some general considerations in the nutritional management of patients.

GENERAL CONSIDERATIONS RELATED TO NUTRITION IN CANCER PATIENTS

The ingestion of food, in general, is a highly socialized process with great cultural and ethnic variances. Within the broad framework of acceptable social norms, there are individual styles and different degrees of significance attached to nutritional habits and needs. In attempting to deal with nutritional problems in any patient, these influences must be considered, both for the sake of the patient's right to individual consideration and for the success of the approach. It is exceedingly difficult, if not impossible, to drastically alter long-standing behavioral patterns or value systems unless they are in conflict with higher values of more firmly implanted behaviors. Therefore, in attempting to motivate patients, one must appeal to the patient's own values and operate as much as possible within existing patterns of behavior.

In addition to customs and values associated with the act of eating, both social and personal values also affect one's acceptance and concept of his body. Inanition may result in drastic changes in body texture, shape, or size which may be very difficult for a patient to accept.

In working with any patient, one must also consider how diminution in one area of interest or pleasure may affect other types of gratification. If a major source of personal esteem or fulfillment is removed, the significance of this loss may be so overwhelming that the resulting depression may curtail enjoyment of lesser sources of gratification, such as eating. On the other hand, the loss of one outlet for pleasure may intensify interest in other areas. For example, a hospitalized patient deprived of many diversionary stimuli may focus much more than usual on food. Thus, the nurse may be faced with patients whose attitudes toward nutrition range from total disinterest to intense preoccupation. At times, too, food intake, as well as other aspects of care, can become the battleground for patients who need to maintain some kind of control when it has been deprived of them in this or in other areas. Complaints related to food may also be merely safe outlets for hostilities stemming from other, perhaps more threatening and less conscious, feelings or conflicts. One should be alert to these possibilities.

Health professionals must be aware that their own beliefs and values do not always coincide with those of patients. They must also keep in mind that patients and their families do not always have enough background or information to make sound decisions or to focus on significant problems. When this is the case, the choice may be either to supply the information necessary to prepare patients to make the most appropriate decisions for themselves or to appoint ourselves or family members as guardians, and thus decision makers, regarding the patient's best interests. For those who firmly believe in the individual's right to determine his own destiny, insofar as possible, the former is more desirable. To fully comprehend the meaning of this issue in cancer, one must look at what informed consent means, at how much free choice patients are permitted, and at the distinction among cure, palliation, and prolongation of life.

Free choice is an illusion without truly informed consent. The patient must have access to all pertinent information to choose his own alternatives. Often the goals pursued during illness are a reflection of the value-orientation and outlook of persons treating the patient rather than those of the patient. Much health practice is permeated by a philosophy of aiming for a cure at any cost and of salvaging as many days of life as possible, regardless of the quality of the remaining life. Obviously there are many exceptions to any general statements, but many patients seem unaware of all the consequences of particular courses of action, or, even when they are well informed, they do not have the personal strength to withstand the subtle and overt pressures from a prestigious and powerful medical group to conform to prevailing practices rather than to deviate for the sake of personal needs or beliefs. Nutritional concerns do not lend themselves to the best illustration of all aspects of this discussion, as there are other more highly charged threats to a person's values, such as sexual impairment or physically visible mutilation, but there are some situations where personal choice in relation to nutritional problems can become an issue. An elderly person who has lived a full life and is ready to face the possibility of death with equanimity may prefer to live with palliative treatment for an extensive esophageal or gastric tumor rather than face the cost, the stress, the handicaps, and the slim chance for cure entailed in major curative treatment for these tumors. If, however, he is unaware of any of the above implications, he may submit to treatment out of ignorance or even because of the forcefulness with which any option is presented. He may not even fully realize that he has the right to choose.

In the distinction between cure, palliation, and prolongation of life, nutritional aspects of care may be a pivotal focus. In patients in whom cure is attempted and seems likely, optimum nutrition is a nearly indisputable goal. When one comes to considerations of palliation and prolongation of life, however, nutritional concerns can become clouded by conflicting issues. When used in reference to the cancer patient, palliation implies the relief of distress or maximization of the ability to live life as fully as possible in a patient with a malignancy believed to be incurable and thus almost inevitably fatal (allowance must still be made for spontaneous regression, even though it is extremely rare and may be interpreted either scientifically or divinely, depending on one's religious, emotional, and intellectual predisposition). Palliation is not to be equated with prolongation of life, but humane attempts at reduction of suffering may result in the extension of a life which no longer holds any joys. To use an extreme but commonly occurring example, the patient in an advanced stage of a gastrointestinal malignancy, who is often unable to ingest food or fluids by mouth, is often given intravenous fluids and nutrients. Even this minimal intake is often enough to sustain an otherwise unsupportable life for days to weeks. For a bedfast patient incapable of participating in or enjoying any aspect of life other than stark, unembellished existence, this may seem cruel. What happens, though, if the patient is still conscious and able to talk and interact with loved ones? Does one permit dehydration with such attendant discomforts as dry, cracked lips, parched tongue, thirst, renal shutdown, and mental confusion to intervene, or does one supply fluids and permit other, perhaps more tolerable but perhaps slower, terminating events to occur? It is difficult at times to determine which courses of action are actually most humane, and both patient and family feelings and wishes might be taken into account. These issues are pointed out here to enable the reader to keep them in mind throughout the rest of this discussion. For ease in approaching nutritional aspects, all management discussed in this chapter is based on the premise that optimal nutrition is the goal. Additional factors which may conflict with this assumption must be viewed on an individual basis with each patient.

NUTRITIONAL ASPECTS OF MALIGNANCIES

Nutrition can be viewed as relevant to cancer in two ways. One is the effect of nutritional aspects on the initiation and growth of tumors. The other is the effect of the tumor or its treatment on the nutritional status of the host.

Nutrition in Tumor Etiology

Numerous studies have concentrated on the relationship between various nutritional factors and the etiology of tumors.[1] Such studies attempt to correlate the development of malignancies with various metabolic variables ranging from broad states, such as obesity, to very specific conditions, such as certain vitamin deficiencies. In general, these studies have been rather inconclusive. Most investigations have dealt with laboratory animals, and it is not known if the same results would be obtained in human beings. Eating patterns and habits have also been investigated in regard to tumor etiology, mainly on the evidence from epidemiologic studies showing significant differences in the incidence of various tumors in different locales. Since the etiology of cancer is not within the scope of this text, this aspect of nutrition and cancer is not considered here.

Nutrition in Tumor Growth

Nutritional factors may also affect neoplasia by influencing either progression or regression of tumors which have already developed. In general, tumor growth seems much less responsive to dietary variation than does tumor genesis. Most studies have shown that caloric, protein, or vitamin restrictions do inhibit tumor growth, but the health of the host is equally impaired. Dietary manipulation of specific nutrients, such as vitamins or amino acids, has recently been suggested as a possible therapeutic measure, particularly in conjunction with chemotherapy, but this area has not yet been explored very far.[2] In general, the nutritional therapy for cancer patients currently consists of attempts to promote a normal, well-balanced, optimal nutritional intake. Specifically, the purpose of therapy may be preparation for treatment, either surgery, chemotherapy, or radiotherapy, support in recovery from treatment, or maximum function between treatment phases, during disease-free intervals, or even in far-advanced or terminal illness. In pondering the value of nutritional therapy, one must not overlook the common meanings attributed to food. Food is often comforting and nuturing: to eat may mean to be getting better, while to offer food may mean to care.

OBSERVATION AND RECORDING OF NUTRITIONAL PROBLEMS

Anticipation of nutritional problems with institution of appropriate prophylactic measures is the ideal approach to management. This obviously requires a good basic understanding of which physiologic processes are operating. Nearly all of the measures available to correct nutritional imbalances will also help to prevent them if instituted early enough. However, since not all abnormalities are predictable, identification of their existence becomes crucial. There are numerous measures of nutritional status available to the nurse, and nurses should be able to make use of them in order to help evaluate the problems and approaches.

Total body weight is a staple in the techniques of nutritional evaluation. To be maximally useful it must, of course, be accurate. Even accurate weights are only gross indicators of the patient's nutritional state, as they fail to reflect fine disturbances, and they are easily misleading when fluid and electrolyte disturbances exist. However, they do give a good general measure of overall progression or regression of difficulties related to maintenance of sufficient caloric intake.

Measurement and recording of how much, what, and by what route a patient is taking in and putting out fluids and solids can be a very valuable aid in identifying and correcting problems. Patients and families can, in many instances, be taught to reliably record or report such data themselves.

Laboratory data often give much information about the nature of nutritional problems. Identification of types of anemias, protein levels, electrolyte levels, and a wide array of other chemical, serologic, and hematologic examinations often serve to indicate the basis and severity of problems.

General observations on the appearance of patients also serve as a rough guide to nutritional status. The condition of skeletal muscles, presence or absence of subcutaneous fat, color and tone of skin and mucous membranes, the condition of the mouth, edema, vital signs, speech, behavior, and effectiveness in masticating or swallowing are all observable areas which can yield significant clues as to the existence and extent of nutritional problems.

NUTRITIONAL PROBLEMS AND APPROACHES TO THEM

Understanding the potential for nutritional problems and some of their causes should aid the nurse in assisting with and planning care for the cancer patient. Anorexia, impaired food ingestion, malabsorption (and diarrhea), constipation, nausea and vomiting, fluid and electrolyte imbalance, sensory impairment, and anemia are the major nutritional problems which occur in cancer patients.

Anorexia

Anorexia, and its offspring, cachexia, are perhaps the commonest nutritional problems seen in cancer patients. There are a variety of situations in which diminished appetite and consequent loss of body weight occur in cancer patients.

Weakness and decreased activity may cause anorexia when they occur as a result of anemia or muscle wasting. Anemia is discussed on pages 150–153. Muscle atrophy is seen in numerous instances, often associated with Cushing's syndrome, which may be induced either iatrogenically (steroids are used for both symptomatic and definitive treatment in many types of malignancies, notably in leukemias, lymphomas, and breast cancer) or by excess hormone production from the tumor itself (most often oat cell carcinoma of the lung). Weakness is also a result of anorexia which is caused by other mechanisms.

Anorexia may also be related to emotional depression, nutritional deficiencies, such as thiamine or protein deficits, or alterations in the physiologic food intake regulatory mechanisms. Protein deficits may arise because of high demands caused by tumor growth, and it is postulated that tumor cells trap nitrogen.[3] Another theory explaining the unexpected appearance of anorexia in cancer patients proposes that the tumor produces a lipid-mobilizing factor which acts upon fat depots, mobilizes lipids, and thus frees nutrients for tumor utilization. The released lipids cause an elevation in serum lipid levels. Since the appetite-regulating center in the hypothalamus is believed, in the lipostatic theory of appetite control, to respond to blood lipid levels, hyperlipemia may cause the anorexia. This theory helps to explain why even very small tumors with no apparent effect on nutritional processes may cause anorexia.

In addition to the pathophysiology of the tumor itself, treatment of the tumor sometimes causes anorexia. General malaise, fatigue, and anorexia commonly occur in patients receiving high doses of chemotherapy or radiotherapy. Large numbers of cells are being destroyed with these treatment methods, and there is a general toxic effect from the breakdown of so many cells in the body. It is very important for these patients to understand that it is normal for them to "feel worse before they feel better" with these types of treatment. Otherwise they may become unduly discouraged.

Nonspecific anorexia and cachexia can be approached in several ways. Management is, however, often tedious and frustrating and requires much patience. Nutritional problems in patients should be treated early before debilitation, with its attendant risks, becomes severe. The regimen prescribed should be based on all available data regarding the patient's existing nutritional state and the goals to be attained. Careful patient preparation and explanation, at a level comprehensible for each individual, should be an integral part of any form of management. Teaching and self-care should also be a goal in appropriate situations. The inclusion of family members in all instances is desirable, provided they are interested, helpful, motivated, and capable.

PRESENTATION OF FOOD.   A diet history is often a very valuable aid in planning approaches to combat anorexia. Determination of food preferences as well as patterns and behaviors related to food intake can provide a basis for trying to make eating as desirable and enjoyable as possible. For acutely ill or debilitated patients, foods they associate with illness may be appealing to them. They may eat what they usually eat when they are sick or what they ate when they were sick as children even when their appetite for most other foods is greatly diminished. Soups, broths, tea, toast, and other foods often fall into this category. Providing these foods or engaging families in the provision of them may increase food intake. Families should never be burdened, pressured, or made to feel guilty if they do not seem able or inclined to prepare or bring in special foods for patients, but they are often eager to help and can be made to feel more useful by participating in this aspect of care.

The aesthetics of food and its ingestion become more significant when natural hunger is absent. One must strive to eliminate any factors which detract from the desire to eat and enhance any factors which entice a patient to eat. Generally speaking, eliminating potentially detrimental factors means that the patient should be physically clean, comfortable, rested, relaxed, free of pain, and his immediate environment should be conducive to a pleasant meal. Unpleasant sights, sounds, and smells should be minimized. For many cancer patients, the attainment of these objectives requires careful recognition of the desired results and a great deal of planning. For example, to have a hygienically clean patient one must plan to complete bathing, dressing changes, ostomy care, linen changes, and so on prior to the arrival of food. Routine mouth care prior to all meals is particularly essential. Washing patients' hands and face prior to meals will also help to refresh them.

To enable a patient to be rested enough to take some interest in eating, one may have to perform tasks for the patient which he could possibly do himself if the goal were not to conserve energy for high priority functions. For example, a patient who is severely fatigued from the performance of his daily ablutions is not likely to eat well.

Striving for freedom from pain should be an ongoing concern, but pain cannot always be completely controlled. Some thought should be given to achieving maximum relief of especially troublesome pain before mealtime. Painful or upsetting procedures might be done well enough in advance of meals to permit relaxation to return for mealtime. Pain medications might be timed to achieve peak effect during meals, providing that drowsiness does not interfere with eating. Positioning is a crucial aspect of comfort as well as ease of ingestion. A sitting position, if comfortable, provides for the least amount of effort in chewing and swallowing. Many patients, however, must be helped into a sitting position to enable them to eat.

Obviously, when a patient's food arrives, he must be assisted in all necessary ways to eat it. Both patient and food must be positioned for easy ingestion. Ingenuity is sometimes required in devising methods and utensils which assist patients with a variety of handicaps to eat. Some patients may have to be fed, but sometimes simple things, such as putting soup into a cup rather than a bowl so that the patient can drink it rather than ladle it, may make a great difference in ease of eating. And the power of positive suggestion or the very directive approach, both of which work very well with some patients, should not be overlooked. An affirmative but gentle "You are going to drink your eggnog now" may be much more successful than the timid or uncertain approach, especially in withdrawn or depressed patients, who are not interested in making minor decisions anyway.

If the patient associates meals with companionship, he may eat better if mealtimes can be made more social. There are several ways this can be accomplished. Few institutions have patient dining rooms, but many have solariums or recreation rooms where several ambulatory patients could be assisted to eat together. Families could be encouraged to visit during mealtime and could perhaps even eat meals with the patient. Either the hospital could provide the food for both, the family member could bring in his own food, or the family could bring in food for both themselves and the patient. It should be certain, though, that the presence of others does not distress the patient or distract him from eating. Very loquacious persons, for example, may expend more energy in talking than in eating if they have company during meals.

If it is the patient's custom, taking a cocktail or wine before or during a meal may stimulate the appetite and also provides a source of many calories. Since hospital personnel often demonstrate a teetotaler attitude while on the job, it is usually much less complicated to keep these little libations as private as possible.

Clearly the appearance of the food itself and the manner in which it is served affect appetite. While it is difficult to control the preparation of institutional food, the manner in which it is served can often be altered. A single flower on a tray, a bouquet of flowers on the overbed table, attractive napkins, small decorative favors, hard utensils (rather than plastic), and other minor changes can often be implemented either by the institution or by the family.

The quantity of food served may also affect appetite. Large portions are often unappealing or discouraging to debilitated patients, and they frequently get over-tired in attempting to eat too much at one time. They seem to manage better with smaller, more frequent servings. Also, finishing a serving may have the effect of a success experience and can thus be rewarding and reinforcing.

Obviously the nature of the foods served is of paramount importance in treating anorexia. The most therapeutic foods are those which provide the most of the specific nutrients the individual patient needs, but providing adequate calories, proteins, and vitamins is usually challenging enough without becoming concerned about more specific nutrients. Unless nonprotein calories are supplied in sufficient quantities, body protein will be depleted, and protein intake must be adequate to maintain positive nitrogen balance. Various conditions in cancer patients, such as draining fistulas or weeping ulcerations, will greatly increase normal protein requirements. Therefore, high-protein, high-calorie foods are usually most therapeutic, and any manner in which caloric intake can be increased is helpful. Cream, butter, or dry milk can be added to many soups. Sugar can be added to fruit juices. Gravy can be added to meats. Patients can be advised to drink juices or other caloric beverages instead of water when they are thirsty. Some nurses have filled bedside pitchers with orange juice or have carried juice or milk with them when administering oral medications. Noncaloric foods and beverages (coffee and tea included) should be discouraged unless the patient is particularly fond of or dependent on them.

Attention, too, should be given to providing nontiring foods or those which do not require much masticatory or swallowing effort. Whole steak, for instance, is more tiring than ground steak; a hard roll is more tiring than a soft one. Institutional soft diets, however, tend to be quite monotonous and unattractive, so that careful selection of a general diet may prove more beneficial than provision of a soft diet.

MEDICATIONS.   Multiple vitamin supplements should be given if there is long-term nutritional deficiency or when the patient is not eating a well-balanced diet. Specific vitamins should be ordered when there is an obvious deficit or increased metabolic need for them.

Certain medications may improve a patient's appetite, usually as a by-product of altering the patient's mood. Adrenal corticosteroids, for example, enhance appetite, but in a framework of generalized improvement in outlook, the sense of well-being which is a characteristic effect of these compounds. Androgens exhibit a protein-sparing effect on body tissues but have other rather serious side effects and thus probably should not be used solely for their anabolic effects. Tranquiliz-ers may improve food intake by promoting relaxation and decreasing anxiety. Mood elevators may help combat the devastating effects that severe emotional depression has on appetite.

Depression is a nearly universal problem in various stages of cancer. Optimally, the etiology rather than the symptoms of depression should be dealt with. An overall and overwhelming disinterest in nearly everything is a hallmark of profound depression, and appetite is decreased as much as sleep, libido, and other vital functions. It is nearly impossible and perhaps even of questionable value to try to convince someone to take an interest in nutrition when he may be struggling to combat the monstrously devitalizing effects of depression. Mention has been made earlier of emotional reactions to altered body image. Part of the depression in cachetic patients may be due to changes in feelings of physical attractiveness, self-worth, and wholeness related to physical changes in the body. Anything which can sincerely be done to reassure patients of their continued worth and to positively enhance their feelings about their physical selves may be very helpful.

Generally speaking, many of the above approaches to nutritional problems can be more easily accomplished with the patient in his own home, provided that the patient and family have a sound understanding of the purposes and goals to be achieved. The home situation is usually much more flexible and allows for greater selection of foods, easier provision of food preferences, and more variable timing of meals. In addition, the patient's emotional outlook may be greatly improved at home. There is usually much more at home to stimulate, to pique interest and joy in living, and, consequently, to decrease depression and apathy. Ongoing assistance with nutritional problems in the home may be provided by the visiting nurse.

INTRAVENOUS FEEDINGS.   Intravenous administration of fluids and nutrients may be necessary to supplement the intake of patients who cannot take adequate quantities of these by mouth. Because hypertonic solutions infusing into peripheral veins cause phlebitis and thrombosis, the number of calories delivered by this method is limited by the ability of the circulatory system to tolerate the fluid load, and renal or cardiac impairments may compromise the body's usual ability to handle fluid loads. Adequate carbohydrates, electrolytes, vitamins, and water can be supplied intravenously without difficulty. Proteins can be covered by the use of blood, plasma, amino acid solutions, albumin, or protein hydrolysates. But proteins and crbohydrates provide only 4 calories per gram and cannot fulfill caloric needs in an isotonic solution without the addition of higher caloric nutrients, such as fats, which give 9 calories per gram. Unfortunately, safe intravenous fat emulsions have not yet been developed. Those tested have resulted in dangerous circulatory and respiratory complications. The addition of alcohol to intravenous mixtures may be a partial solution, as alcohol provides 7 calories per gram, but alcohol is not tolerated well by some individuals, particularly elderly patients. Therefore, even though peripheral intravenous administration of nutrients may be useful as a supplement to oral intake or other routes of alimentation, especially if hydration is the main concern or as a short-term measure to tide the patient over a period of impaired ingestion, it is inadequate as a sole mode of alimentation for an extended period of time.

PARENTERAL HYPERALIMENTATION.   Another technique used within the last ten years in selected cases of nutritional impairment is parenteral hyperalimentation. Through a catheter which is inserted through the chest wall into the subclavian vein, hypertonic solutions can be infused. Rapid dilution of the solutions in the central venous system overcomes problems related to osmolarity. Adequate amounts of calories can thus be provided by this route, and patients with a variety of disorders have been maintained for long periods of time at normal weight or have even gained weight on this regimen. The indications for use of this procedure in cancer patients may be somewhat limited, as it seems to be significantly successful only in patients whose nutritional problems may be transient or correctable by other methods. Preparation for definitive treatment or assistance in toleration of or recovery from treatment may be enhanced by this procedure. The far-advanced or terminally ill patient seems to gain little long-range benefit from parenteral hyperalimentation, although temporary nutritional palliation, sometimes a worthy goal, may be obtained. Hyperalimentation may be indicated in patients with disseminated malignancies treated with chemotherapy. They may tolerate the chemotherapy better, and poor-risk patients may be converted to good risk if hyperalimentation is employed.[4] Patients with far-advanced malignancies show improved performance status with the institution of this procedure and life may be prolonged up to several months, but eventually such patients become unresponsive to nutritional support and begin to regress again.[5] If the majority of complications can be controlled in patients with disseminated malignancies, parenteral hyperalimentation may be valuable in enhancing the quality of remaining life.

Use of parenteral hyperalimentation requires skillful management, and calculated risks are taken. Infection is a hazard with any indwelling intravenous catheter, and the solutions infused with parenteral hyperalimentation are excellent media for the growth of infectious organisms. Careful sterile technique is required for preparation and administration of solutions. In some institutions solutions are prepared in laminar air flow rooms. Since few commercial preparations are entirely suitable for the individual patient's needs, the pharmacy usually mixes the solutions in accordance with the prescribed formula. Millipore filters are used on intravenous lines to filter out organisms and particles, and the sterile intravenous setup and tubing itself should be changed every 24 hours. Routine antiseptic management of the catheter insertion site with use of skin-defatting agents, antibacterial cleansers, antibiotic ointments, and sterile dressing changes helps to prevent bacterial entry at this point. It has been shown that the risk of infection increases with the length of time a catheter remains in place, but the number of veins suitable for insertion of the catheter is limited, and it is usually desirable to maintain a given catheter as long as possible. Catheters may remain in place for many weeks without infection if proper precautions are taken.[6] In spite of all precautions, however, septicemia is a serious, omnipresent possibility, especially in cancer patients, many of whom are predisposed to infection.

Placement of the catheter can of itself result in complications. Strict aseptic technique is obviously mandatory to help prevent sepsis, but air embolism and pneumothorax must also be avoided. Since the catheter ultimately rests within the superior vena cava and since venous pressure is lowest in this area (central venous pressure), allowing the catheter access to atmospheric pressure may result in air embolism. Placing the patient in Trendelenburg position and having the patient perform the Valsalva maneuver during insertion of the catheter will raise central venous pressure and dilate the subclavian vein, aiding in catheter insertion as well as helping to prevent the possibility of air embolism. Placing a rolled towel under the vertebral column and having the patient turn his head to the opposite side also permit easier access to the subclavian vein. Pumps are available which accurately deliver a specified amount of solution over appropriate time intervals, but care must be taken with or without their use to keep the solution running freely at all times. A dry or empty bottle of intravenous solution may result in air embolism or a clogged catheter. Since the catheter passes so closely to the lung during insertion, pneumothorax can occur. A chest x-ray is taken shortly after insertion, before solution is allowed to infuse very rapidly, to document correct catheter placement. Once placement has been verified, the infusion rate can be increased.

Patients receiving parenteral hyperalimentation must be very carefully monitored. The amount of dextrose delivered is usually increased gradually over a few days to permit the patient's endogenous insulin production to keep pace with glucose being absorbed. If the patient's own insulin production is inadequate, exogenous insulin may be supplied in the infusion. Fractional urine testing should be done routinely every four to six hours to determine the adequacy of glucose absorption. Spillage of large amounts of sugar in the urine requires the addition of insulin or the reduction of glucose administered, or both. Because of the need for regulation of insulin, the rate of infusion should be kept constant. A sudden increase in rate may result in severe hyperglycemia. Daily weights should be taken to evaluate the patient's progress and, along with intake and output records, to determine fluid balance. Because of the high risk of drug incompatibilities, medications should not be added to the infusion without consultation with the pharmacist. All solutions are usually refrigerated until 30 minutes prior to use to decrease potential bacterial proliferation. For the same reason, no one bottle of solution should be allowed to infuse for longer than eight hours. Solutions should be examined for clarity and color before infusing to detect precipitation or incompatibilities. For an excellent, very detailed discussion of many of the technical as well as some of the emotional problems of nursing management of patients receiving parenteral hyperalimentation, the reader is referred to the amply illustrated article by Colley and Phillips.[7]

TUBE FEEDINGS.   Tube feedings may be used temporarily in the anorexic patient to combat debilitation until the patient is again able to ingest adequate quantities of nutrients, but they also have a number of drawbacks and should be used cautiously. If there is permanent impairment in food ingestion, which will be discussed on pages 142–145, long-term tube feedings may be necessary. If tube feedings are necessary, they should be instituted early to avoid the vicious cycle which develops with anorexia and weakness.

Perhaps one of the main disadvantages in the use of tube feedings is the nearly total obliteration of oral intake with all its attendant meanings and comforts. Nasal and pharyngeal irritation develop quickly with the tube in place and, combined with a narrowed esophageal lumen, create difficulty in swallowing. The feedings usually sate whatever appetite the patient has, so there are very major obstacles to promoting any oral intake. Problems also arise with the concentration, storage, and rapidity of administration of the feeding mixture. Mixtures which provide more than one calorie per millimeter or those which are administered too rapidly can result in nausea and diarrhea. The latter may cause excessive fluid and nutrient loss. Cardiovascular symptoms may appear if sudden changes in blood volume are brought about. Should these symptoms develop, feedings should be stopped to allow the patient to rest. The feeding mixture should then be adjusted by dilution, slower rate of administration, decrease in the fat content, or any combination of these. Diarrhea may be controlled by decreasing the fat content or by giving antidiarrheal agents.[8] Mixtures which are not handled or stored properly can harbor bacteria. Feeding mixtures should be refrigerated constantly and should not be allowed to warm between uses.

The tube itself should be flushed with water after usage to prevent souring or clogging within the tube. The tube should periodically be changed from one nares to the other to prevent nasal ulceration. The nares should be cleaned routinely to prevent excessive encrustation. The use of mineral oil and cotton-tipped applicators is usually sufficient to remove secretions. The tube should be anchored to avoid pull. Frequent mouth care is imperative. A lubricant or cream can be applied to the lips if they are dry. Stick preparations specifically designed to coat and protect the lips, though more expensive, may be more effective than mineral oil or glycerin.

These, then, are some of the approaches to nonspecific cachexia. The ingenious, concerned nurse can doubtless think of many other ways to improve the nutrition of cachetic cancer patients. The authors believe that a deep, fundamental respect for the comfort, worth, rights, and dignity of every human being must be at the core of all approaches to treatment.

Impaired Food Ingestion

Cachexia in cancer patients may also be caused by impaired food ingestion. Tumor bulk which obstructs some portion of the gastrointestinal tract is the commonest cause of impaired ingestion in cancer patients. Stenosis or adhesions from previous surgical or radiotherapeutic treatment may be other causes. Surgically created handicaps in chewing or swallowing and toxicity from chemotherapy or radiotherapy to the upper gastrointestinal tract may result in difficulties with oral intake.

Surgical resection and radiotherapy are the most definitive procedures to alleviate tumor bulk. These procedures may be either palliative or curative. Palliative resection or radiotherapy, even for patients with far-advanced malignancies, may be highly justified if the patient is expected to survive any length of time, as the misery and extremely unpleasant death from gastrointestinal obstruction are significant considerations. For purely palliative treatment, surgical bypass procedures often provide dramatic relief from distressing symptoms. They may also be used as supportive measures to improve the patient's nutrition while other therapy is in progress or to increase tolerance to other therapy. Intravenous feedings and parenteral hyperalimentation are also sometimes used when obstructing gastrointestinal lesions are present.

A variety of surgical bypass procedures are done for alimentary tract lesions.[9,10] Feeding ostomies anywhere below the obstruction establish a route of alimentation. Cervical esophagostomies for cancers anywhere above the upper third of the esophagus or gastrostomies for those below that level may be formed. Feeding jejunostomies may be suitable for obstruction of the upper portion of the stomach. Although jejunostomy feedings have often not been well tolerated, careful management can provide for satisfactory nutritional balance.[10]

The management and care of a patient receiving ostomy feedings are essentially the same as that described earlier with nasogastric tube feedings. In addition, attention to the skin around the opening of a feeding stoma is essential to prevent excoriation, especially with gastrostomy or jejunostomy stomas, as pancreatic enzymes in the intestinal contents digest proteins and are thus extremely irritating to the skin. Skin may be protected with a variety of water-insoluble agents, such as zinc oxide, aluminum paste, or Desitin ointment. To deter leakage around the tube, patients should lie flat after feedings. After several weeks, most ostomy tubes can be removed and inserted only at the time of feeding.[8]

For patients discharged on ostomy feedings, food blenders are useful in preparing mixtures. They pay for themselves by allowing the family to use regular foods rather than expensive special commercial preparations.

For lesions in the lower portion of the stomach and in the small intestine, anastomosing procedures may be helpful. Gastrojejunostomy may relieve blockage at the lower level of the stomach, cholecystojejunostomy may relieve obstruction caused by cancer of the head of the pancreas, and resection with end-to-end anastomosis or enteroenterostomy may relieve involvement in the small intestine. Lesions below the small intestine may be resected with anastomosis of the two portions of the intestine, they may be merely bypassed with anastomosis, or for very low lesions, intestinal contents may merely be diverted to the abdominal wall by the creation of a colostomy.

The most distressing of these procedures are those which require permanent dependence on tube feedings or fecal diversion. Oral and anal needs and habits are highly charged with emotions and socially prescribed customs. At best, adjustment is difficult, and many patients never seem to adjust. Careful evaluation of the problems and thoughtful analysis of approaches to resolving them may do much to ensure maximum rehabilitation. Many of these considerations are discussed in Chapter 8.

Irritation or edema of the oropharynx or esophagus may be another cause of impaired ingestion. This may be due to radiotherapy, chemotherapy, or the disease process itself. Large doses of radiation to the oropharyngeal area reduce the production of saliva and cause irritation and edema. Irritation and edema are also seen in the esophagitis which results from esophageal or mediastinal irradiation. Stomatitis may also occur as a manifestation of toxic chemotherapy or of acute leukemia when infection has developed. All these causes result in painful or difficult chewing and swallowing.

When stomatitis or esophagitis occurs, topical anesthetics will reduce the discomfort of eating and are thus sometimes very helpful. Unfortunately, they also eliminate the sense of taste. For patients with a very dry mouth, liquids, purees, or very soft foods are often the only types of food that can be swallowed, and dry foods are nearly impossible to eat. Extremes in the temperature of foods are not well tolerated, nor are very heavily seasoned, spicy, or highly acidic foods. Tobacco and alcohol may also aggravate the irritation. Patients and families should be assisted to select appropriate foods and to plan for optimum nutrition until therapy is terminated or the disease process is controlled, at which time the symptoms rapidly disappear.

Severe handicaps in food ingestion may result from surgical resection for head and neck tumors, as also may disfigurement and speech impairments. Removal of portions of the tongue, mandible, palate, and sinuses and radical neck dissections all present major obstacles to adequate nutrition. Tube feedings are often prescribed until healing has progressed. When oral intake resumes, the patient sometimes literally has to learn once again to eat. Mastication and swallowing may be awkward. If a radical neck dissection has affected muscles of the dominant arm (hand), the seemingly simple task of getting food from plate, bowl, or glass to mouth may be embarrassingly and painfully tedious. For a poignant and revealing personal account of these and other adjustments associated with this type of surgery, the reader is referred to *The View From a High Bed* by Max Hampton.[11] Discouragement, depression, anger, and social withdrawal are all common and expected patient reactions. Newer methods of surgical and prosthetic reconstruction have helped to repair many of the defects, but the usual reactions to this type of surgery are still profound. Physical therapists, nutritionists, speech therapists, and perhaps a variety of other health team members should be intimately involved in the management and planning of the care and rehabilitation of these patients.

Good oral hygiene is imperative for any patient experiencing oral trauma, irritation, or ulceration. In addition to patients undergoing surgery or radiotherapy to the oral areas, those patients with leukopenia or bleeding tendencies require special mouth care (leukemic patients and those with severe systemic reactions to radiotherapy and chemotherapy). Meticulous cleansing of the oral area helps promote comfort and deters the development of infection in all these patients.

Mouthwashes help to loosen secretions as well as cleanse, but care must be taken in their selection, as some are very irritating. Water piks may help to remove particles between teeth and keep gums in healthy condition. Soft bristled toothbrushes, cotton swabs, or small gauze squares may be used to clean teeth, tongue, and gums, as gentleness is necessary to avoid further irritation and to reduce the chance of bleeding. Irrigation of the oral area is often instituted after oral surgery. As far as possible, teeth and gums should be kept in good repair, as poor dentition may result in serious infection. Ideally, dental repair should be considered for any patient with dental problems prior to the initiation of chemotherapy or radiotherapy or surgery of the oral area. It is no longer general practice to extract all teeth prior to initiation of radiotherapy to the oral area. Weight loss or other changes in oral tissues may result in ill-fitting dentures, which not only make eating difficult, but also add to the likelihood of ulcerations developing. In general, dentures or partial plates should not be used in patients who have stomatitis.

Antibiotic therapy as well as decreased immunologic responsiveness may alter normal oral flora and result in oral monoliasis (candidiasis). Mycostatin or gentian violet preparations will combat this particular infection. The patient's oral cavity should be closely inspected regularly to detect this or any changes. Notation of progress should be made, as stomatitis and certain other conditions may be an indication for discontinuing certain chemotherapeutic drugs, such as 5-FU, which may have a peak activity several weeks after the last dose has been administered. It is imperative that baseline data concerning the condition of the mouth be obtained prior to the initiation of chemotherapy so that preexisting lesions will be documented and will not erroneously halt essential therapy.

Many of these patients have dysphagia, and aspiration of food into the lungs may be a hazard. Patients should be observed for or questioned about choking. If it seems likely that they are aspirating or will aspirate, oral intake should be postponed until that danger is eliminated. Proper positioning and instruction in ways to prevent aspiration may reduce the possibility of its occurrence.

Malabsorption

A wide array of alimentary absorptive derangements may also cause nutritional problems in cancer patients. These may be either a result of treatment methods (chemotherapy, radiotherapy, or surgery) or effects from the tumor itself. Certain types of chemotherapy and radiotherapy to the bowel may affect absorption by their toxic effect on the rapidly proliferating gastrointestinal mucosa. Edema and irritation of the bowel lead to diarrhea and decreased absorption of fluid and nutrients. Radiotherapy to the intestinal tract may also affect absorption by causing sclerosis of blood vessels, fibrosis of tissues, or fistula formation. These side effects of radiotherapy may not appear clinically until months or years after cessation of therapy. Various surgical procedures may interfere with absorption in several ways, including decreasing or increasing peristalsis or gastric stasis, altering the production of gastrointestinal secretions, especially enzymes, and reducing the absorptive surface of the gastrointestinal tract. For example, esophagectomy and esophageal reconstruction usually include bilateral vagotomy, which causes gastric stasis. Stenosis or fistula formation may also occur after esophageal surgery. Total gastrectomy removes gastric secretions, including intrinsic factor which is essential to vitamin B_{12} production, and results in rapid delivery of food to the intestine with reduced time for food breakdown and absorption. Resection of the small intestine reduces the total absorptive surface. Total removal of the ileum or the ileocecal junction may result in vitamin B_{12} deficiency. Pancreatectomy eliminates digestive pancreatic enzymes and causes diabetes mellitus. Hyperchloremic acidosis may occur with uterosigmoidostomy or ileal bladder construction. These complex problems can occur with treatment for malignancy.

The tumor itself can often cause problems similar to those resulting from treatment. Tumors affecting the exocrine functions of the pancreas or obstructing secretion of its enzymes (amylase, lipase, trypsin) inhibit the breakdown of complex starches, fats, and proteins, thus hampering their absorption. Small bowel epithelium secretes enterokinase, which is necessary to activate pancreatic trypsin. Since the mucosa of the small bowel contains numerous patches of lymphatic tissue, infiltration of this tissue by lymphoma or metastatic tumor may either obstruct or interfere with the secretory or absorptive functions of the small bowel. Tumors may cause fistulous bypasses of the small bowel. Certain noninsulin-secreting tumors of pancreatic islet cells are associated with intractable peptic ulcer, diarrhea, and steatorrhea (Zollinger-Ellison syndrome). These tumors produce an enormous quantity of gastrin or a gastrinlike substance which causes excessive stimulation and production of gastric acid and results in numerous gastric ulcerations. Steatorrhea seems to be caused by decreased fat digestion in the small bowel. The great outpouring of gastric juices renders the food so acidic that the action of fat enzymes is inhibited. Diarrhea is believed to be the result of secretion of another, unidentified hormone which specifically causes the diarrhea. Certain types of bronchogenic tumors, mostly oat cell carcinomas, and carcinoid tumors may secrete excessive amounts of biologically active serotonin or kinin peptides and result in a carcinoid syndrome with steatorrhea as one of the many troublesome symptoms. Gastric carcinomas or lymphomas may cause protein-losing enteropathies. Since protein digestion begins in the stomach under the influence of pepsin, which is produced by the chief cells in the fundus of the stomach, and since hydrochloric acid, necessary for the activation of peptic enzymes, is also produced in the lining of the stomach by the parietal cells, widespread gastric involvement may greatly impede protein digestion and, thus, absorption. Impaired fat digestion and absorption (steatorrhea), possible with several types of tumors, may lead to a deficiency in fat-soluble vitamins, notably vitamins D and K, both of which may require supplemental administration.

The diagnosis and management of problems related to malabsorption obviously may be very complex. Surgical resection, bypass, or repair may be indicated in some cases. Oral replacement or supplementation of digestive enzymes may be indicated. Parenteral or oral supplementation of certain vitamins may be necessary. Careful alteration of feedings to selectively replace or control problems with carbohydrate, fat, or protein digestion or deficiency may be indicated. In many cases, smaller, more frequent feedings may be necessary. Patients with greatly reduced food storage or absorptive capacities may find that they must eat almost continuously to maintain normal weight.

In addition to these measures, management of diarrhea itself deserves careful attention. Since diarrhea contributes to fatigue, often the patient may require more rest than usual. Anything which slows intestinal motility, including rest, may alleviate diarrhea. Measures which reduce anxiety (tranquilizers, a restful environment) and specific medications to decrease peristalsis (usually anticholinergics or opium derivatives) may help. Foods which previously caused loose stools in particular patients and high roughage foods, such as raw fruits and vegetables and whole grain foods, should be avoided. Coffee, tea, nicotine, and alcohol may be poorly tolerated. Cold liquids seem to be more stimulating than warm ones. All oral intake may be eliminated for a time, as the intake of any food or fluid stimulates peristalsis. The patient may be placed on total parenteral therapy to allow the bowel to heal, rest, or until more specific treatment is instituted.

Most patients who have diarrhea for even a short time develop anal excoriation. Careful cleansing after each bowel movement, use of local anesthetic ointments or protective creams or oils, and sitz baths may all help to reduce discomforts. Easy access to a toilet or bedpan reduces chances of accidental evacuations, which are so embarrassing to patients. Pads may be used to protect the bed from soiling. Recording of the nature and amount of the movements in diarrhea may be necessary for proper diagnosis of the cause, replacement of fluid, evaluation of progress, and administration of antidiarrheal medications.

Constipation

Constipation is sometimes considered a nutritional problem. This may occur in cancer patients who are receiving large doses of opium-derived narcotics for pain and in patients receiving the plant alkaloid vincristine (Oncovin) as chemotherapy. The constipation resulting from the neurotoxicity of Oncovin can be very serious. High fecal impactions, inaccessible to digital removal, can occur and can become so intractable as to require surgical intervention. Patients' bowel function should be followed closely to prevent constipation from becoming a major problem. Prophylactic measures are indicated with Oncovin administration. Stool softeners, mineral oil or another laxative daily, and enemas as necessary can be used to avoid constipation. High fluid intake, natural laxatives (prune juice, high roughage foods), and physical activity may also help to prevent constipation.

Nausea and Vomiting

A nutritional problem seen in a wide variety of cancer patients is nausea (and vomiting). It is seen often with the systemic use of certain chemotherapeutic agents, with radiotherapy to the upper intestinal tract, with surgery or tube feedings which cause dextrose or fats to be rapidly absorbed in high concentrations, and in many other situations, including anxiety.

Most of the drugs used in cancer chemotherapy cause gastrointestinal toxicity. Alkylating agents, antimetabolites, antibiotics, plant alkaloids, and female sex hormones can all cause nausea, although the nausea from estrogen or progesterone therapy is not due to gastrointestinal toxicity. Some of these drugs cause an acute but transient nausea shortly after drug administration (usually when the drug is given in an intravenous bolus), nitrogen mustard being the classic example. Others cause a less acute, longer-lasting nausea.

Although it is the authors' opinion, in general, that the best-informed patient is the one most capable of coping with his disease and that people have a right to know what to expect in the course of their treatment, informing patients beforehand about nausea and vomiting as a possible side effect in any situation may be one exception to this basic operating principle. Nausea seems to have a strong supratentorial component, and the power of suggestion may work to a disadvantage here. It may be possible that patients who expect to become nauseated do become nauseated, while those who are unaware of its possibility may be less prone to develop it. For this reason, the authors do not routinely forewarn patients that nausea may develop in the course of chemotherapy or radiotherapy. Patients are, however, watched very closely for signs of its occurrence, and some are treated prophylactically for nausea when it is highly likely to occur. The power of suggestion has other applications in nausea and vomiting, similar to those with pain (p. 70). Basically, it has been fairly well documented that a strong, positive approach to nearly any form of symptomatic treatment will do much to ensure the success of that particular treatment. As with the management of pain, the patient must have confidence that a method will work. Asking patients what they have found in their own experience to be helpful with certain symptoms and then utilizing their methods (if they are sound) may help more than all other traditional measures. If one is introducing or suggesting a particular method, a confident "This should help your nausea" seems to have a detectable effect on the actual success of the method, particularly in trusting patients.

The use of nitrogen mustard so univerally causes acute, transient nausea that a rather standard protocol has been established with its use. An adequate dose of an antiemetic and a sedative are given at least a half-hour before the Mustargen is injected. Ideally, since the drug is given only once during any day, it should be given late in the evening to enable the patient to ingest and absorb his meal without discomfort and to allow for the possibility that, with sedation, the patient may sleep through the hours when nausea is most likely to develop. It is illogical to administer this drug near mealtime. Estrogens also notoriously cause rather protracted nausea. Sometimes a gradual increase in dosage will help to control this annoying side effect.

For patients with less predictable nausea, certain patterns can sometimes be seen to develop. If peak times of nausea can be pinpointed, treatment, drugs, and meals may be planned to provide for satisfactory oral intake. For example, if a patient seems to be consistently nauseated after a dose of chemotherapy or radiotherapy, the treatment time may be altered to avoid interference with meals, antiemetics may be given prior to treatment, or meals may be ordered earlier or later than usual to avoid confronting the patient with food at the peak of his nausea. Nearly continuous nausea may require administration of antiemetics at specified intervals, but even with great ingenuity, an anorexic patient with protracted nausea is rarely enabled to maintain an interest in eating.

Anything which helps reduce anxiety will probably have a beneficial effect on nausea, too. Most antiemetics are also tranquilizers, but additional psychopharmacologic drugs may be indicated. Once again, it should be stated that removing or alleviating the source of anxiety or dissipating it through more definitive methods is usually more desirable than masking it.

Certain seemingly small details in nursing care may diminish nausea or make it more tolerable. Position, for example, may have an effect on nausea. Elevation of the upper torso or sitting may be more tolerable than lying flat. Cleansing of the mouth often, especially after each episode of vomiting, and use of sour balls or breath fresheners will help to remove unpleasant tastes and odors. Objectionable sights and smells should be eliminated insofar as possible from the immediate environment. Emesis basins should be within easy reach, although it is a good idea to keep them out of direct sight. Aspiration is a hazard, especially with weak patients, and patients should be taught how to help avoid this danger. Distraction may help greatly to diminish the awareness of nausea.

Since few patients who are nauseated or vomiting can or should be induced to eat, every effort should be exerted to provide adequate control of these symptoms. Careful measurement of intake and output will enable more accurate evaluation of needs for fluid and nutrient replacement. Food and fluids should be withheld until patients are able to retain them, as continued vomiting may only result in aggravated fluid and electrolyte disturbances, and patients may become strongly conditioned against food intake. Parenteral fluids and nutrients may have to be instituted until nausea and vomiting subside.

Fluid and Electrolyte Imbalance

Another complex area of nutritional concern affecting a great many cancer patients is fluid and electrolyte balance. Every known fluid and electrolyte derangement is possible in cancer patients, but some imbalances occur more commonly. Many imbalances are obviously possible with the previously discussed problems. Sodium, potassium, and chloride levels are most often altered by problems relating to food ingestion, malabsorption, diarrhea, and vomiting. In addition to effects already noted, certain tumors may secrete substances which alter electrolyte balance, such as those which produce antidiuretic or adrenocorticotropic hormonelike hormones (notably oat cell carcinomas). Patients with breast cancer, osseous metastases, and certain other types of malignancies, as well as those on estrogen therapy, may develop sudden, severe hypercalcemia, the mechanism of which is not well understood. Death may result unless the effects are reversed with administration of corticosteroids, the cautious use of phosphates or sulfates, or the more recently used drug, Mithramcycin. Fluid and electrolyte disturbances may also occur with cardiac, renal, or hepatic dysfunction, which may be either primary or secondary results of either primary or secondary tumors. Due to the complexity and scope of all these problems, further discussion is not possible here. Careful record-keeping, monitoring of laboratory data, and evaluation of clinical evidence is necessary for selective replacement of deficits or reduction of excesses. The patient's caretakers should be aware of potential disturbances in particular situations and should institute the appropriate corrective measures.

Sensory Impairments

A somewhat unique nutritional problem occurs in some patients who undergo surgery or radiotherapy to the head and neck—their sense of taste may be severely impaired. This is particularly acute in the mouth blindness which perseveres for a long time after high dosage radiotherapy to the mouth. Laryngectomy detours the passage of air from the nares to the tracheal stoma, thus preventing inspired air from passing the olfactory end bulbs in the upper air passages. Since the greater part of taste is smell, laryngectomized patients are limited to the sensations registered by the taste buds on the tongue—sweet, salt, sour, and bitter. These four tastes may be intensified due to lack of competitive tastes. For both groups of patients, this problem seems to subside over time but may be very distressing initially. More careful attention to other appealing aspects of food, such as appearance, may help somewhat to pique the patient's appetite when taste is hampered.

Anemia

As mentioned earlier, anemia is intimately related to the nutrition of cancer patients in a number of ways. Anemia in cancer patients may be due to loss or destruction of red blood cells, altered or abnormal erythrocyte production, or a deficiency of the precursors necessary for erythrocyte production. Chronic blood loss is seen often in gastrointestinal and some other malignancies. Acute blood loss can occur anytime a tumor invades a major blood vessel or when clotting mechanisms are incompetent. Frequent episodes of bleeding from nearly any part of the body occur with decreased thrombocyte availability (leukemia, bone marrow depression from high dosages of marrow-toxic chemotherapy, or high dosage radiotherapy to large areas of functioning marrow). Marrow abnormalities in leukemia or marrow metastases and depressed marrow functioning from chemotherapy or radiotherapy may result in decreased production of adequately functioning red blood cells. For example, patients who have received total pelvic irradiation will usually never again produce normal supplies of red blood cells. Marrow function normally diminishes with advancing age, and since many cancers are primarily diseases of the elderly, mild anemia may exist in a great number of cancer patients as a normal consequence of aging. Another cause of anemia may be hemolysis of red blood cells, associated with lymphomas, especially Hodgkin's disease. And, finally, vitamins and minerals necessary for erythrocyte production may be deficient because of decreased intake, excessive loss, or inability of the body to manufacture them. Iron deficiency, for example, is to be expected in chronic blood loss without iron replacement, or in malabsorptive syndromes. Vitamin B_{12} deficiency eventually develops after total gastrectomy, and it also occurs after resection of the terminal ileum.

Correction of anemia is a vital concern in cancer patients. Without sufficient numbers of erythrocytes to transport oxygen to tissues and remove carbon dioxide, the chemical reactions necessary to metabolize nutrients to usable energy cannot proceed properly, and various potentially dangerous compensatory mechanisms are initiated (eg, increased heart rate and respirations and acid-base alterations). The weakness and fatigue seen in anemia make any activity, including eating, a chore, and proteins taken in by the anemic patient will be used in erythrocyte production at the expense of protein deposition.[9] In addition to these concerns, patients undergoing radiotherapy should be well oxygenated, as oxygenated cells and tissues are more susceptible to most types of radiotherapy than are hypoxic cells.

Correction of anemia obviously depends on the cause. If the basis is blood loss, the factors lost can be replaced while the cause of the bleeding is being determined or treated. For chronic blood loss, packed red cells are usually preferable, as blood volume is usually normal. Chronic blood loss may also have depleted the body's iron stores, necessitating iron replacement. For acute blood loss, transfusion of whole blood is necessary to replace both blood volume and cellular components.

If thrombycytopenia is the cause of bleeding, platelet transfusion may sustain the patient until platelet production increases. If the cause is decreased prothrombin production, as may occur with hepatomas or liver metastases, vitamin K may have to be administered. With leukemia, the cause of bleeding and anemia is the disease process itself, and treating the disease aggressively is the best approach to these problems, even though treatment may temporarily aggravate the symptoms. Chemotherapy or radiotherapy for malignancies other than leukemia, however, may be suspended, when either anemia or thrombocytopenia becomes marked, until marrow function recovers.

With severe thrombocytopenia, precautions to prevent trauma should be taken. All measures necessary to avoid cuts, bumps, bruises, or falls should be instituted. Injections should be avoided if possible, but if they are absolutely necessary, they should be given with needles with the smallest possible bore, and strong pressure should be applied to the site for several minutes after the injection has been administered. To minimize episodes of spontaneous nasal bleeding, patients should try to avoid blowing their nose or sneezing forcefully. Stool softeners may be given to reduce the need for straining during bowel movements. Thrombocytopenic patients should also be observed for bleeding. Skin, stools, urine, gums, vomitus, sputum, and nasal secretions should be checked for bleeding. Females who menstruate may have a problem with menorrhagia. Drug protocols which induce amenorrhea may be used. Medroxyprogesterone (Depo-Provera) given intramuscularly once a week in combination with a daily dose of Premarin will cause amenorrhea and alleviate problems with menorrhagia.[12]

If the cause of bleeding is ulceration or necrosis of tumor tissue, resection, irradiation, cautery, or treatment of the tissue with either topical or systemic chemotherapy may control bleeding. If the cause is vessel rupture, ligation of the vessel may be necessary. For instance, carotid blowouts, which sometimes occur in patients with advanced head and neck tumors or after radical neck dissections, can sometimes be treated successfully if the vessel is clamped immediately. Cautery, local application of pressure, or packing may help control bleeding from accessible sites, such as the nose. Application of ice and topical administration of Adrenalin may also help reduce bleeding by causing small vessel constriction, especially with epistaxis or bleeding from vessels in mucous membranes. Iced saline may be instilled through nasogastric tubes to help control gastric bleeding or given by enema for rectal bleeding. Ice may also be applied in bags to active bleeding sites on the skin (hematomas). In general, reducing bleeding tendencies or eliminating sources of blood loss will help correct anemia.

Some general measures are appropriate for all actively bleeding patients, whatever the cause may be. Physical and emotional rest will generally help to control bleeding, as this lowers the pulse rate and blood pressure and allows clots to form. Since acute bleeding is often a very frightening occurrence for patients, calm reassurance and support are essential. Sedation may be necessary, and staying with the patient may help to reduce fear. Few events are more terrifying to patients than seeing themselves lose large quantities of blood. They may derive comfort from the physical presence of a quietly competent person who is ready to take any action necessary to assist them. Disruptions of the patient's rest should be minimized to encompass only essential activities. Priorities may need to be revised, for example, it may not be wise to bathe a patient or perform other nonessential functions while serious bleeding is a hazard. With careful planning, even essential functions can be grouped together to cut down on the number of times a patient must be disturbed. Families may need help in understanding and abiding by these precautions. In some cases, if they are behaving detrimentally to the patient or his wishes, their visits may need to be restricted.

The anemia of patients who are hemolyzing their own erythrocytes is not well understood and is more difficult to treat than the anemia resulting from active bleeding. Seen most often in patients with lymphomas, this autoimmune phenomenon is usually treated with adrenal corticosteroids. Anemia resulting from altered or decreased red blood cell production is generally treated by infusion of red blood cells. Occasionally, depressed marrow may be stimulated with androgens to produce more blood cells. Anemias resulting from leukemias and marrow metastases are treated by treating the underlying disease process; the anemia is treated symptomatically until therapy controls the disease. Anemia caused by deficient supplies of metabolites, such as iron, necessary for erythrocyte production, are treated by supplying these compounds by a utilizable route (orally or parenterally).

Since anemic patients are tired patients, their expendable energy should be reserved for the most important activities. It may be more important, for example, for them to eat than to bathe themselves, and their caretakers may need to take over some of their activities until they have more energy. They may still need to be active to some extent, but activity should be balanced with adequate rest, which usually requires planning for hospitalized patients.

Long-standing anemia may result in certain cardiac irregularities, which present additional reasons for carefully monitoring physical activity. Tachycardia occurs early, but heart enlargement and congestive failure are later possible sequelae of the body's attempt to oxygenate tissues with decreased blood viscosity and an inadequate supply of red blood cells. One should be alert for these occurrences.

In summary, it should be obvious that the entire spectrum of nutritional abnormalities is possible in the wide variety of cancers seen in patients and with the forms of treatment available. Adequate nutrition is the sine qua non of life processes. Nursing measures can be very influential in maintaining or restoring optimum nutrition in cancer patients, and this is one of the areas in cancer nursing where the aspect of hope can prevail. Hope undergoes constant revisions during the lifetime of any human being. It may be necessary for nurses to revise their own hopes for patients to coincide with the hope a patient has for himself, or nurses may assist patients in revising their own unrealistic hopes to more realistically attainable ones. The crux of the authors' belief is that patients never relinquish hope altogether—they merely revise it. They hope for different things in different circumstances. Thus the corollary belief that there is always something which can be done for cancer patients comes alive and becomes workable as an operating philosophy, and it can be a rewarding philosophy rather than a depressing one. One fails or lacks rewards only when one strives to reach impossible goals. This discussion of nutritional problems in cancer patients should be an illustration of a few of the many things which can be done to help cancer patients.

References

1. Shils ME: Nutritional and dietary factors in neoplastic development. CA 21:399–406, November-December 1971
2. Bertino JR, Nixon PF: Nutritional factors in the design of more selective antitumor agents. Cancer Res 29:2417–2421, December 1969
3. Maxwell A: Cachexia of malignancy: Some possible factors. New Physician 12:40–44, November 1963
4. Schwartz GF, Green HL, Bendon ML, Graham WP, Blakemore WS: Combined parenteral hyperalimentation and chemotherapy in the treatment of disseminated solid tumors. Am J Surg 121:169–173, February 1971
5. Dudrick SJ, Rhoads JE: New horizons for intravenous feeding. JAMA 215:939–949, February 1971
6. Shils ME: Guidelines for total parenteral nutrition. JAMA 220:1721–1729, June 1972
7. Colley R, Phillips K: Helping with hyperalimentation. Nursing 73 3:6–17, July 1973
8. Given BA, Simmons SJ: Nursing Care of the Patient With Gastrointestinal Disorders. St. Louis, Mosby, 1971
9. Hickey RC, Tidrick RT: Nutritional support in cancer palliation: General concepts and palliative surgical aids. In Hickey RC (ed): Palliative Care of the Cancer Patient. Boston, Little, Brown, 1967
10. Michaelis LL, Horsley JS, Fairweather WE: Bypass surgery: Nutritional palliation for alimentary tract cancer. CA 22:74–79, March-April 1972
11. Hampton M: The View From a High Bed. Indianapolis, Bobbs-Merrill, 1969
12. Schumann D, Patterson PC: The adult with acute leukemia. Nurs Clin North Am 7:743–761, December 1972

Bibliography

Benoliel JQ: Care and Cure: Problems and Priorities. Paper presented at program, Quality of Survival and the Cancer Patient. University of Pittsburgh School of Nursing–Western Pennsylvania Regional Medical Program, Pittsburgh, Pa, June 13, 1973
Cheraskin E, Ringsdorf WM, Clark JW: Diet and Disease. Emmaus, Pa, Rodale, 1968
De Wys W: Working conference on anorexia and cachexia of malignant disease. CA 21:72–76, January-February 1971
Dudrick SJ: Intravenous feeding as an aid to nutrition in disease. CA 20:198–211, July-August 1970
Everson TC, Cole WH (eds): Cancer of the Digestive Tract. New York, Appleton, 1969
Grant JN, Moir E, Fago M: Parenteral hyperalimentation. Am J Nurs 69:2392–2395, November 1969
Grenvik A: Prolonged Parenteral Alimentation. Lecture presented at Sixth Annual Symposium on Critical Care Medicine, Pittsburgh, Pa, May 25–27, 1972
Mayer J (ed): Nutrition and cancer 1: Problems due directly to tumors and associated diseases. Postgrad Med 50:65–67, October 1971
———: Nutrition and cancer 2: Problems caused by drugs, radiation and surgery. Postgrad Med 50:57–59, 1971

McNeer G, Pack G: Neoplasms of the Stomach. Philadelphia, Lippincott, 1967

Reed GF: The long-term follow-up care of laryngectomized patients. JAMA 175:132–137, March 1961

Shils ME: Nutritional problems arising from the treatment of cancer. CA 20:188–196, May-June 1970

Trainex Corporation. Parenteral Hyperalimentation. Instructor's Guide and Script, 1971

7
Elimination

In Chapter 8, the meaning of various organs and their functions to the integrated psychologic functioning of the individual will be explored. A change in elimination poses a threat not only to gastrointestinal integrity but also to the character, the personality, and even the identity of the person involved.

OSTOMIES

Since cancer of the bowel is the second most commonly occurring type of cancer in the total population, the nurse working with cancer patients often encounters patients who must undergo a surgical procedure creating a diversion of urine or feces. Because of the tremendous potential for patient improvement and the personal satisfaction that can be gained from working closely with these patients and watching nursing assessment, planning, and implementation of care work out, this is an area where nurses can readily see the value of the nursing process. However, this is not always true, and many, if not most, ostomy patients are discharged from the hospital ill-prepared to begin functioning at home. Unless physicians and nurses obtain the necessary skills and show a greater disposition to concern themselves with the total and continuing care of these patients, patients will continue to spend long periods of their postsurgical lives struggling for information and assistance from other sources. The positive attitude and practical realistic approach which could and should have been provided during the immediate crisis may never be attained once the patient has been subjected to the fears and frustrations of trying to go it alone.

One of the solutions to this dilemma has been the development of ostomy specialists and technicians. It has been a resounding success. The authors in no way want to detract from the tremendous contribution made by these dedicated people to the care of the ostomy patient. The failure has been that of nursing in seeing the ostomy specialist as justification for not learning about ostomy care and not becoming involved with ostomy patients. The patient is confronted with yet another specialist who treats another *part of him*. Someone must begin again to see the total being! Total patient care has been proposed for years, yet the patient continues to be parcelled out to one after another specialized technician. The other problem inherent in complete reliance on ostomy technicians is that it tends to foster the belief that this ostomy is a strange and complex thing—even the well-trained nurse or doctor cannot handle it.

This chapter does not intend to make ostomy technicians of the readers. It may be seen as the background information needed by the practicing nurse in order to fully extend to the ostomy patient the assistance to which he is entitled. Emphasis is on helping the patient gain control of his ostomy so that he may lead a normal life. The two major subdivisions within the realm of surgery affecting elimination patterns in cancer patients are procedures creating fecal diversions and those creating urinary diversions. Of the two, fecal diversions are more commonly encountered. The first part of this chapter deals with fecal diversion and considers the nurse-patient relationship in the preoperative phase, surgery, the immediate postoperative phase, including possible complications, care of the wounds, and skin care, and finally, the postoperative period of patient involvement in care. This last section includes the content and skill areas which ideally should be mastered by all patients capable of learning them. The second part of this chapter uses essentially the same approach and covers the same aspects of care for patients undergoing urinary diversions. The third portion of this chapter deals with other problems of elimination. This section includes consideration of fistulas, constipation, obstruction, bladder insufficiency, and uremia.

Fecal Diversion

Most cancer patients who require some form of fecal diversion have a primary malignancy somewhere in the intestinal tract. Since primary lesions in the small bowel are very rare, the great majority of patients undergo surgery on the large intestine. Depending on the location of the tumor, various portions of the large bowel may be removed. Those fortunate patients who have tumors of the cecum, ascending colon, transverse colon, or descending colon may be successfully treated by resection of the tumor with end-to-end anastomosis of the remaining bowel. This group, however, accounts for only about 30 percent of the people who develop colon cancers. The remaining 70 percent develop tumors further down the large bowel in the sigmoid colon or rectum, and these tumors usually necessitate removal of the anal sphincter, with diversion of feces by way of a colostomy. Obviously, the nurse working with these patients must have her facts clear. One cannot assume that all patients undergoing surgery for bowel cancer will have a permanent colostomy. Some patients may have no colostomy at all, and some may have temporary colostomies created at the time of tumor resection. Temporary colostomies are usually performed to allow the suture lines of the anastomosed bowel to heal. Patient management and adjustments are quite different in these various situations.

There are two conditions believed to predispose to cancer which sometimes necessitate total colectomy with the creation of an ileostomy. There is a type of hereditary intestinal polyposis which is mendelian dominant and progresses to colonic malignancy in a high percentage of cases. Chronic ulcerative colitis is the other condition believed to be a possible predisposing factor in the development of intestinal malignancy. For both of these conditions, total colectomy is sometimes performed (much more often for familial polyposis, however). With the exception of these two conditions, though, the nurse working in the field of cancer prevention or treatment rarely encounters patients with an ileostomy. Therefore, the following discussion of the management of the patient undergoing a procedure for fecal diversion is specific for colostomy patients. Ileostomy management is somewhat different, although much of the information regarding ileal conduit is relevant to the ileostomy patient. Should additional information about ileostomy be needed, references in the bibliography should provide some resources.

PREOPERATIVE CARE. It is essential that the nurse who desires to enable the patient and his family to adapt maximally to an ostomy begin working with both the patient and his family as soon as possible after the decision is made to have surgery. During the preoperative phase, the nurse should establish a relationship with the patient which is based on honesty, trust, confidence, understanding, and mutual respect. All of these factors are essential, and none come quickly and easily—they must be earned.

The nurse can achieve many goals by working with the patient before surgery. While discussing, explaining, and answering questions regarding the various diagnostic tests, she is establishing herself as a knowledgeable, helping person. She can begin working toward rehabilitation and acceptance of the surgery by her attitude, support, and explanations. She can provide the necessary assurance of eventual return to normal life, and, equally important, she can sort out the unrealistic fears which the patient almost always has. She can identify factors and problems which may be influential in recovery. She can also begin to formulate a plan for postoperative nursing management of the patient. The degree to which each of the aims is realized will, of course, depend on many variables in each individual patient—his physical and emotional status, his intelligence, the meaning of the surgery to him. It is before surgery that the patient must be shown that he will receive the help he needs in coping with the situations which will be necessitated by the surgery. Families, especially spouses, should be included in as much of the preoperative preparation as possible. The nurse and physician need to work together from planning the approach to telling the patient of the need for surgery and a description of the procedure throughout planning for care and rehabilitation. The nurse must know the physician's plan for care, his philosophy regarding the care of patients, and the particular surgery involved. She can then be confident in giving information and reinforcing the physician's efforts. Even if the physician takes little part in the process, the nurse who understands the surgery and is sensitive to people will be able to work with the patient. The nurse can provide the necessary information and support independently.

Preoperatively, attention must be given to both the physical and the psychologic preparation of the patient. The feelings associated with a change in the method of elimination are firmly established. Early training in bowel control is not easily ignored. The patient needs to begin to cope with these problems preoperatively if at all possible. This means that the patient must know and understand what the surgical procedure means. In this day of informed consent it is uncommon that a patient would be unaware of the type of surgery he is facing. However, knowing that an abdominal-perineal resection is scheduled is insufficient. Even when the patient says that a colostomy will be the result, it cannot be assumed that the patient understands what will happen. He may be repeating words that are meaningless to him. The complete information should be given by the physician in gradual doses as the patient adjusts to the impact of the idea. It is never the responsibility of the nurse to be the first person to tell the patient the type of surgery intended. This can be traumatic to the patient and a hindrance in the nurse-doctor-patient relationship. If the nurse knows what information the physician has given the patient, it may be necessary for her to clarify the results of the surgery with the patient one or more times. All teaching must begin at the point where the patient is.

Use of teaching aids in preparation for surgery will depend on the individual patient. Illustrations, diagrams of the nature of the surgery, and samples of the mechanisms of control may be helpful. It is useful for the patient to understand basic anatomy and physiology relevant to his condition. A visit from a person who has had similar surgery is often recommended, but the authors agree with others who feel that a preoperative visit may not always be helpful. At this time the patient is often so overwhelmed and confused by all that is happening that the visit only serves to add to his confusion. After surgery when the patient better comprehends the nature of his situation and is more highly motivated to relate to an ostomy visitor, he is better able to profit from such a visit.

Explanation of the surgical preparation should be given. Preparation invariably includes some method of partially sterilizing the bowel. This is done to help avert intraperitoneal and wound infection and to facilitate viability of the mobilized bowel. Caution must be exercised that the preparation of the bowel does not result in undue dehydration and loss of nitrogen and electrolytes. Standard bowel preparation includes antimicrobial agents, dietary restrictions, enemas, and cathartics.

Antimicrobials used for bowel preparations are given orally and consist of drugs which are not absorbed from the gastrointestinal tract. Sulfonamides, which have a specific effect on gram-negative organisms, are frequently used. These are started three to five days before surgery. One to two days preoperatively, neomycin, streptomycin, Kantrex, or Chloromycetin may be used. The hazard inherent in suppression of intestinal flora is the overgrowth of resistant strains such as *Pseudomonas* and *Proteus*.

Dietary restrictions for a bowel preparation often include a low-residue diet for three to four days prior to surgery, then liquids only on the day before surgery, then nothing by mouth. In addition, the diet is purposely planned to be high in caloric, carbohydrate, and protein content. Vitamin therapy including vitamin K, vitamin C, and multivitamins may also be ordered. Every effort to maintain or improve the patient's nutritional state prior to surgery is worthwhile. Fluid intake should be 2,500 to 3,000 ml daily.

Mechanical cleansing of the bowel often includes a cathartic usually given several days before surgery. This may be followed by cleansing enemas every evening for several days until surgery.

THE SURGICAL PROCEDURES.   Colostomy procedures vary. The stoma may consist of bowel from either the ascending, transverse, descending, or sigmoid colon, depending on the location of the area of the colon to be removed or bypassed. When the surgery is done for cancer of the rectum, a sigmoid colostomy with only one opening, a single-barreled colostomy, is performed. If however, the colostomy is done for other reasons (to allow a rectosigmoid anastomosis to heal or to prevent or relieve obstruction), a double-barreled or loop colostomy is done. The loop colostomy is formed by pulling through the abdominal wall a loop of bowel which is temporarily held in place by a glass or plastic rod, which is removed in several days. After the skin sutures beneath the loop have begun to heal, the loop is opened surgically or with cautery. The opening formed has two portals—one to the proximal portion of the bowel and one to the distal portion. The double-barreled colostomy is formed by dividing the bowel and bringing each end through a separate tunnel onto the abdomen. Both openings are sutured onto the abdomen and are separate from one another. The loop or double-barreled colostomy is most frequently a transverse colostomy. Figure 7.1 illustrates the various sites for colostomies.

The higher the colostomy is formed the more liquid is the drainage which is expelled. A transverse colostomy generally requires that the ostomate wear an appliance, although Katona has reported success with irrigation and control of both transverse and ascending colostomies.[1] Patients with sigmoid colostomies can usually achieve fecal continence. The excreta from a sigmoid colostomy no longer contains digestive enzymes and is not nearly so destructive to the skin as that of an ostomy higher in the intestine.

IMMEDIATE POSTOPERATIVE PERIOD.   For the first few days after surgery, priorities in nursing care are physical and metabolic needs. The observations for signs of blood loss and shock and respiratory difficulty are well known. A review of the observations related to the general response to surgery will be treated here. The patient would be expected to have a slight tachycardia and hypertension due to increased epinephrine. Gradually over a period of several days these should return to the patient's normal level. Failure to return to normal levels for that patient may indicate continued sympathetic stimulation or failure of the liver to meet the need for detoxifying these products. A slowly falling blood pressure with stable tachycardia warns of impending shock.

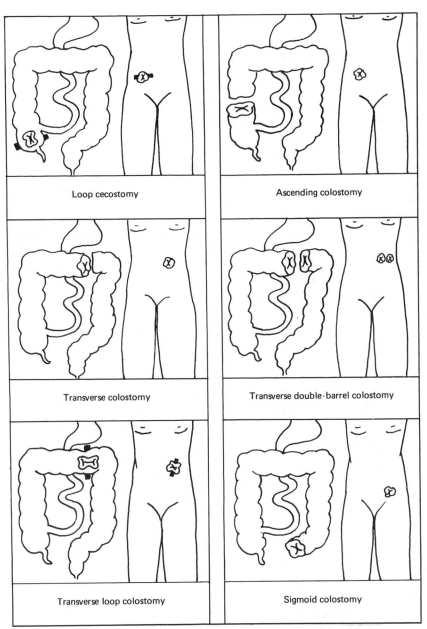

Loop cecostomy

Ascending colostomy

Transverse colostomy

Transverse double-barrel colostomy

Transverse loop colostomy

Sigmoid colostomy

FIG. 7.1.   Various colostomy sites. Left view. Relationship of colostomy to internal organs. Right view. Skin placement of stoma.

Because of the acid by-products of cellular destruction and the elevated metabolic rate, a slight increase in body temperature is expected. A subnormal temperature, one greater than 101 F, or one which persists signals trouble, and measurement every two hours is indicated.

Since the increased production of aldosterone, cortisol, and antidiuretic hormone (ADH) combine to produce oliguria with sodium retention and potassium excretion, the urine output needs to be monitored hourly. In the first 24 hours it is not unusual for it to be as low as 500 ml. The possibility of damage to the ureters or bladder makes observations of the character and amount of urine especially important after radical pelvic surgery. At the time of this oliguric state, the urine output is a reflection of renal blood flow, not glomerular filtration, and as such, it is a valuable tool in evaluating circulatory function.[2]

The interaction of cortisol, immobilization, and starvation contribute to increased protein catabolism. After extensive surgery, the patient may excrete nitrogen wastes of 150 g of protein per day. This loss of protein and the potassium loss previously mentioned contribute to the weakness noted in postoperative patients. The loss of potassium in a patient with heart disease or in a person who for some reason was deficient in potassium preoperatively can predispose the patient to cardiac complications. The hypovolemia and pulmonary diffusion impairments which attend major surgical procedures intensify this problem. Any alterations in pulse rate, volume, alterations in muscle turgor, or tremors should be noted and reported.

In most malignancies there are alterations in liver function even without metastasis. This may be the result of chronic stress or increased cellular waste load. Combine this with the transient hepatic malfunction produced when the cardiac output decreases during surgery, and the liver has a reduced capacity to detoxify materials postoperatively. Yet it is just at this time, when large amounts of protein are deaminized and anesthetic agents are still being detoxified, that medications of all types are given. The effects of all medications may be intensified and prolonged due to the demands already placed on the liver. Consequently the patient may need less analgesia in the first 24 to 36 hours postoperatively than he will during the following two to three days.

The hyperglycemia and glycosuria which result from increased gluconeogenesis, glycogenolysis, and impaired peripheral utilization of glucose contribute to the acidosis produced by an elevated metabolic rate with reduced pulmonary diffusion. Observations of respirations should be made with full realization of this acidosis. As the factors causing this situation are removed from the body, the individual's insulin production will hasten to lower the blood sugar. The diabetic who is controlled by diet or the prediabetic may have difficulty coping with this hyperglycemia. Routine urine reductions done on the second and third postoperative days may be valuable in screening for latent diabetes.[2]

Sodium and water retention with the pooling of large quantities of fluid in the operative site complicates the problem of fluid balance. There is constant danger of overhydration, especially when the third space fluid begins to be mobilized. This often occurs about the second day after surgery.[2]

Hypercoagulability is a special problem. Hemorrhage and shock, even when corrected, malignancies with cellular destruction, and the surgical destruction of tissue and interference with venous plexuses all contribute to high levels of thrombokinase and the consequently high risk of thromboemboli.[2]

If the colostomy has not been opened at surgery it is usually opened on the second or third postoperative day. For a few days it discharges only mucus and a little fluid. About the fifth day after surgery liquid stool begins to be expelled. Gradually this becomes more solid. Drainage from the perineal wound accounts for much greater fluid loss than drainage from the stoma itself. After the first few days the perineal drainage begins to subside, but it is not unusual for the patient to have some drainage for weeks to months. Patients who have had extensive blood replacement are particularly prone to profuse oozing of blood from the perineal wound because of a deficiency of clotting factors in the stored blood used for transfusion.

Nutrition is extremely important after surgery. Calories, carbohydrates, and proteins should be present in maximum quantities. When the nasogastric tube is removed the patient begins to take clear liquids. As soon as possible, low-fiber, nonirritating items should be introduced. The patient then progresses to a low-residue diet and often to a general diet. Between-meal supplements are often indicated, as anorexia may persist for some time after extensive surgery. Vitamin therapy is recommended for nearly all patients with ostomies, although this is not as important in the colostomate as in the ileostomate.

Antibiotics are given for five to seven days postoperatively to cope with the peritoneal contamination which is inevitable in this type of surgery.

Complications.   There are several postoperative complications which are likely to be seen with this type of surgery. Thromboembolic complications and fluid and electrolyte imbalances have already been cited. Bloody urine after surgery may indicate damage to ureters or bladder. Pelvic dissection may be extensive enough to cause temporary or permanent neurogenic bladder. In either case, a Foley catheter remains in the bladder until function can be assessed. Spontaneous voiding does not generally occur until 10 to 14 days after surgery. Prolapse, stenosis, recession, fistula formation, and ulceration of the stoma are all complications that require surgical correction. Mechanical bowel obstruction is the most frequent major complication after ostomy surgery. This is usually caused by adhesions either to the pelvic floor or between intestinal loops. The symptoms are those of bowel obstruction, and surgery is required.

Care of the Wounds.   The abdominal and the perineal wound will require attention. The stoma itself should be covered with a temporary appliance as soon as it is opened to help avoid contamination of the abdominal incision and to prevent the emotional revulsion associated with fecal leakage. Once the initial dressing is changed by the surgeon, dressing changes become the responsibility of the nurse. She must be careful to remember that care of the incision calls for sterile technique; care of the stoma does not. Sometimes the abdominal wound is separated from the stoma by plastic sheeting or waterproof tape to prevent contamination. This is unnecessary if care is taken to assure that a tight seal is maintained on the appliance covering the stoma. It may be necessary to shape the adhesive backing of the appliance to avoid the retention sutures. The retention sutures are generally removed about the tenth postoperative day.

The perineal wound requires some ingenuity in management. For one thing, it makes sitting very uncomfortable for the patient. If the wound is left open to granulate, packing is usually inserted, and management involves daily wound irrigations and dressings. Irrigation is usually done with half-strength solution of hydrogen peroxide. With the open type of wound, healing is usually very slow, the patient is quite uncomfortable, and oozing is profuse. Sitz baths may be used later to promote healing and to help to keep the area clean. T-binders or sanitary belts are very helpful in holding dressings in place. These perineal dressings should always be sterile. If the perineal wound is closed, frequently the procedure of choice, a drain is left in place. Sometimes a drainage tube is inserted into the wound and allowed to drain into a collection system. The drain is shortened daily and removed altogether in a few days. Healing is more rapid with closed perineal wounds. Occasionally there may be some fluid collection which requires incision and drainage, and at times the healed wound opens and drains. Heavy scar tissue which may cause persistent pain has been a problem. Katona notes that several of her patients have also developed intractable itching which was refractory to traditional treatment.[1] All perineal wounds are very sensitive and must be handled gently. Perineal sutures are usually removed by the tenth postoperative day, but dressings will be needed until the drain tract closes.

Skin Care.   One area of concern in the management of stomas begins immediately after surgery and continues as long as a stoma remains. This perpetual problem is peristomal skin care. Attention to details is essential if skin integrity is to be maintained. Creativity may be needed to solve some specific problems, but several general principles apply to all situations. These include (1) gentleness and an appreciation for the delicacy of the skin, (2) cleanliness, including thorough rinsing and drying of the skin, (3) protection from irritants, and (4) an appropriate, well-fitting appliance.

An adhesive type of appliance may be needed when the colostomy first begins to function until the stool begins to solidify. Adhesive appliances must never be pulled from the skin without use of a solvent between the appliance and the skin. When they are, they often take the horny layer of the skin with them, and breakdown is underway. The appliance is peeled off only as the adhesive material dissolves. A medicine dropper, a cotton wad, or cotton swabs soaked in solvent are handy for dripping the solvent. Some of the solvents are irritating to the skin, and all should be used sparingly. Rubbing should be avoided as much as possible. It is better to leave some adhesive on the skin than to rub briskly to remove it and damage the skin in the process. The solvent itself should then be washed off the skin and the area rinsed well and gently dried.

Protection of the skin may also be accomplished through the use of various gums and solutions. These prevent the discharge from coming in contact with the skin. Application of tincture of benzoin beneath an appliance is a common practice. It toughens the skin and increases adhesiveness. Care must be taken that only *plain* tincture of benzoin be used. The tincture of benzoin compound has factors in it which initiate a dermatitis in a significant proportion of the population. The increased adhesiveness provided by the compound is never justification for assuming the risk of a severe skin reaction. Silicone sprays or solutions and karaya powder or paste are two other substances which may be used under an adhesive bag to protect the skin. Zinc oxide, aluminum paste, silicone paste, Desitin, Brewer's yeast paste, and Kenalog spray with Mycostatin powder prevent adherence of the appliance, so they are generally used with nonadhesive bags, absorbing dressings, and to protect and heal skin to which an appliance will not adhere.

Appliances. Essential to the maintenance of healthy peristomal skin is a properly fitted appliance. If too much skin is left exposed because of a large opening in the bag, this area will break down. Because the stoma shrinks quite rapidly after surgery, temporary appliances with a starter hole which can be enlarged are popular. Care must be taken that the appliance does not fit so tightly around the stoma as to cause irritation. In order to provide a close fit without irritation, the karaya seal bags have become popular. Karaya has been a great discovery for ostomy patients. It has marvelous protective and healing properties, and it also has adhesive properties. Karaya comes in various forms: commercial preparations of the powder under a variety of names, karaya washers or seals in various sizes, and sheets of karaya gum. Karaya ring appliances are expensive, as is the use of a karaya ring with any disposable appliance. However, as a temporary appliance, because of the protective value of the karaya ring and the ease with which they can be cared for by the patient, they have a definite value. Moistening of the karaya gum washer is generally not necessary, as body heat and moisture are usually sufficient to ensure softening and stickiness. Once the stool begins to solidify, the use of karaya gum is seldom justified in a colostomy patient, and if an appliance is needed, a nonadhering type usually suffices.

Any appliance must be changed frequently enough to prevent leakage and certainly at the first sign of leakage, but too frequent changing of the appliance is a common cause of skin irritation. Bags can often be emptied rather than changed when they become full. In the immediate postoperative period a drainable appliance is less expensive for the patient, more gentle to the skin, and easier to care for than a bag which may require changing five or six times daily.

Appliances which rely primarily on karaya for adherence and the nonadhering bags require a belt. The belt needs to be snug but not tight. Some patients feel more secure when wearing a belt with an adhering appliance, and for some the belt seems to have a definite impact on the control of leakage.

Once skin breakdown has begun, management becomes difficult. Weeping, oozing skin does not tolerate well the various agents used to help an appliance adhere, and the appliance then fits poorly, resulting in more leakage. It is far easier to prevent excoriation by prompt accurate fitting of a bag with appropriate care of the skin than to try to heal even the smallest area of skin breakdown once it has occurred.

POSTOPERATIVE PERIOD OF PATIENT INVOLVEMENT. The aforementioned aspects of care are those which will likely concern the nurse before the patient has recuperated enough to begin taking an active role in his own care. Explanation of care and procedures during this time as well as the preoperative preparation already accomplished will form the groundwork for the patient's introduction to self-care.

The patient's reaction to his surgery must always be taken into account. Psychologic influences related to the loss of bowel control and alteration of body image are monumental. Altered body image brings about a grief reaction. During the immediate postoperative period, it is useless for the nurse to expect the patient to learn new and complicated techniques. Patients are seldom ready to get involved until at least three to four days after surgery. It is well to remember what Katona has said of patients' attitudes toward colostomy.

> The patient's original attitude toward his colostomy is in part due to the amount of discomfort he has prior to surgery. When the symptoms are few and cause little discomfort, the procedure appears to be out of proportion to the disease. The patient is usually irritable, demanding, and complains constantly of many things. But when he has had weeks and months of agonizing pain, or frightening bouts of rectal bleeding or diarrhea, he looks forward to the procedure as a welcome relief, and thus he is able to accept the colostomy as helpful. This patient is usually cooperative, willing, eager to learn self-care, and grateful for his survival.[3]

The patient who has had a sigmoid colostomy for rectal cancer has generally had few symptoms to prepare him. The patient who must have a colostomy for bowel obstruction or a fistula is more likely to have had distressing symptoms for a long time, so that even though a transverse colostomy is harder to care for, the patient may initially do better than the patient with a controllable sigmoid colostomy. One must never forget, however, that most of this information refers to what is happening to the patient when we have the most contact with him, while he is hospitalized immediately after surgery. As studies with other cancer patients have indicated, this may be no measure of what the patient's long-term reaction will be. Possibly when the memory of the pain and fear have faded all patients face the same problems: adapting to an altered body image, self-hatred, self-pity, fear of death, fear of rejection, anger, depression, isolation.

The nurse must also keep in mind that in our society elimination is a very private function. The patient must be allowed as much privacy as possible in the management of his excreta. Dressings, irrigations, and discussions should take place in private and should involve only the essential people.

Throughout the patient's recovery, the nurse must be patient. She must encourage but not push the patient into looking or doing too soon. She must have the ability to perceive when the patient is physically and emotionally ready to begin caring for himself. She must work out his teaching plan according to the level and amount of information he wants and is able to understand. Visual aids and written instructions, booklets, and lists should be used when appropriate. Information is best absorbed if conveyed in small bits, and repetition and testing for recall as well as return demonstration are essential. Even the patient who remembers everything while in the hospital will have lapses of memory when he is at home on his own. Careful recording of methods used and progress achieved is done as needed. Transmission of this information to the public health agency which will follow the patient after discharge will reduce the confusion to the patient of being introduced to varieties of technique when he is having difficulty coping with one.

It needs to be repeated that families should be incorporated into the recovery program as much as possible. Careful coordination of visiting time with instruction and care is usually necessary if the family is to be included. A word of caution about families is required. Not all families are able to be supportive and helpful. If the family is disinterested or overwhelmed, they may be more destructive than helpful.

The exact points which will need to be included in a particular institution with a particular patient will vary somewhat. An attempt is made to present general information with some specific techniques which the authors have found helpful in enough situations to warrant general application.

The first aim in patient rehabilitation is *control*. The patient's feelings of helplessness, the unpredictability of his stools, and his feelings of being dirty must be dealt with quickly. The patient who has never had to experience uncontrolled fecal leakage will have fewer problems to cope with than the patient whose postoperative course was one incontinent episode after another. For all ostomy patients, control, increased independence, and relative cleanliness can all be initiated with the use of an effective appliance for the collection of drainage. The bag must be sturdy enough to be effective—to provide the patient with security that it will stick and will not leak. Because of the importance of adequate collection of excreta and the relative simplicity of this process, this is probably the best place to begin allowing the patient to take over his own care. He should have been receiving instructions in skin care and bag changes while the nurse was doing these things for him. Obviously, the patient's ability to look at and handle the stoma are prerequisites to his assumption of these responsibilities. The way should have been paved for this by a frank, matter-of-fact approach and great care in assuring the patient that he and his ostomy are acceptable and in no way repulsive. The simple act of looking at the stoma for the first time is invariably upsetting to all patients. For some patients viewing a colored picture of a stoma lessens the shock of seeing his own stoma. It is also often helpful to show patients pictures of stomas as they appear weeks or months after surgery. The edema and sutures are gone and the stoma has shrunk. This is much less shocking to the patient than the large, bulky, red, unsightly stoma he has immediately postoperatively. With understanding and support, the patient is usually able to quickly overcome this initial crisis and learn to care for his skin and appliance with little assistance. This is the patient's first step back into the world of independent functioning—a very important step.

Control.   For many patients, learning control further involves eventual regulation of the fecal discharge itself. Some specialists advocate that patients with sigmoid colostomies never wear a bag over the stoma, that they use only dressings and early irrigation. Others believe that this emphasis on continence is detrimental and prefer the use of the appliance even to the exclusion of irrigation. Yet another regimen includes control using diet and medication with or without the need for an appliance. In some areas there is a growing interest in nonirrigation control. The advocates of this system feel that it is more natural and less restrictive than daily irrigations. The exact dosage and timing of medications, diet, and suppositories need to be manipulated under close supervision in order to find the appropriate combination for a particular patient. Such drugs as tincture of opium, paregoric, codeine, belladonna derivatives, and diphenoxylate hydrochloride (Lomotil) are often used for their constipating effects.

Obviously, control has different implications for different patients. In the United States, at this time, control for most patients with sigmoid colostomies is achieved through mild dietary restrictions and irrigation of the ostomy. According to a survey conducted in both the United States and in England, irrigation is superior to dietary/medication control in most patients. Nonirrigation methods of control are recommended in specific situations: (1) when hypermotility causes irrigation failure, (2) when toilet facilities are inadequate, (3) when fairly regular natural control has been achieved without irrigation, (4) when the ostomy is of the transverse or ascending colon, and (5) when the patient is unable to irrigate, as in advanced age, illness, or certain living conditions.[4] Again it must be reemphasized that each situation must be assessed, and the appropriate solution for that individual at that particular time must be determined. Not all colostomates can or should irrigate. Not all should or can be controlled by diet/medication regimens.

A few fortunate individuals achieve a natural control over their stoma. Elimination may spontaneously occur on a reflex basis at regular, predictable intervals. Mild stimulation, such as drinking juice, coffee, or a mild laxative food, may help promote this kind of reflex.

Some authorities advise the use of suppositories to achieve regular evacuation. Although movement is usually initiated, many patients find that evacuation is incomplete, and spillage occurs.

Irrigation.   If irrigations are to be used, they are begun between the second and the tenth postoperative days. The physician usually does the first irrigation, but in some cases the physician orders the amount and type of solution and the frequency of irrigations, and the nurse is expected to initiate the procedure. For double-barreled or loop colostomies, the nurse must know which is the proximal opening for irrigation. If the distal bowel is irrigated, the fluid will be expelled rectally. Though not a catastrophe, this is alarming to the patient and lessens his faith in the nurse.

Before irrigations are begun, it is necessary to determine when the patient will be doing them at home. He needs to consider various factors: the time he leaves for work if he will return to work, the needs of other members of the family for the bathroom, the time of day large meals are eaten. The half-hour to hour after ingestion of a large meal is often optimal for bowel evacuation, providing all other factors are equal. It must be kept in mind that the time required for irrigation may be from 30 to 90 minutes. Once the time for irrigation is determined, consistency must be maintained. Scheduling in the hospital unit needs to take into account the fact that most colostomates will need to irrigate either early in the morning or late in the evening. This practice must be begun in the hospital. If control by irrigation is ever to be realized, this schedule must be adhered to within an hour's leeway whether at home or away, whether done by the patient or for the patient.

From the beginning, irrigation should be done with the equipment which the patient will be using after discharge. Everything is new to the patient, and he is in no position to make the transition from one setup to another.

It is useful to explain to the patient that the irrigation is like an enema and that the purpose is to allow him to gain control over his bowel movements. It may be necessary to clarify several times that this is not an effort to clean out the entire bowel, but an effort to stimulate evacuation of the stool in the lower part of the colon on a regular basis. One periodically is made aware of the number of colostomates who spend a large part of their lives in the bathroom, trying to ''clean out all that dirt.'' Warm tap water is usually used, although cold water may be used and is a better stimulant. Some recommend adding a teaspoon of salt to a quart of water to reduce the electrolyte loss from a practice which is repeated daily. Hot water must never be used, and soap solutions are to be avoided, since they are harmful.

The amount of solution required for irrigation varies with the individual but may range from 1 pint to 2 to 3 quarts. The proper amount is attained by trial and error. Initially the use of 1 quart seems to work well, and the amount may be altered as needed. The use of more water is not generally harmful, but it encourages the tendency of some patients to irrigate for unnecessarily long periods of time. Use of less than a pint delays control because of increased spillage.

A number of companies supply ostomy appliances and irrigators. Often the choice of which to use depends on physician preference, availability within a given hospital, or chance. The set must include an enema bag, tubing, insertion catheter, backflow dam, shut-off valve, drainage sleeve, and a method of attaching the drainage sleeve to the patient. Care should be taken that the portion of the tubing or the insertion tip which will be put into the stoma is soft and flexible to reduce the chance of perforating the bowel. Also the shut-off valve should be readily accessible to the patient and easily worked with one hand. Having met these criteria, cost, estimated life of the equipment, and ease of cleaning should be determined if possible. With all this information and knowledge of the patient, one can make the best decision. This is not always possible, and an interested nurse might do her patients a great service if she were to look into these matters and choose a set which could act as a standard for her particular hospital. Some physicians prefer to handle this aspect of the patients' care themselves, but a nurse who is sure of her information and honestly concerned about her patient should not neglect talking with the physician about changes in his routine. The physician is often happy to relegate this task to someone else. Uncooperative or disinterested physicians can be a stumbling block to the execution of an orderly plan of care. It behooves the nurse to improve her powers of persuasion and her basic knowledge and skills to convince these physicians that the above points regarding patient care are necessary for the well-being of their patients. Many physicians have had only bad experiences with hospital care of ostomy patients; good care can convert them.

To return to the subject of the irrigation itself, the nurse explains and demonstrates the first few irrigations as she does them for the patient. Many patients are then able to begin irrigating with supervision. One basic procedure for colostomy irrigation follows.

1. The irrigation bag is filled with 1 to 2 quarts of warm or cool water.
2. The flexible tubing or a soft rubber catheter is lubricated. All the air is expelled from the system.
3. The bag is hung on a hook so that it is 18 to 24 inches above the stoma, about shoulder height.
4. The patient is seated on the commode or a comfortable chair facing the commode. The stoma bag or dressing is removed and replaced with the irrigator drain.
5. The irrigator drain is held in place with a belt and the end placed in the commode.
6. The lubricated catheter is directed into the stoma with a rotating motion for a distance of 4 to 6 inches. It is easier to insert the catheter if the shut-off clamp is partially open and some water is running through the catheter.
7. The water is allowed to run in slowly over a period of approximately 10 minutes.
8. The catheter is removed when all of the solution has been instilled or when symptoms indicate that the irrigation should be terminated.
9. The irrigation solution is allowed to drain back into the commode for 10 to 20 minutes.
10. The patient rinses out the drain, folds up the end, and moves about freely for about 30 minutes to allow complete return of all of the irrigant and fecal material before applying a dressing or stoma bag.

It is helpful to keep the irrigation equipment in a box which can easily be carried into the bathroom. The procedure is easier for the patient if done in the bathroom whenever possible. Patients find it easier to learn if they are helped to do the procedure in steps starting with the crucial step of inserting the catheter into the stoma. More often than not, the patient spends days learning to fill the irrigating bag and to clean up the equipment while his anxiety about inserting the catheter and controlling the flow of water mounts. Once this crucial step is behind the patient, learning can proceed at a more predictable pace. Force must never be exerted when inserting the lubricated catheter into the stoma. If resistance to the easy introduction of the catheter is met despite lubrication and a free flow of solution during insertion, it may be helpful to insert a lubricated, gloved finger into the stoma to dilate it prior to irrigation. As some physicians object to dilation of the stoma, this technique should be used only with a physician's knowledge and consent.

Abdominal cramping may occur during the irrigation if the reservoir bag is hung too high, the solution is allowed to run in too fast, or the temperature of the water is too cold. If this happens the tubing should be clamped for several minutes until the cramping subsides. When the cause of the cramping has been corrected, the irrigation can be completed. Flushing, diaphoresis, chills, tachycardia, or cramping indicate water overload, and either the amount or speed of irrigation needs to be reduced. Some patients prefer to have two irrigation sleeves ready and to switch from one to the other after the initial 10 minutes of drainage rather than trying to wash out and dry the original before folding it up to allow freedom of movement. Reading, cooking, showering, or preparation for the day or for bed are all common activities carried on while the ostomate is waiting for complete returns. Standing, walking, and change of position aid in assuring a complete evacuation.

The bulb-syringe method of colostomy irrigation has not been discussed here, as it is not widely used. The principles are essentially the same, but the equipment used is very different. For more specific information regarding irrigation the reader is referred to the bibliography.

Common Problems.   Certain problems are often associated with colostomy irrigation. These include retention of irrigation fluid, return of clear water without stool, spillage, backflow, bleeding from the stoma, and mucous discharge. Retention of the irrigation fluid is usually the result of one of three factors: (1) dehydration, (2) bowel spasm caused by emotional upset or trying to hurry, or (3) insertion of the catheter too far. If the fluid does not return, no harm will result. The fluid will either be absorbed or expelled later. Some authorities recommend inserting the catheter and siphoning back any fluid remaining in the bowel. As spillage is a possibility, the patient should wear a stoma bag after an irrigation with retention of fluid.

Return of water without stool indicates an ineffective or unnecessary irrigation. This may occur when there has been a movement prior to irrigation when the bowel is free of stool, or the bowel may be ready for less frequent irrigation. Clear returns may also occur with backflow, when water runs in and out simultaneously. In this case, as in the use of insufficient water, there is not enough water entering the bowel to stimulate evacuation. Though irrigation is usually begun as a daily procedure, most patients progress to irrigating only every second or third day. Katona presents the following guideline for this progression.

> Daily irrigation is continued until there is no spillage after the irrigation for 24 hours. Once control is established for one day, the schedule is adjusted to irrigation every 48 hours, again maintaining the same hour of irrigation. By observing returns, the day to skip irrigation will become self-evident. One day the spillage will be copious; the next day, slight. Finally, there will be little or no fecal drainage with the return of fluid, and that will be the day to skip the irrigation. There may be a slight movement on the first day the irrigation is omitted; however, frequently there is only a slight mucous discharge, which is to be expected. The use of a temporary ostomy bag will help allay fear of a fecal accident.[5]

Estimates as to when a patient can expect control from irrigations vary from three days to several months. Some will never feel safe without an ostomy bag.

The problem of spillage is usually caused by inadequate cleansing of the bowel or by insertion of the catheter too far, causing retention of fluid. Alterations in the length of catheter insertion, increasing the volume of fluid, or prevention of backflow usually correct this problem. Many authorities recommend irrigation of the colostomy until the final returns are clear. The authors object to this as a general rule. If one remembers that irrigation is not an end in itself but a method to provide the patient with the best possible chance of returning to a normal productive life, one must also consider the results of too great an emphasis on irrigation. The patient who irrigates to cleanse the bowel but has some spillage and continues to wear a bag at all times but who goes about his business confident that there is little chance of an accident is closer to the ideal than the patient who spends three to four hours a day trying to wash out any sign of fecal material from "that thing." It is essential to remember always that the goal is *living*, not doing a particular procedure.

Backflow often occurs when the catheter has not been inserted far enough, when the reservoir has been hung too high, or when a dam is not used. The current trend is to insert the catheter only as far as needed to assure adequate flow of water when using a dam. Most commerical appliances come with some sort of damming setup. A catheter threaded through a baby bottle nipple or a Foley catheter with a 30 ml bulb inflated also works well.

The bowel is insensitive to most painful stimuli. Therefore, manipulation of the stoma is not uncomfortable. Also, perforation of the bowel is not always noticed until abdominal pain and symptoms of shock occur. At times small areas of bleeding may occur on the stoma, which may be the result of pressure and irrigation and should not cause concern. Bleeding from within the bowel itself merits prompt medical attention. Both patient and nurse need to be aware that the color of the feces is dependent on the types of food ingested. Beets, for instance, will cause reddish stool.

Discharge of mucus can be alarming to the patient if he does not expect it. A Patient whose rectum has not been removed will also have mucous discharge into the rectum associated with an urge to defecate. The patient with a loop colostomy may periodically expel feces per rectum. This may be only mucus, it may be feces not eliminated prior to surgery, or some fecal material may be passing the opening in the transverse colon. This can alarm a patient if he is not prepared for it.

Appliances.   Patients who need or want to wear a bag at any time must have one which fits properly. For several days after surgery all stomas are edematous and large. Loop colostomies are unusually big and unsightly. Patients must be assured that the stoma will shrink in size with time. They also need to know that the appearance of the stoma (size, protrusion, and color) will vary somewhat with position and temperature. Immediately after surgery, the trend is to use temporary disposable adhesive-backed plastic bags. The correct stoma opening is cut with a measuring guide (supplied by all manufacturers of ostomy equipment) or by cutting a round hole the size of the stoma in a piece of cardboard and measuring the size of this hole. The correct stoma opening is approximately one-sixteenth to one-eighth inch larger than the stoma to allow for changes in the stoma. If appliances with precut stoma openings are used, care must be taken to measure the stoma and use the proper size bag instead of resorting to a standard size. At least six to eight weeks are needed for the stoma to reduce to its eventual size, although some stomas continue to shrink for many months. Permanent bags are generally not suitable for colostomates. If the drainage is somewhat liquid, as from an ascending or transverse colostomy, a drainable temporary or permanent appliance with a karaya seal is most effective. For the patient with a sigmoid colostomy who does not irrigate, one of the appliances which consists of a ring to which inexpensive disposable plastic bags are attached and which is held tight to the body with a belt is usually sufficient and the least expensive. Even when a patient has achieved satisfactory continence, he may find use of a small, lightweight protective device comforting. Some require a stoma protector to prevent undue irritation to the stoma. Many commercial manufacturers have products specifically designed for these situations. For the patient who does not need a bag, a small piece of gauze, tissue, a piece of a plastic-lined disposable diaper, a dressing held in place with tape, a belt, or underclothing is all that is needed. Most patients should have some karaya seal or adhesive bags available for inopportune bouts of diarrhea.

Figures 7.2 illustrates the variety of temporary and permanent appliances for colostomates. The cost per month varies from $1.50 to $20.00. Where price is no object and convenience is of the upmost importance, the disposable karaya seal bags have become popular. Their price makes them an unnecessary burden for most patients past the initial postoperative stage or when the colostomy is temporary.

The specifics of any given appliance are beyond the limits of this chapter. However, some general principles apply to all. Either the bag must be odorproof, or some form of deodorant must be used. If the stool is solid, the skin requires only normal cleansing with soap and water. If the stool is liquid in nature, a properly

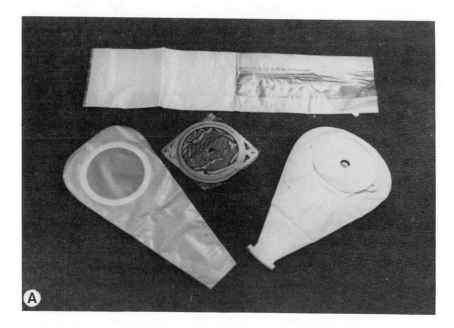

FIG. 7.2.   A. A variety of large stoma colostomy appliances. Left to right. Hollister loop ostomy set, Atlantic, and Nu-Hope.

fitting adherent appliance is an absolute necessity to keep the stool from excoriating the peristomal skin. Karaya is an excellent material to heal and protect peristomal skin, but it is an unnecessary expense in the patient with formed stool. The appliance must be emptied or disposed of promptly when soiled. The cheapest appliance which meets the patient's needs for collection of fecal material, odor control, and convenience is the best one for that patient. The reader is referred to the manufacturers of ostomy supplies for specifics pertaining to their individual appliances. A list of ostomy suppliers is provided at the end of this chapter (p 203).

Diet.   Special low-residue diets are still routinely ordered for some colostomy patients. The more recent trend is to progress the patient to a general diet while he is still in the hospital, with some special teaching about how to decide which foods to choose and which to avoid. Some foods are almost universally troublesome. Onions, beans, melons, vegetables of the cabbage family, carbonated drinks, and concentrated sweets cause flatulence in many people. Uncooked fruits and vegetables and fruit juices frequently cause diarrhea. The patient is the best judge of what he can eat. It is easier for him to decide if there are some foods he must avoid if he adds one food at a time in moderation and evaluates the results. Any food he could not tolerate before surgery is generally eliminated. It is important to remind the patient to eat slowly, to chew food well, and to swallow with the mouth closed to

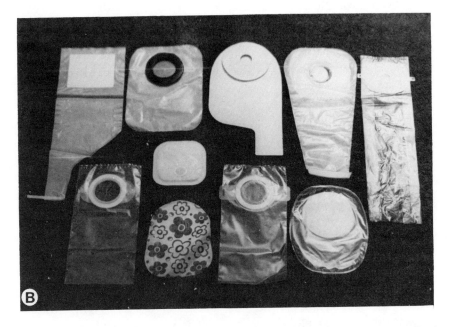

FIG. 7.2.   B. A variety of colostomy appliances. Left to right. Top row. Coloplast/Bard, Hollister, Permatype, Hollister, and Bongort (United Surgical). Middle row. Hollister. Bottom row. Greer, Coloplast/Bard, Marsan, and Dansac (Greer).

avoid swallowing excessive amounts of air. Fears of foods are minimized if the patient realizes that he can control the results. Trying new foods early in his rehabilitation before he has many social commitments will reduce the chance of having a bad experience at his first outing. Deodorants can control odor. And the patient who has to have his sauerkraut and spareribs can eat them some night when he is going to be at home alone. It is often very important to repeatedly tell the patient that refraining from eating or drinking is not the way to control the ostomy. Dehydration and improper nutrition will make control more difficult and will lead to a variety of medical problems for the patient.

Diarrhea.   Diarrhea and constipation are two occurrences requiring some dietary adjustments. Diarrhea is most often treated by a low-residue or diarrhea diet. It is wise for every patient to have a prescription for an antidiarrheal medication when discharged from the hospital. Paregoric or Kaopectate are most often prescribed but should not be taken regularly without consulting a physician. Diarrhea is not a normal occurrence, and its cause should be determined. Most often it is the result of dietary intolerances or indiscretions, medications such as antibiotics, diuretics, or tranquilizers, illness, or emotional upsets.

Constipation.   Constipation is frequently the result of inadequate food or fluid intake. Some medications, such as narcotics, also produce constipation. Increasing the bulk in the diet, eating laxative foods, and irrigation may help alleviate the problem. If persistent, the problem should be discussed with the surgeon, as it may signal problems of stenosis or obstruction. The physician may recommend certain changes in the patient's routines. It is best not to take a laxative or a stool softener without the advice of the surgeon.

Flatulence.   Increased flatulence is another problem related to diet. Everyone expels some gas, but excessive amounts may come from swallowed air, gas-forming foods, constipation, or unsatisfactory irrigations. Spicy foods, carbonated drinks, and beer are common offenders. The United Ostomy Association reports that Mylanta or Mylicon tablets taken orally reduce flatus in most patients. A small piece of damp cotton (or a junior tampax) inserted into the stoma will help to muffle the noisy discharge of gas. Also for the patient who does not wear a bag, there are devices sold commercially which muffle the noise. Whether these are more effective than the inexpensive innovations mentioned about is questionable.

Odor.   Some foods cause exceptionally offensive odors in feces. Eggs, fish, coffee, and garlic are among the worst. Some medications cause malodorous stools. Odor can be combated with oral medication, bismuth subcarbonate and bismuth subgallate being among the most effective. As many as 10 tablets may be needed initially to control the odor, and then the dosage may be reduced to a maintenance level of 1 tablet after each meal or heavy snack. Since a colostomate should take no medication without the knowledge of his physician, and since both of these preparations tend to be constipating, the surgeon should be consulted before a patient elects to take either of the bismuth preparations mentioned. Oral preparations of chlorophyll and activated charcoal are also effective in reducing the odor in feces and do not have the constipating side effects. For many ostomates certain foods when eaten at each meal help to control odor. These include oranges, orange juice, parsley, cranberry juice, or buttermilk. Sodium benzoate or several crushed aspirin in the pouch may control odor. There are a variety of commercial deodorants specifically for ostomies. One may work better for a particular patient than another, and expense is no measure of effectiveness. Deodorizers may be used in the room, but this tends to call attention to the problem rather than eliminating it and should be used as a last resort. General personal cleanliness, meticulous cleaning of appliances and equipment, and the use of the appropriate nonodor-retaining equipment are essential in odor control.

Other Areas of Teaching.   The practice of dilating the stoma may need to be explained to the patient. Since this is a controversial practice, the physician should indicate whether or not this is to be done, how, and how often. Dilatation is usually done by gently inserting a finger covered with a well-lubricated finger cot or rubber glove into the stoma as far as it will go and rotating the finger several times. Dilatation, when done, should precede irrigation. Some authorities feel that dilatation should be done with caution and only by a physician, and that the need for dilatation signals the need for stoma revision.

A few other bits of advice are often helpful to patients. Time and energy may be saved at home by the use of a rubber or plastic draw sheet until full control is attained. Patients need their sleep, and measures to prevent worry over soiling the bed need to be made available. Frequently a patient wears a bag at night long after he is confident with only a small dressing during the day. Bathing, showering, and swimming may be undertaken safely with or without an appliance as soon as the incisions are healed. Patients often expect that they will need much special equipment and a totally new wardrobe. They need to be assured that neither of these are necessary. Before discharge they should have all the equipment they need to begin functioning at home and a written list of all the supplies that will be needed and where to obtain them. The cost of various types of equipment should have been considered in relation to the patient's financial solvency. If the patient is unable to bear the expense of needed materials, the social worker and various community agencies should be consulted as to the availability of financial assistance.

Travel should pose no problem, but it is suggested that patients take along enough materials to see them through their trip and to provide for unexpected accidents. Many patients carry small emergency kits at all times. The amount of physical activity permitted, such as participation in sports, depends on the patient's general physical condition not on the presence of an ostomy.

If vocational retraining is necessary, this is available through state rehabilitation services and should be discussed with the patient. However, it is rare that a patient need change his occupation because of an ostomy. Many healthy workers as well as patients think that an ostomy will require such changes.

The influence of emotions on ostomy function should be explained to patients. They should know that emotional stress is intimately related to physiologic functions. Many bowel abnormalities are associated with psychologic factors, and ostomy regulation may be difficult if patients are not relaxed and tension free.

Patients are often concerned about whether or not to tell others about their ostomy. This is an individual decision, but it seems wise not to mention the ostomy unless necessary. If it becomes necessary to mention the ostomy, it should be discussed openly without embarrassment. Family and close friends will, in most cases, already know. If the ostomate sees himself as a normal person living a typical life, there seems to be no need to call attention to this alteration in body function.

Ostomy Associations. Before the patient is discharged from the hospital, he should be informed of the ostomy associations. These societies are dedicated to rehabilitating ostomates through moral support, education, and the sharing of practical information. In addition, the national organization provides a quarterly magazine, lecture material, audiovisual aids, and new information in the ostomy field. The patient would ideally have met an ostomy visitor in the postoperative period, but he should in any event know the location of the nearest club, whom to call for information, and the dates and times of the meetings. Information about local clubs can be obtained from the United Ostomy Association, 1111 Wilshire Boulevard, Los Angeles, California, 90017.

Home Care.   Regardless of the teaching program in the hospital, patients with ostomies can benefit from the services of a visiting nurse. Referrals should take place before discharge so that the visiting nurse may be ready to visit as soon as the patient is at home. To prevent misunderstandings and failure to follow a uniform teaching regimen, clear communication between hospital and the visiting nurse is required. Whenever possible the assigned visiting nurse should make a hospital visit to meet the patient and review the procedures *as the patient has learned them.* This enables the hospital staff to acquaint the nurse with other areas to consider and possible problems, and it enhances the likelihood that the nurse will in turn keep the hospital informed of the patient's progress. One must always remember that no matter how well one thinks a patient has been taught, home is very different from the hospital. One can never really know how effective one's teaching has been unless there is postdischarge follow-up and evaluation. Patients should also know when and where to return for follow-up medical care, whom to contact, and what to do if they have any problems or questions upon their return home.

Sexual Activity.   One area of great importance which is infrequently discussed with patients and families is sexual activity. Most health professionals are too uncomfortable or ill informed to handle the topic well, and patients are reluctant to bring it up. The basis for this reluctance is twofold: (1) even in our liberated society, sex remains a taboo subject for most people when discussed personally, and (2) when confronted with a life-or-death situation, sexual activity becomes a secondary concern. It is, however, one of the areas of greatest adjustment for ostomates. Sexuality in general is handled in more depth in another chapter, but a few points regarding ostomy patients need to be made here. The question of male potency is very closely related to ostomy surgery. Radical cystectomy and abdominal-perineal resection nearly always affect potency to some extent. Various sets of statistics infer complete loss of potency in 20 to 90 percent of males undergoing radical pelvic surgery. There is insufficient information available at this time to be certain of any figures. Women are generally not as concerned as men are with their ability to perform sexually. Except for exenteration procedures which involve vaginectomy, ostomy surgery should not affect a woman's ability to participate in or to enjoy sexual relations. However, the effect of an ostomy on a woman's feelings of acceptability and desirability are often detrimental to satisfactory sexual functioning.

Marital problems which arise from lack of understanding can be prevented. However, there may exist actual rejection on the part of either spouse, and the ostomy may be used by either person as an excuse for abstinence when sexual experiences are undesirable for other reasons. Both partners need to know when sexual relations can be normal in every respect without inhibition of either partner. It is also imperative that both partners understand what problems are likely or inevitable and what alternatives or substitutes are available. Vaginoplasties and penile implants have not yet become common, but they are available to the patient and spouse who need them to maintain their relationship and who are self-confident and forthright enough to demand them.

Physicians and health workers in general have ignored sexual problems in patients undergoing surgery for cancer. They have allowed themselves to be satisfied with the knowledge that a better chance for a longer life was given the patient. Before and immediately after surgery, this is usually satisfactory for the patient and his spouse. However, with time it is very difficult, and for some apparently impossible, to reestablish a relationship without what was previously a major part of that relationship, sexual relations. Some adjust well, others adjust poorly. Little help has historically been available to aid anyone in this area of coping. The United Ostomy Association has recently published three excellent pamphlets dealing with sex and the ostomate.[6-8]

Clean, odorless bags, an attractive bag cover, deodorants, fancy underclothes, and the cover of darkness have all been proposed as aids for the ostomate in coping with lovemaking. Frank discussion between sexual partners, knowledge of the help available, and understanding and helpful health-care personnel can do far more than these little tricks. All the aids in the world will not make the adjustment possible without frankness and the willingness to work toward a solution. For a fuller discussion of problems pertaining to sexuality, the reader is referred to Chapter 8.

That we are not meeting these many and complex needs of ostomates is evidenced by the results of various studies which indicate that the first year after colostomy is one of disability and that the majority of these patients suffer a deterioration of social relationships primarily from fear of producing odor. Follow-up on patients whose surgery was done several years previously and for whom the threat of the diagnosis is waning shows the recurring themes of isolation, chronic depression, and low self-esteem.

Urinary Diversion

Although fecal diversions are more commonly encountered in cancer patients, there are a variety of conditions which require surgical diversion of urine. Ureteral obstruction, invasion of the bladder with a malignancy, or permanent damage to the bladder, as with a persistent vesicovaginal fistula, are the principal reasons why urinary diversion is employed in oncology. It must be remembered that several noncancerous conditions also necessitate urinary diversion. These conditions generally require far less extensive surgery than in the case of malignancy, and, of course, the meaning to the patient is very different.

THE SURGICAL PROCEDURES.   There are three surgical procedures commonly employed to divert the urine stream: (1) ileal conduit, (2) cutaneous ureterostomy, and (3) ureterosigmoidostomy. Nephrostomy and other procedures which may be seen in nonmalignant conditions are less frequently seen in the patient with cancer. Currently the ileal conduit (also called "ileal bladder," "ileal loop," or "Bricker's procedure") is the preferred form of permanent urinary diversion in the United States. In England, the ureterosigmoidostomy is more popular. For emergency situations or conditions which preclude more extensive surgery, the cutaneous ureterostomy continues to be used. Table 7.1

TABLE 7.1
Comparison of Common Procedures for Urinary Diversion

ILEAL CONDUIT	URETERO-SIGMOIDOSTOMY	URETEROSTOMY
Procedure		
A portion of the ileum is resected, taking care to preserve its attachment to the mesentery through which flow the blood vessels. The proximal end of the isolated ileal segment is closed, the ureters are anastomosed to this segment, and the distal end is brought through a skin incision to form the stoma	The ureters are implanted into the pelvic colon	The ureters are brought through a skin incision and sutured at the skin line
Advantages		
Peristalsis prevents the backflow of urine and reduces the risk of retrograde infection

One pouch is needed even if both kidneys are functioning

The short ileal segment acts as a conduit rather than a reservoir, eliminating the problem of hyperchloremic acidosis due to reabsorption by the intestine

The ureters and conduit are out of the field of pelvic radiation | The patient has control via the anal sphincter

There is not an unnatural orifice

No appliance is needed | The procedure is brief and simple |
| **Disadvantages** | | |
| The procedure is long and complex

Multiple anastomoses increase complications

Radical change in body image is necessitated

Fitting difficulties are a problem | Retrograde infection is common. Reabsorption by the colon leads to hyperchloremic acidosis

Stenosis of ureters occurs at anastomosis; Corrective surgery is often required | If both kidneys are functioning, two pouches will be required

Fitting difficulties are common

Radical change in body image is necessitated |

compares these procedures, their advantages, and their disadvantages. No matter which procedure is performed, control of the urine flow with an appropriate appliance is the first and most influential step to full rehabilitation of the patient.

PREOPERATIVE CARE.   Preoperatively attention must be given to both the psychologic and the physical preparation of the patient.

Psychologic Preparation.   Although urinary diversion does not elicit quite the revulsion which accompanies fecal diversion, the feelings associated with a change in the method of the elimination of body wastes are similar. Early training in bladder control is not easy to ignore. It is important to try to help the patient begin to cope with the meaning of this change preoperatively. It is seldom enough for the patient to know that "My bladder will have to be removed." Many people will assume that some sort of substitute bladder will be devised. After all, we replace hearts, why not replacement bladders! Even the information that the urine will come out of his side is insufficient. The complete information should ideally be given by the physician in gradual doses as the patient adjusts to the impact of the idea. More likely, however, the physician will tell the patient that it is possible that he will have to remove the bladder and that he will make a new opening for the urine. In the experience of the authors, the only other information which is routinely given is to inform the male patient that this will render him impotent. Under these circumstances it is essential that the nurse ascertain what information the patient has regarding the surgery. Sometimes this is not easy. Only after discussing the more routine aspects and fears regarding surgery in general and returning to the subject of the results of this particular surgery in several different ways will the nurse lead the patient to saying or to recalling what he denies, that "he might have to change my urine." From this information the nurse can begin her teaching. Occasionally a patient's denial is such that he does not remember being told the effects of the surgery. In this case each encounter must be prefaced with a clarification of what the patient remembers is going to happen and what in essence is being discussed. Again, as has been said before, the important thing is not so much what the physician said as what the patient heard. It is from this point that all teaching must begin.

Both the patient and his family need preoperative instruction and support. Once the patient begins to comprehend that removal of the bladder means wearing an appliance to collect the urine for the rest of his life, his greatest need is for those about him to portray a hopeful, matter-of-fact attitude. False cheerfulness has no place. Katherine Jeter says that it behooves the nurse to be aware that all patients and their families have one or more of the following fears: (1) fear of the disease, (2) fear of death, (3) fear of surgery, (4) fear of pain, (5) fear of inability to manage postoperatively, (6) fear of family rejection, (7) fear of altered sexuality, (8) fear of unemployment, and (9) fear regarding the quality of their survival.[9] A nurse who has seen many other patients adjust to the surgery and deal with these fears is a tremendous asset to the patient and his family. She can help differentiate the real problems from the unrealistic ones, can help the patient develop a realistic attitude toward his ostomy and what it will mean to his life, and can help the patient and his family understand and help one another.

Preoperatively most patients look upon the ostomy as a lifesaving measure and may be hesitant to examine any further meaning. Usually they are better equipped preoperatively to deal with their emotional responses than they are postoperatively, when pain, healing, and prolonged hospitalization are also vying for their energies. However, not all patients are able to begin this process of adjustment when it seems best. Some steadfastly refuse to discuss the implications of the surgery preoperatively, saying, ''It has to be to save my life. I'll handle it when it happens. Right now I don't want to.'' Many people would predict that these patients should have a harder time postoperatively, but that does not seem to be the case. Some do very well, and others have a variety of problems, as do the patients who are taught in detail preoperatively. Obviously, individuals have a variety of ways of coping with this stress, and it behooves the nurse to honor these defenses unless she is certain that they are interfering with rehabilitation. For instance, a patient who completely denies that he will have anything to adjust to after surgery is not ready for the surgery. He must at least recognize that adjustments will be necessitated by the operation whether or not he is willing to discuss them before they occur. The patient's need for information is unique to him. He may want only a vague idea of what is to be done with assurance that this will be to his benefit, or he may seek a detailed explanation of every segment of the surgery, its implications, and the routines involved. To fail to assess this difference assures a difficult course for the patient and for his nurse-teacher.

Physical Preparation.   Preoperative preparation also includes a certain routine of testing. Depending on the particular surgeon, the tests may vary somewhat. They may include intravenous pyelogram, cystoscopy, barium enema, and proctoscopy, none of which is pleasant for the patient. A thorough explanation of the test and the necessity for it needs to be given in time for the patient to assimilate the information and ask questions. Although it has been said that telling a patient about these tests increases anxiety, every patient must be told that he will have a particular test performed. He then discussses it with other patients, visitors, family, and the cleaning lady. From these people he obtains misinformation and the fears of the informant. It is only reasonable that the patient also be given valid and positive information. It is especially important to stress that though the test will be somewhat uncomfortable, the patient's ability to relax and cooperate with the physicians and technicians can minimize the discomfort. Conditioned relaxation and distraction techniques are a valuable tool at such a time. When a patient is transferred from another institution or referred from another physician, these tests may have already been done. If the tests are to be repeated or more tests are required, it is necessary to explain the reason for this to the patient.

If the previous diagnostic work-up is adequate, the patient may enter the hospital shortly before surgery. It is important for this patient to receive extra attention. He will be in the hospital a much shorter time before surgery and will have few needs that absolutely must be met by nurses. It is easy to forget his need to develop a trusting relationship with his nurse-teacher and his needs for support, understanding, and education. One must be careful not to try to force the patient to assimilate all the necessary information in too short a time. Frequent short visits beginning with the least threatening information and progressing as the patient is able are more worthwhile than one long stressful encounter. In the event that this gradual progression is not possible, it is usually more important to develop a relationship based on trust and competence than to impart specific information.

Physical preparation includes preparation of the bowel, including laxatives, antibiotics to sterilize the bowel, low-residue and then liquid diet, and enemas. This usually begins two to four days preoperatively. When a patient is to have only cystectomy, he may be very anxious about all of this attention to his bowel. He should be told of the necessity to obtain the ileal conduit from the ileum and therefore the necessity of thorough cleansing of the bowel.

The entire family need not know the particulars of the patient's problem and rehabilitation needs. But the spouse or another responsible party should be included. This serves two purposes: first, there should be someone who understands and can assist the patient in all aspects of his adjustment at home, including care of the appliance if the patient should require it at any time; second, a family member can be extremely valuable in tempering the patient's response to the change in body image. The patient may feel totally changed, repulsive, and ugly. If the family member, knowing all, can remain loving, caring, and unrepulsed, it will do much to help the patient realistically integrate the stoma into his changed body image. A female patient refused to let any but a select few nurses care for her because she felt that her stoma would make others sick. She showed an abrupt change in her attitude when her daughter, whom she defined as a fussy girl with a weak stomach, assisted in changing both her urine and fecal appliances without any show of disgust.

Site Selection.   In order to select an appropriate site for creation of the stoma, some sources recommend that the patient wear the postoperative appliance for a day preoperatively. This is not necessary if care is taken to examine the patient's abdomen for scars, bony prominences, and other defects which could interfere with adherence of the appliance. It is essential that this be done in a reclining, a sitting, and a standing position. A patient who had recently lost a great deal of weight and had a number of surgical scars was examined, and an appropriate site was selected to avoid the scars. This was done in a reclining position. Unfortunately, the patient had such poor underlying muscle tone that when she stood this ideal site fell to the area of the inguinal canal. This posed many fitting problems which could have been avoided had an unusually high site been selected.

Care must be taken so that the area of adherence of the appliance is not disrupted by scars, wrinkles, depressions, bony prominences, the belt line, or free body movement. Figure 7.3 shows how to choose the correct site for a stoma. A triangle is drawn from the umbilicus to the anterior superior iliac spine to the symphysis

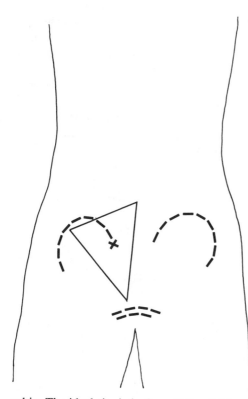

FIG. 7.3. Selection of stoma site. An imaginary triangle is drawn from the umbilicus to the anterior superior iliac spine to the symphysis pubis. The ideal site is in the center of this triangle, taking into consideration all skin folds, scars, or irregularities. The site is confirmed in the standing and sitting positions. (Adapted from Jeter: Management of the Urinary Stoma, 1970. Courtesy of Katherine Jeter. Photograph courtesy of Magee-Women's Hospital, Pittsburgh, Pennsylvania)

pubis. The ideal site is in the middle of this triangle. With the patient in a sitting position and standing, note is taken of any scars, skin folds, or other factors which may interfere with a watertight, flat bonding surface between appliance and skin. The chosen site is revised as needed. To allow for bending, the stoma site must be at least 2 inches below the belt line. The site so chosen is marked with indelible ink, and the surgeon should be alerted to the need to use this site.

Appliances which require some manual dexterity to assemble should be given to the patient to handle preoperatively. The patient should be observed assembling the various parts. The nervous individual, the elderly patient, or the arthritic patient may be unable to assemble a particular appliance. Another appliance should then be chosen (Fig. 7.4).

Skin Testing. Skin testing of the various solutions which will be used on the skin should be done preoperatively. This *must* be done when a patient has a history of dermatologic allergies or a specific allergy to adhesive products. Tincture of benzoin compound enjoys a reputation as an all purpose skin-protector, but it is also the solution which is most likely to cause a sensitivity reaction. Its routine use will lead to frequent skin reactions. The authors have found it best to avoid entirely using compound tincture of benzoin. Plain tincture of benzoin has many of the

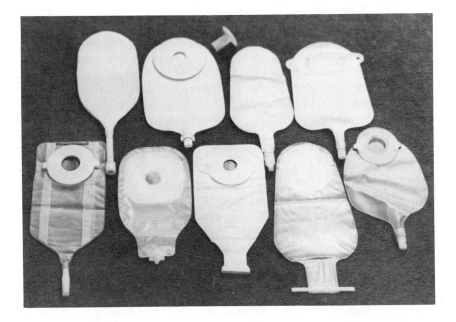

FIG. 7.4   A variety of urostomy appliances. Left to right. Top row. Grick, Permatype, Perry, Marlen, and Davol. Bottom row. Mason, Hollister, Nu-Hope, Coloplast/Bard, and Torbot

properties of the compound, namely, it toughens the skin and increases adherence. It does these less effectively than the compound, but it does them without the danger of severe skin reaction. Nothing is more detrimental to a patient's rehabilitation than having to spend the second week postoperatively clearing up a skin reaction caused by the use of tincture of benzoin compound in the first week. The multiple problems, including leakage, complex procedures, and pain involved in healing the skin convince the patient that he will never be able to cope with this new body fixture.

SURGICAL PERIOD.   Since the operative procedure is generally lengthy, the patient will usually go to surgery early in the morning. Arrangements may be needed so that the family can stay close to the hospital or can arrive early enough to see the patient before surgery. Occasionally a patient does not want to see his family before going to surgery. After discussion of this matter with the patient and his family, the nurse should be able to assist all concerned in accepting the decision which is mutually beneficial. If both the patient and his family are comfortable with the decision, it should not matter to the staff whether the family arrives and is supportive, arrives and cries openly, or stays away.

While the patient is in surgery, the family will need some consideration. They should have been given an honest estimate of the length of surgery. They frequently expect to see the patient in one or two hours and become panicky when hours pass without word. They should be able to obtain food without fear that they will miss the opportunity to speak with the surgeon or see their family member. The exact mechanisms for these kinds of help must be set up according to the policies and needs of a given institution. The value in patient and family satisfaction and cooperation is immeasurable.

IMMEDIATE POSTOPERATIVE PERIOD.   Immediately postoperatively, the patient's physical needs take precedence over the continuing psychologic needs. The multiple surgical procedures included in the construction of an ileal bladder and the resulting multiple anastomoses make this period one of observation for various complications. The patient who has an ileal bladder because of cancer is a much sicker patient than is the patient who requires an ileal bladder for a benign condition. Often the former has not only had construction of an ileal bladder but also a radical cystectomy and possibly also a colostomy. This may include en bloc excision of all or most of the contents of the pelvic cavity. The fluid losses from severed tissues into this space may be considerable, as evidenced by the large quantities of vaginal drainage which many women complain of after this surgery. An adequate system for draining the pelvic space is provided either by packing the wound or by insertion of drains. Observation of the amount and character of the drainage is performed with the knowledge that infection, hemorrhage, and fluid imbalances are possible complications.

Complications.   The general response to surgery as discussed previously in this chapter in relation to colostomy surgery (p. 160) occurs with construction of an ileal bladder. The effects of epinephrine, aldosterone, cortisol, and antidiuretic hormone (ADH) must be considered. The nitrogen and potassium losses, as well as liver and cardiovascular changes, are essential considerations. With three or four anastomoses in the bowel and urinary tract, the danger of fistula formation is great. The urine is bloody for several days postoperatively, clearing gradually. Should gross bleeding occur, the urine output fall, or a sudden increase in drainage appear from the incision or perineum, a defect in one of the anastomoses is suspected. Such information should be conveyed to the surgeon immediately. Since some obstruction to the free flow of urine often has preceded surgery, a compensatory polyuria is expected postoperatively. Evaluation of renal function is essential. Accurate intake and output is important both to prevent dehydration from the polyuria and to warn of impaired renal functioning. Many of these patients are operating on less than 40 percent of normal renal capacity, as indicated by an elevated blood urea nitrogen (BUN) and creatinine, and any further insult will be poorly tolerated. A fall in urine output below 25 ml per hour indicates inadequate renal blood flow, since immediately postoperatively urine output reflects renal perfusion rather than glomerular filtration. Position of the tubing, fluid intake, central venous pressure, vital signs, other output, and previous renal health need to be evaluated in order to determine whether this symptom results from dehydration, renal damage, or obstruction. Mannitol is frequently used to differentiate the oliguria of acute tubular necrosis from prerenal causes. It also prevents the accumulation of debris in the renal tubules. Use of vasopressors is contraindicated, as the resulting vasoconstriction leads to reduced renal perfusion and further renal impairment. Isuprel or digitalis may be used to increase the cardiac output. In prolonged oliguria, the principles of caring for the patient in renal failure apply. These include (1) maintenance of hydration (intake 500 ml greater than total output), (2) minimization of catabolism, (3) prevention of acidosis, (4) prevention of potassium intoxication, and (5) prevention of infection.

With the amount of surgery undertaken and the often poor operative status of many of these patients, infection is a significant problem. The urine in an ileal conduit is generally contaminated with a variety of bacteria. Over time, these individuals tolerate this contamination with minimal difficulty. In the immediate postoperative period, however, urine contamination may rapidly lead to clinical infection and even septic shock. Urine samples must be taken directly from the stoma or from a catheter inserted into the stoma after thoroughly cleansing the stoma and the surrounding tissue. A program of obtaining urine specimens at specific intervals as well as when temperature curves indicate infection has proven beneficial.

Contamination of the incision by urine in the presence of a poorly fitting appliance, while not as serious as fecal contamination, does impair healing and predispose to wound infection. In a patient previously irradiated, a debilitated patient, or a patient who has had previous surgeries, poor wound healing with dehiscence or evisceration is a distinct possibility. Increased drainage from the wound, redness, or tenderness should alert the nurse to this problem.

In addition to the observations mentioned previously, it is essential to observe the stoma. Is it healthy or becoming ischemic? It should be deep pink to red in color and firmly attached to the skin. The surrounding skin should appear healthy and should not be reddened, weeping, denuded, or otherwise irritated.

Control of Urine. Protecting the skin from urine leakage is one of the primary goals in the patient with a urinary diversion. To assure this, a properly fitting appliance is essential. (When ureteral catheters are used, they may be left in place for as long as a week. Since the urine does not always drain only through the catheters but also around them, it is often necessary to fit the patient with his appliance even though he has ureteral catheters in place. In this case the catheters are threaded into the appliance and rest in the bottom of the pouch.)

The patient is generally fitted with some type of disposable temporary appliance immediately after surgery. The majority of these disposable appliances are totally inadequate and should be replaced with a permanent or semipermanent appliance at the first sign of leakage. Certain of the disposable appliances are meant to be used on a permanent basis, but their expense has precluded their extended use when another appliance would suffice. However, for some patients they adhere so much better and for such a long period of time that the expense may actually be less than for a permanent appliance using cement or adhesive discs. If the pouch of the permanent appliance is clear or the pouch can be removed without disturbing the faceplate, so that the stoma can be inspected regularly, the permanent appliance may be fitted soon after surgery. In the event that the patient will be wearing a permanent one-piece appliance, fitting of the appliance should be delayed at least one to two weeks to allow the stoma to shrink. To fit this patient immediately would usually mean purchasing an appliance for the immediate postoperative period, purchasing one for the period from two weeks to approximately three months postoperatively, and then purchasing another set of appliances to accommodate stoma shrinkage. This is a tremendous expense when one is dealing with permanent one-piece rubber pouches (15 to 25 dollars per pouch). There are a number of appliances available, and certain facts may help decide the suitability of each for an individual patient (Table 7.2, Fig. 7.4).

If the site for the stoma has been well chosen, fitting the appliance entails measuring the stoma and bonding the appropriate urostomy device to the skin in a manner which will allow it to remain leakproof for at least 48 hours. To measure the stoma, a measuring guide is helpful. The opening in the guide which allows one-sixteenth to one-eighth inch more than the exact diameter of the stoma is the correct size.

A solution to protect and toughen the skin is often used. It is not always essential, but it is a useful precaution until the patient's skin becomes accustomed to being sealed beneath the faceplate for extended periods. Among the materials currently used to provide protection to the skin are dry karaya powder, plain tincture of benzoin, and a variety of silicone preparations in both liquid and spray form.

No matter what method of urine collection is used, the major principle remains constant—an appliance must fit properly and remain in place without leakage for a minimum of 48 hours. This is essential for maintenance of skin integrity, for healing of the incision, and for rehabilitation of the patient. In the immediate postoperative period, this can be accomplished by (1) fitting the patient with a permanent appliance as soon as possible, (2) measuring the stoma and obtaining an appliance with an opening no larger than one-eighth inch larger than the stoma, (3) removing the appliance only with solvent, (4) changing the appliance at the first sign of leakage, and (5) washing the peristomal skin with warm soapy water, rinsing well, and drying thoroughly at each appliance change.

POSTOPERATIVE PERIOD OF PATIENT INVOLVEMENT. Application of Permanent Pouch. The later postoperative period is a period of patient involvement and patient teaching.

One procedure which can be used both by nurses in changing urinary appliances and as a guide for teaching the patient follows.

1. Assemble all equipment: faceplate, pouch, solvent, skin protector solution, adhesive disc or cement, washcloth, soap and water, small bottle, scissors, cotton balls, guide strips, and waterproof tape.

TABLE 7.2
Characteristics of Urostomy Appliances

LIFE OF APPLIANCE

Permanent — One to three years depending on care and type of urine—cost $30–$100 per year

Semipermanent — Permanent faceplate (five years plus) with disposable pouches (two to eight weeks)—cost $30–$50 per year

Disposable — Easiest to use—cost $30–$150 per year

TYPE OF MATERIAL

Vinyl — Odor resistant, easy to maintain, inexpensive

Rubber — Durable, develops odor and calcium deposits producing maintenance problems, allergies to rubber, expensive, durable

NUMBER OF PIECES

One — No assembly, rubber or totally disposable, larger pouch necessitates larger faceplate

Two — Rubber or vinyl, may change pouch independently of faceplate, pouch size and faceplate size independent, must be assembled

FACEPLATE

Flexible — Most easily worn, least likely to be loosened by fat folds, activity, etc, flexibility varies

Rigid — Variety of convexities to choose from for depressed stomas, flabby musculature, oval stomas, etc

SIZE OF FACEPLATE

The smaller the diameter, the easier it is to find a spot on the abdomen which avoids scars, folds, incisions, bony prominences

METHOD OF ADHERENCE

Adhesive discs — Easy to use, many manufacturers, some allergies develop with time

Cement — Seal is generally most durable, many manufacturers, many people develop allergies, more difficult to use

Relia-Seal — Easy to use, many outlast adhesive discs, manufacturer claims no allergies, expensive

Karaya — Urine causes rapid disintegration

2. Assemble appliance. (If a belt is to be worn, be certain that the belt hooks are horizontal.)
3. Cut proper size hole in adhesive disc if necessary.
4. Remove paper from one side of adhesive disc and smooth over faceplate. Be careful that stoma openings are aligned.
5. Remove paper from other side of adhesive disc and set appliance aside. (Insert guide strip.)
   NB: If cement is used, apply a thin coating of cement to the entire faceplate. Let dry at least the time indicated by the manufacturer. Apply a second thin coat of cement and again allow to dry as before.

6. Moisten cotton ball with solvent and wedge gently between the skin and the faceplate to allow the solvent to dissolve the adhesive and permit the faceplate to come away from the skin without discomfort. NEVER PULL OFF WITHOUT SOLVENT. NEVER ALLOW ANYONE TO PULL THE APPLIANCE OFF WITHOUT SOLVENT.

7. Remove adhesive remaining on the skin by wiping gently with a cotton ball moistened with solvent. Do not rub briskly. It is better to leave a bit of adhesive on the skin than to scrub it off and damage the skin in the process.

8. Wash the area with soap and rinse thoroughly. Dry well. (The stoma may bleed slightly when washed.) At least once a week, bathe without the appliance.

9. Hold a small bottle filled with cotton over the stoma to collect the urine.

10. Apply a thin coating of skin protector solution to the skin. (Keep the stoma covered with small bottle.) If the urine drips, blot the area dry and reapply solution to that area. Allow to dry.
    NB: If using cement, apply a thin coat of cement to the area to be covered by the faceplate. Let dry at least the time indicated by the manufacturer. (The cement will not feel dry, but all irritating substances will have evaporated in this period of time.) A second thin coating of cement may often be needed. It is applied in the same manner and allowed to dry.

11. Stand or lie flat so that the skin is taut and without folds or wrinkles. Coughing just before removing the bottle and applying the pouch will often prevent leakage at this crucial point. Hold appliance so that drain can be easily opened into a commode. Line up guide strips with the stoma and press appliance into place. (A guide strip is a small piece of paper which is rolled into a cylinder and inserted into the stoma opening so that it extends out and can be used to guide the appliance over the stoma. It is specially treated to dissolve in the urine.) Holding appliance firmly in place with one hand, snap the belt into the belt hooks or frame the faceplate with waterproof nonallergic tape.

Anyone who works with the patient and his appliance must follow *exactly* the same procedure. This is especially important in the early weeks after surgery. Until the patient is confident of one method, he cannot be expected to judge the merits of variations in that method. There is no one procedure which is universally the best. The steps outlined above have proved satisfactory in a majority of situations, and they are easily adapted to the use of cement, as noted. Despite the type of appliance used, the major steps and the principles remain the same.

When the patient is in bed most of the time, as immediately after surgery, it is helpful to attach the appliance in such a way that it drains to the side of the bed rather than inferiorly. Then the drainage device can be attached directly over the side of the bed to the floor. Once the patient is up a great deal of the time, it is better for him to wear the appliance in the usual manner with the drain toward the inner aspect of the thigh. With the appliance in this position, when using a vinyl pouch one must take care in attaching the night drainage, as it tends to twist. If the drainage tubing is run down the inner aspect of the leg and over the end of the bed, the patient can move freely without twisting the bag and having it fill with urine and leak. Some people also prefer to put a piece of tape or tie a wide band around the drainage tubing and their leg at two or three places to assure that neither the tubing nor the pouch twists. Still other ostomates prefer to awaken themselves every two hours and empty the pouch rather than be hooked up every night. It is essential to find a process which allows the person a restful sleep without fear of wetting himself, his bed, and his mate. Since there is always a small danger of leakage, it is wise to have a waterproof covering put on the mattress. Washing linen in an inconvenience, but replacing a mattress is an unnecessary financial burden. Two drain tubes should be sent home with the patient. However, a gallon bleach bottle set in a wastebasket (so it will not tip) is a no-cost, no-maintenance, easy-to-replace receptacle. For travel, the collapsible type receptacle is preferred.

Maintenance. Several facts need to be known about maintenance of the equipment. Cleanliness is essential; sterility is not necessary. All adhesive should be removed from the pouch, and it should be washed and dried promptly after removal. Deodorants are rarely necessary if proper cleansing of the appliances has been carried out. All manufacturers sell deodorants, but it is questionable whether they are any more effective than household products, such as Lysol, vinegar, or baking soda. The appliance can be soaked in a solution containing one tablespoon of a household disinfectant or one-half cup of vinegar in a quart of warm water. After thorough washing it is rinsed and dried. The night drainage tube and collection device should receive daily care. They should be washed each morning with warm soapy water and rinsed. They may also be soaked in a solution containing a household disinfectant for 15 to 20 minutes and then rinsed if odor is a problem. Belts and rubber appliances may be washed with the family clothes.

Rubber appliances develop an odor and crystal deposits quickly if they are not cared for properly. After washing and rinsing, they should be soaked in a solution of one-half cup white vinegar to a quart of water. Care must be taken that the pouch is filled with this solution while soaking. Leaving this solution in the pouch for 30 minutes at each appliance change not only prevents odors but also dissolves the calcium deposits which accumulate opposite the stoma. These deposits can abrade the stoma when the appliance is in place. After soaking and rinsing, the appliance is hung to dry with the spout open and a washcloth or hanger placed within the pouch to prevent the rubber from sticking together. When a rubber appliance becomes soft and sticky it is time to replace it. How often this is necessary varies with the appliance, the composition of the individual's urine, and the care given the appliance. Vinyl appliances are two-piece appliances. This is necessary because the vinyl pouch is a semidisposable part which lasts only a few weeks. The faceplate is the most expensive part and is considerably more permanent. Once the pouch and faceplate are assembled, they can be treated as a one-piece appliance until it is time to replace the vinyl pouch, that is, it need not be disassembled for routine cleansing. After each wearing, the adhesive should be removed, and it should be washed in lukewarm soapy water and rinsed thoroughly. The manufacturers recommend replacing the vinyl pouch every two weeks to prevent leakage due to old age. If the pouch is replaced this often, odor is not a problem. Some patients who wear the pouch considerably longer than two weeks have found it necessary to soak the appliance in a vinegar solution for 20 minutes at each change to reduce odor. It would also be possible to get this same deodorizing effect by using a household disinfectant instead of detergent when washing the appliance. Calcium will tend to deposit on the threads of the drain assembly and will need to be scraped off occasionally.

Skin Care.   A properly fitted appliance which is leakproof for at least 48 hours will prevent almost all skin problems. Should irritation or excoriation occur, treatment is begun at once, and the cause is identified and eliminated promptly. Following is a list of treatments for skin irritation. In general the simplest is listed first. It is usually wise to employ the simplest effective measures while eliminating the cause of skin problems.

Mild Excoriation

1. After washing and drying the area as usual, expose the area to the heat of a 60 watt light bulb held at 18 inches for 20 to 30 minutes and/or the cool setting of a hair dryer before replacing the appliance. (Cover the stoma with a cotton ball whenever it is exposed to heat or a dryer.)
2. Cleanse the area and rinse and dry as usual. Dust with karaya powder. Wait one minute and brush off excess powder and apply pouch as usual.
3. After cleansing and drying area, apply a thin coating of a systemic antacid to the sore areas. Let dry thoroughly. Since adhesive discs bond poorly over this coating, it will be necessary to affix the appliance with cement.
4. Cleanse and dry area as usual. Apply calamine lotion to the sore areas and allow to dry. If area is small, cover with Micropore tape and affix appliance as usual; if area is large, affix the appliance with cement.
5. Cover small areas of excoriation with a piece of karaya gum, and cover the karaya gum with a piece of Micropore tape. Affix appliance in the usual manner.

Severe Excoriation

1. Use heat lamp (60 watts at 18 inches) and dryer (on cool setting) for 15 minutes every two hours until the skin begins to heal. Ostomate lies on his side with urine draining onto pads beneath the body. The stoma is covered with tissue or a cotton ball. This generally produces an adequate bonding surface within 24 hours. Then affix appliance.
2. After using the heat lamp and dryer, spray the area with a corticoid

preparation three times daily until appliance can again be worn. (This requires a prescription.)

3. After use of the heat lamp and dryer, spray area with a corticoid preparation and dust with nystatin powder. Wipe off excess and cement appliance in place. (Prescription rerequired.)

4. Moisten giant karaya washer (size of faceplate). Apply a corticoid spray and nystatin as above (No. 3). Dust with karaya powder. Place moistened karaya washer over stoma (use no adhesive). Tape pouch and faceplate in place with Micropore tape. (Prescription required.)

5. This is the most complex procedure but very effective.
    (a) Cleanse skin with large amount of saline.
    (b) Apply heavy coat of Maalox (or any antacid) by pouring onto the skin and spreading with finger.
    (c) Apply light layer of karaya powder over the moist Maalox.
    (d) Moisten skin side of faceplate and affix over the karaya and Maalox. A belt must be worn. Leave in place for 48 hours. A crust will form. Do not remove the crust. Remove appliance and clean it. Repeat steps (a) through (d), taking care to remove no more of the crust than falls off of its own accord.

Obviously it is easier to prevent skin excoriation than it is to repair the damage when it has occurred. During the treatment of the skin, it is imperative that the cause of the excoriation be determined in order to prevent recurrences. The common causes are (1) an ill-fitting appliance, (2) harsh treatment of the skin, and (3) sensitivity to one or several of the substances used on the peristomal skin.

Encrustations on the stoma and surrounding skin are caused by calcium precipitating out of an alkaline urine. Often ingestion of a pint of cranberry juice daily and/or placing one pulverized aspirin tablet into the pouch after each emptying will acidify the urine enough to prevent further encrustation. If the appliance fits properly, encrustations cannot form on the peristomal skin because it is not exposed to the urine. Proper fitting of the appliance is essential. To dissolve the encrustation already formed, the patient should inject 2 ounces of a vinegar and water solution (one-half cup of white vinegar to one quart of warm water) into the bottom of the pouch twice daily. Lying down for 20 minutes so that the vinegar solution bathes the affected area will eventually dissolve the precipitate. Collection of these salts on the appliance and the stoma often signals precipitation of salts throughout the urinary tract, that is, stone formation.

Urinary Tract Calculi.   Renal stones are the result of insoluble particles precipitating out of the urine and collecting on the wall of the kidney pelvis. These particles accumulate gradually until they form a distinct entity, a stone. A factor which frequently contributes to stone formation in the patient with a urinary diversion is the tendency to limit fluid intake in order to produce a scantier output. The resulting concentration of the urine only increases any preexisting tendency to form stones. It is essential that the material of which the stone is formed be identified so that the appropriate measures to minimize recurrences can be taken.

Inorganic materials, such as the calcium salts, are more soluble in an acid urine. Ingestion of at least a quart of cranberry juice daily or ascorbic acid (1g three times a day)[10] is sometimes useful in acidifying the urine. However, the most effective measure is strict adherence to a regimen of dietary restrictions and increased fluid intake (to 4 liters daily). Organic precipitates, such as uric acid, are more soluble in alkaline urine. The production and, therefore, the precipitation of uric acid are largely prevented by the judicious use of allopurinal. Dietary restrictions are less effective.

The chronic low-grade infection common in patients with urinary diversion also contributes to stone formation. Many common bacteria are urea-splitters. By releasing ammonia, these bacteria produce an alkaline urine in which the solubility of calcium salts is reduced. Other contributory factors which are present in many patients with a malignancy are deficiency of vitamin A, increased intake of vitamin D or other large vitamin supplements, and immobilization.

Due to the structure of the urinary tract, there are three narrow points at which a stone tends to become lodged: (1) the ureteropelvic junction, (2) the point at which the ureters cross the iliac vessels, and (3) the ureterovesicular junction. Accurate assessment of the pain experiences will help to localize the area of involvement. A ureteropelvic stone causes pain at the costovertebral angle (CVA) and spasm radiating along the ureter into the vulvar/testicular area. A stone further along the ureter produces some CVA tenderness but primarily low abdominal pain. A stone at the ureterovesicular junction produces symptoms of bladder irritation and vulvar and scrotal pain, which may or may not occur in conjunction with the forementioned CVA tenderness and abdominal pain. The patient with a urinary diversion has a point of narrowing at the ureteroileal junction. A stone at this point produces pain very similar to that of acute abdominal obstruction, from which it must be differentiated.

LONG-TERM REHABILITATION.   Control of urine is the first and indispensable postoperative goal for the patient with a urinary diversion. However, rehabilitation does not cease when the patient leaves the hospital with a well-fitting appliance. Home is never like the hospital, and follow-up assistance to bridge this gap is important. The ostomy visitor who visits the patient postoperatively will keep in touch with the patient, will encourage him to participate in ostomy society activities, will bring him the newest ostomy information, and will remain a resource as the patient confronts the inevitable problems of adjustment to such a radical change in body function. A good working relationship with the community nursing service provides continuity in teaching and support of the patient at discharge. Again, it must be pointed out that everyone involved in teaching the patient must follow *exactly* the same procedure. Conferences with the community nurse, hospital visits, and a written care plan including the step-by-step procedure are methods for attaining this continuity. The patient needs to know whom to contact with questions, concerns, or problems. In a given situation this might be the surgeon, the enterostomal therapist, the nursing specialist, the community nurse, or the ostomy society. The patient needs to know (in writing) how, where, and when to seek assistance.

The long-range problems of rehabilitation have not been considered here, and, in general, they have not been dealt with in the population. These include sexual adjustment associated with impotency, vaginectomy, and altered elimination, the threat of a recurrence of the malignancy, and the problem of a person defined as different or sick in our society.

Therapeutic modalities to deal with these problems are only beginning to be developed. Penile prostheses and vaginal reconstruction techniques are used for other conditions, but the patient with cancer in his medical history may have to be quite persistent to find a physician who will perform these reparative procedures. More family service agencies are becoming aware of the problems of the ostomate, and hopefully this awareness will give birth to worthwhile programs of therapy.

The American Cancer Society has taken on a new goal, that of not only improving the quantity of life after cancer treatment but also the quality of that life. This chapter has explored some of the problems of living with an altered method of elimination. Now the task is to help minimize or overcome these problems so that the ostomate need never say, "I'd rather that I had died."

OTHER PROBLEMS OF ELIMINATION

Colostomies and urinary diversions represent the most common intentional adjustments in the area of elimination demanded of a patient with cancer. However, other problems do occur either intentionally or as a side effect of the disease or its treatment. These include fistulas, diarrhea, constipation, bladder insufficiencies, incontinence, bowel obstruction, and uremia.

Fistulas

A fistula is an abnormal passage within body tissue. It may result from invasion of the tissues by disease or destruction by radiation or surgery. The disease process need not be a malignancy, but fistula formation secondary to a malignancy is not uncommon. The most common cause of a fistula is surgical trauma. The radical surgery associated with cancer increases the likelihood of fistula formation, as do poor nutrition and the loss of elasticity and vascularity produced by radiation.

There is continuing debate as to the best treatment for fistulas. The conservative approach is to nourish the patient orally and parenterally while waiting for the fistula to close of its own accord. The activist approach is to return the patient to surgery as soon as possible for surgical closure. Factors such as the health of the surrounding tissues, the surgical risk to the patient, and the area of the fistula are considered in either approach. The care given to the patient whose fistula cannot be surgically closed or in whom surgery must be delayed is an extension of the preoperative care given the patient who is quickly returned for surgical closure. In either case, care is directed toward three goals: (1) maintenance of nutrition/hydration, (2) protection of the skin, and (3) prevention/control of infection.

Maintenance of nutrition poses little problem in the ambulatory patient with a rectovaginal fistula, yet it is a major problem in the postoperative patient with a high ileocutaneous fistula. Measures to reduce losses and to replace calories, water, protein, and electrolytes must be considered. Parenteral nourishment, including hyperalimentation, may promote healing and eliminate the need for surgical closure.

The magnitude of the problem of maintaining skin integrity varies with the origin of the discharge. Basically, the solution depends on isolating the drainage by an occlusive ointment and containment of the drainage in a receptacle. Enterocutaneous, enterovesicular, and enterovaginal fistulas produce the most urgent problems, as the enzymes present rapidly digest all unprotected tissues. Intubation of the fistula with a catheter and connection to suction may be possible. When appropriate, this is the cleanest and most effective protection for the perifistular skin. Insertion of a needle into the catheter at skin level provides a vent and eliminates the major cause of system failure, catheter obstruction.

In many cases an ileostomy appliance may be affixed over the cutaneous fistula. Care must be taken that the opening in the appliance corresponds to the size of the fistula. Regular emptying of the pouch or attachment to a collection device is often necessary, as a small bowel fistula may discharge 3 to 4 liters of fluid per day. Protection around the fistula can be enhanced by the use of karaya powder, a karaya washer, or karaya paste. When no appliance is effective, success has been obtained by applying a thick coating of zinc oxide, aluminum paste, or Desitin. If this is insufficient protection, the following procedure has proven effective.

1. The entire area exposed to drainage is cleansed with normal saline.
2. A thick coating of the thickened portion of a systemic antacid is applied to the entire area.
3. While this coating is still wet, a large amount of karaya powder is applied and allowed to dry (a hand dryer on the cool setting hastens drying).
4. When dry, any excess karaya powder is brushed away and a dressing is applied.
5. This procedure is repeated every two to four hours as needed, removing as little of the crust formed by the karaya and antacid as possible.

This procedure is far from aesthetic. However, strict adherence to this regimen for 55 days prior to surgery allowed an ileocutaneous fistula 5 inches in diameter to heal to approximately a three-quarter inch diameter, assuring an easier surgical closure and sparing the patient much pain in the interim.

Periodic irrigation of the fistula may control drainage, cleanse the area, and aid in healing. The efficacy of this method depends a great deal on the source and amount of the drainage. Very little benefit is derived from irrigating a fistula from which drainage is constantly running freely. The most frequent exception is an infected tract which is irrigated as part of a regimen to control the infection. When all else fails, placement of the patient on a Stryker frame or Circo-Electric bed, with the fistula over the opening for the bedpan to allow for gravity drainage, may provide adequate protection and collection.

Protection is a greater problem with enterovesicular fistulas, since the drainage cannot be directly contained nor the bladder mucosa protected with an occlusive ointment. Continuous bladder irrigation, antispasmodics, and analgesics are of some help. It taxes the ingenuity of everyone involved to prevent a patient with a fistula, who is being treated conservatively, from feeling that everyone has given up on him. Emotional support, scheduled diversion, and social interaction are essential.

All vaginal fistulas pose a problem of protection and containment. The vagina itself has few pain sensors, but the introitus and perineum are very sensitive and excoriate rapidly when subjected to constant drainage of any type. Sitz baths, protective ointments, or insertion of a vaginal cup attached to a collection device (Tassaway Corporation) may be effective for some patients for short periods of time. The absence of any truly effective method of controlling the drainage from a vaginal fistula makes it one justification for surgery in a patient with advanced disease. Diverting loop colostomy or ureterostomy are not complex procedures, and the comfort provided the patient by eliminating this drainage is a valid reason for the attempt.

Fistulas are not sterile openings, and attention needs to be given to preventing cross-contamination. The possibility of massive infection and septic shock should be considered at all times. Cultures of the drainage and treatment with appropriate antibiotics is preferable to broad-spectrum prophylaxis. Fistulas do exist in areas other than the gastrointestinal or genitourinary tracts. They produce problems more closely associated with alterations in body image, respiration, or nutrition. Despite the site of the fistula, adequate care is based on the determination and evaluation of the following: (1) the organs involved, (2) the character of the drainage, (3) the resulting defects in normal body function, and (4) the measures available to minimize or prevent any of the problems resulting from the drainage or the defects in normal body function.

Constipation

The problems of diarrhea, constipation, urinary retention, and incontinence are frequent among patients with cancer. The problems attending excess excretion of feces or urine are primarily nutritional in nature. The fluids, electrolytes, vitamins, and proteins so lost must be identified and replaced. Accurate measurement of intake and output is essential.

Illness predisposes to narcissism. Concern with elimination often becomes a preoccupation reinforced by the medical personnel. Despite this fact, or possibly in part because of this fact, disorders of elimination are frequently overlooked. Dehydration, anorexia, use of narcotics, manipulation of the intestine during surgery, electrolyte imbalances, such as hypokalemia, and certain chemotherapeutic agents contribute to intestinal hypomobility. A daily bowel movement is unnecessary, but a patient who has not had a bowel movement in three days whose normal pattern is not infrequent evacuation is in danger of fecal impaction. Assessment should include the patient's usual pattern of elimination, usual food patterns, recent changes, character of the feces, medications, observation of the abdomen, and, if the nurse is qualified, evaluation of bowel sounds. Dietary alterations, use of stool softeners, and a bowel training regimen utilizing mild laxatives and suppositories or enemas on a scheduled basis may regulate the patient whose pattern has been disrupted. A patient who requires regular doses of a narcotic also needs regular use of a stool softener and possibly suppositories on a prophylactic rather than therapeutic basis.

Intestinal Obstruction

Intestinal obstruction, like fecal or urinary fistulas, produces such distressing symptoms that even when a patient presents with advanced disease, surgery is a consideration. Conservative medical management, consisting of intestinal decompression and intravenous nutrition, is often given an extensive trial before surgery. Some obstructions are spontaneously relieved for a considerable length of time by this method. As with any treatment in which waiting is a primary constituent, the patient and his family need understanding and encouragement, relief of pain, and conscientious attention to care needs.

Bladder Insufficiency

Pelvic surgery and interference with the innervation of the bladder, invasion or compression of peripheral nerves, metastases to the vertebrae with spinal compression, cordotomy for pain control, and brain lesions are some of the causes of problems with bladder control and function in cancer patients. Damage to any of the nerves serving the bladder initially produces a state of complete bladder anesthesia and flaccid paralysis. As recovery begins, reflex cord control of the bladder returns first. The final condition of the bladder depends on whether impulses are partially or totally interrupted and at which level the interruption of transmission occurs. Table 7.3 compares the three major types of bladder insufficiency (neurogenic bladders), their symptoms, and the appropriate therapy.

TABLE 7.3
Comparison of Various Forms of Neurogenic Bladders*

UNINHIBITED	COMPLETE SPASTIC	FLACCID
	Cause	
Lesion of the cortex or pyramidal tracts	More or less complete transection of the spinal cord above S_2	Interruption of sacral reflex arc in cord or peripheral nerves
	Sensation	
Perception of fullness with uninhibited contractions	No perception of fullness or desire to void	No perception of fullness or desire to void
	Motor Response	
Uninhibited contractions, reduced capacity (150 ml), no residual, normal strength of voiding stream	Uninhibited capacity (250 ml), residual urine (125 ml), strength of voiding stream varies but may be initiated by reflex	No uninhibited contractions, capacity constantly increasing, weak voiding stream, residual urine (150 ml plus)
	Symptoms	
Urgency, frequency	Some frequency	Retention with overflow, incontinence
	Therapy	
Control via scheduled voiding, fluid restrictions at night	Control via stimulation of reflex arc by cutaneous stimulation of thigh/perineum	Control via scheduled voiding with suprapubic pressure, catheter if residuals cannot be reduced

*Data from Smith: General Urology, 1969. Courtesy of Lange Medical Publications

Urinary incontinence results from a variety of causes. Stress incontinence is a frequent symptom in multiparous women. Adding illness, weakness, confinement to bed, and sedation can produce a problem of care for nursing and a significant ego threat for the patient. It is essential that the reasons for the incontinence be thoroughly investigated. Reduction of sedatives, scheduled toileting, or perineal exercises may all be of benefit. Despite the reticence of some physicians to resort to catheterization because of the increasing threat of urinary tract infections, the patient whose incontinence cannot be controlled should be relieved of this burden by the insertion of an indwelling catheter. Condom catheters frequently are sufficient for the male patient. It is then the responsibility of nursing to minimize the risks of infection. If the reasons necessitating insertion of the catheter have not been corrected, the patient should be spared needless attempts to eliminate the catheter. Evaluation of a patient's urinary control can be made at the time of catheter change if this is warranted. An indwelling catheter should never be inserted to relieve the team of the responsibility of taking the patient to the bathroom. A catheter should never be refused a patient who is incontinent despite other efforts.

Uremia

Obstruction to the excretion of urine is a common complication of pelvic malignancies. Injury, infection, or spread of the tumor produce obstruction in the form of strictures, compression, or occlusion. The urinary structures above the obstruction dilate, hypertrophy, and eventually decompensate with loss of function. The increased pressure in the system is referred to the renal pelvis. Obviously the higher the obstruction, the more rapid and pronounced is the effect on the kidney itself. As the pressure within the kidney pelvis rises, larger and larger vessels are compressed causing ischemia and necrosis. The cells farthest from the interlobular arteries are affected first and most severely. The closer the pressure within the kidney approaches the glomerular filtration pressure (30 to 40mm Hg), the less urine is secreted. Active transport is lost before passive diffusion so that the blood urea nitrogen (BUN) may remain normal long after changes are evident in creatinine clearance.

Uremia is the syndrome that results when kidney damage progresses to the point where retention of by-products is producing symptomatology. It is frequently viewed as end-stage renal disease. If this syndrome is caused by reduced renal blood flow, acute tubular necrosis, or obstruction, it may be reversible with prompt treatment. Return of function occurs opposite to the order in which it was lost. The most recently damaged cells recover first, and active transport, one of the first functions to be lost, is one of the last functions to be regained. The symptoms of renal failure include any or all of the following: weakness, drowsiness, anemia, capillary fragility with bleeding, anorexia, nausea, vomiting, diarrhea, pruritis, dehydration, uremic frost, hypertension, congestive heart failure, tetany, paresthesias, and edema. Treatment consists of (1) identifying and correcting the precipitating factors, (2) relieving symptoms, and (3) preventing complications. The principles upon which all treatment is based are (1) maintenance of hydration, (2) minimizing catabolism, (3) prevention of acidosis, (4) control of hyperkalemia, and (5) prevention of infection. Table 7.4 outlines the care given a patient in renal failure whether the goal is to maximize recovery or minimize symptomatology.

TABLE 7.4
Care of Uremic Patient

SYMPTOMS	RELIEF OF SYMPTOMS	PREVENTION OF COMPLICATIONS
Nausea, vomiting, diarrhea Hyperpnea, acidosis	Low-potassium, low-protein, low-sodium diet Intake 500 ml greater than total output Scheduled antiemetics Mouthwash hourly NaHCO₃ (based on serum sodium and urine output) Sedatives (short acting)	Intake 500 ml greater than total output
Edema Hypertension	Daily weight Intake 500 ml greater than output Accurate I and O Low sodium intake	Seizure precautions Observe for signs of cerebral edema: level of consciousness, blood pressure, vital signs at least every four hours Antihypertensive medications
Anemia, weakness, bleeding tendency	Scheduled passive range of motion Activity controlled Scheduled rest Turning sheet Narrow-spectrum bactericidal antibiotics specific to the organism At least 400 calories/day Packed cells Androgens minimize trauma	Central venous pressure every two hours Controlled fluids Cultures with sensitivities for fever, swinging hypothermic curve, drainage Thromboembolic stockings Observations for gastrointestinal bleeding-guiac excreta
Dry skin, dehydration, pruritis	Oral hygiene hourly Body lotion Foam or lambswool pad Rinse skin with solution (2 tablespoons vinegar to pint of water)	Turn every two hours Scheduled passive range of motion
Hyperkalemia	Exchange resins Peritoneal dialysis Renal dialysis Low potassium intake. Glucose and insulin Calcium gluconate	Serial ECG every six hours and/or monitoring Daily electrolytes
Hypocalcemia	Gentleness in care Low Phosphorus intake	Observe Trousseau's sign or Chvostek's sign Calcium gluconate IV Seizure precautions Suction
Susceptible to infection (deranged WBC's)		Minimize trauma Reduce contact with pathogens (refer to pp. 124-127)

References

1. Katona E: Learning colostomy control. Am J Nurs 67:534–539, 1967
2. Zimmerman LM, Levine R (eds): Physiological Principles of Surgery. Philadelphia, Saunders, 1964
3. Katona: *op cit,* p 535
4. Grier WRN, Postel AH, Syarse A, et al: Evaluation of colonic stoma management without irrigations. Surg Gynecol Obstet 118:1234–1242, 1964
5. Katona: *op cit,* p 537
6. Binder DP: Sex, Courtship and the Single Ostomate. Los Angeles, United Ostomy Association, 1973
7. Gambrell E: Sex and the Male Ostomate. Los Angeles, United Ostomy Association, 1973
8. Norris C, Gambrell E: Sex, Pregnancy and the Female Ostomate. Los Angeles, United Ostomy Association, 1972
9. Jeter K: Management of the urinary stoma. Uro-Gram 2(1):1–2, 1973
10. ———: Urinary Stomas—A Guidebook for Patients. Los Angeles, United Ostomy Association, 1973

Bibliography

Anatomy of Ostomy. Los Angeles, United Ostomy Association, 1971
Andersen L: Care and management of ostomies. Bedside Nurse 3:24–28, June 1970, 3:15–20, July 1970
Black D: Renal Disease. Philadelphia, Davis, 1962
Calcock BP, Braasch JW: Surgery of the small intestine in the adult, in Major Problems in Clinical Surgery, vol 7. Philadelphia, Saunders, 1968
Campbell JE, Oliver JA, McKay DE: Dynamics of ileal conduits. Radiology 85:338–342, 1965
Coller FA, Regan WJ: Cancer of the Colon and Rectum. American Cancer Society, 1963
Dericks VC: Nursing Care of the Patient with an Ostomy. Proceedings of the National Conference on Cancer Nursing. American Cancer Society, 1973
———: Booklet of Instructions for Persons with a Colostomy. New York Hospital, 1966
Douglas AP, Kerr DNS: A Short Textbook of Kidney Disease. Philadelphia, Lippincott, 1971
Dyk RB, Sutherland, AM: Adaptation of the spouse and other family members to the colostomy patient. Cancer 9:123–138, 1956
Gill N, Miller D: The care of ileostomies. Mich Nurse 44:10–11, January 1971
Grier WRN, Postel AH, Syarse A, et al: Evaluation of colonic stoma management with irrigations. Surg Gynecol Obstet 118:1234–1242, 1964
Harrington JD, Brener ER: Patient Care in Renal Failure. Philadelphia, Saunders, 1973
Honesty H: Essentials of Abdominal Ostomy Care. New York, Springer, 1972
Jeter K: Management of the Urinary Stoma. New York, Columbia-Presbyterian Medical Center, 1970
Katona E: A patient-centered, living-oriented approach to the patient with an artificial anus or bladder. Nurs Clin North Am 2:623–634, December 1967
Kuhnelian JG, Sanders VE: Urologic Nursing. New York, Macmillan, 1970
Lenneberg E, Rowbotham JL: The Ileostomy Patient. Springfield, Ill., Thomas, 1970
———, Mendelssohn AN: Colostomies—A Guide. Los Angeles, United Ostomy Association, 1969

Lyons AS, Brockmeier MJ: Mechanical management of the ileostomy stomas. Surg Clin North Am 52:979–990, 1972

Managing Your Colostomy. Chicago, Ill., Hollister, 1971

Managing Your Ileostomy. Chicago, Ill., Hollister, 1971

Managing Your Urostomy. Chicago, Ill., Hollister, 1974

Murray BS, Elmore J, Sawyer JR: The patient has an ileal conduit. Am J Nurs 71:1560–1565, 1971

Ostomy Review. Los Angeles, United Ostomy Association, 1968

Saxon J: Techniques for bowel and bladder training. Am J Nurs 62:69–71, 1962

Smith DR: General Urology. Los Altos, Cal., Lange Medical Publications, 1969

Sparberg M: Ileostomy Care, Springfield, Ill., Thomas, 1971

Stitt A: When the problem is ileostomy. Emergency Med 2:107–112, 1970

Strauss MB, Welt LB: Diseases of the Kidney. Boston, Little, Brown, 1971

Stryker RP: Rehabilitative Aspects of Acute and Chronic Nursing Care, Chapter 8 Philadelphia, Saunders, 1972

Sutherland AM, Orbach CE, Dyk RB, Bard M: The psychological impact of cancer and cancer surgery. Cancer 5:857–872, 1952

Vukovich V, Scrubb RD: Care of the Ostomy Patient. St. Louis, Mosby, 1973

Winter CC, Barker MR: Nursing Care of Patients with Urologic Diseases. St. Louis, Mosby, 1972

OSTOMY SUPPLIERS AND INFORMATION

Atlantic Surgical Co., Inc., 1834 Lansdowne Avenue, Merrick, New York 11566

Coloplast/Bard, Inc., 731 Central Avenue, Murray Hill, New Jersey 07974

Davol, Inc., Providence, Rhode Island 02901

John F. Greer Co., 5335 College Avenue, PO Box 2898, Oakland, California 94618

Grick, Inc., 202-11 Jamaica Avenue, Hollis, New York 11423

Hollister, Inc., 211 East Chicago Avenue, Chicago, Illinois 60611

Marlen Manufacturing and Development Company, 5150 Richmond Road, Bedford, Ohio 44146

Marsan Manufacturing Company, Inc., 5924 South Pulaski Road, Chicago, Illinois 60629

Mason Laboratories Inc., Willow Grove, Pennsylvania 19090

Nu-Hope Labs, Inc., 2900 Rowena Avenue, Los Angeles, California 90039

Osteolite Company, 842 East 18th Avenue, Denver, Colorado 80218

Perma-Type Company Inc., PO Box 175, Farmington, Connecticut 06032

Tassaway, Inc., Tassette, 195 Shippan Avenue, Stamford, Connecticut 06902

Torbot Co., 1185 Jefferson Boulevard, Warwick, Rhode Island 02886

United Surgical Corp., Largo, Florida 33540

United Ostomy Association, Inc., 1111 Wilshire Boulevard, Los Angeles, California 90017

8

Identity and Body Image

This text approaches the care of the person with cancer from the viewpoint of the problems he encounters, not the disease he has. Certain organ system dysfunctions logically fall into one category more than into another; for instance, cancer of the bladder creates problems related to elimination. Likewise, this chapter dealing with identity will treat, specifically, those cancers which most often and most obviously assault one's view of and comfort with himself. In an attempt to provide some order to this immense subject, some theoretical material regarding identity, body image, and sexuality will be presented. This will be followed by an overview of the information available relating to the effects of illness, disease, or mutilation on identity, body image, and sexuality. Appropriate nursing care based on this information will be discussed in relation to the specific areas of sexuality and cosmesis.

IDENTITY

Identity and the concept of self have been pondered and studied by philosophers and psychologists through the ages. To attempt to summarize even a portion of what has been said would be impossible. The following paragraphs will present some theoretical material and information from a variety of sources which are relevant to the purposes of this text. Much of the material presented can be viewed as a model of identity and identity formation. One must keep in mind that models are not facts. They represent a way of viewing phenomena in a organized way. No individual ever exactly fits any model. To attempt to force perceptions of individuals into models is to forget that all human beings are unique.

For the purposes of this chapter, the terms ''identity'' and ''self-concept'' will be used synonymously. In Freudian terms, the concept of self is an interplay between the ego and that portion of the superego which represents the internalized ideal of what one is striving to become, the ego-ideal. Self-concept can be viewed in terms of a basic striving toward differentiation in mass society. It has also been defined as the sum total of the reflected appraisals of others. More recent models present the self-concept as a fluid product evolving from the interaction of a variety of forces: biologic, social, and experiential. Figure 8.1 illustrates these interacting forces. One's genetic makeup is the foundation upon which an identity is built. One's body build, sex, coloring, and other characteristics compose the baseline from which identity develops. Biologic attributes affect one's perception of himself and others, and, in varying degrees, they influence the reactions of others and the total experiences of life. In addition to physical characteristics, the inner core of identity consists of biologic and psychologic givens and potentials. This initial mass of potential is constantly being molded by the changes which occur with growth, aging, health and illness, forces of the environment, people of significance, the experiences one has, and the accumulative effect of all of these forces on the developing self. One might define the self-concept as all the perceptions an individual has of himself—his attitudes, beliefs, thoughts, feelings, goals, fears, fantasies, what he has been, what he may become, and the worth of it all—constantly being formed by the interaction of his biologic givens, the environment in which he lives, the people with whom he relates, and his perceptions of these multiple interrelationships.[1] Three characteristics of the self-concept which have particular relevance for nursing the cancer patient are (1) a self-concept is fluid, (2) a self-concept is learned, and (3) a self-concept is complex. The most central and inflexible of the perceptions contributing to the self-concept seem to be those pertaining to body image, sexuality, and work.

BODY IMAGE

The body image is the sum total of the feelings and perceptions an individual has about his body. The effects of mutilating surgery and prolonged illness invariably

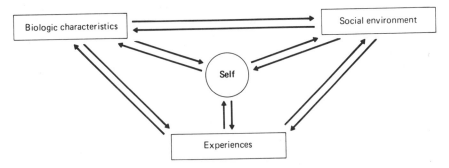

FIG. 8.1.   A model for the development of identity.

assault the specific aspect of an individual's self-concept known as body image. A better understanding of this concept is useful in realistically assisting the patient to cope with assaults upon it.

Though one begins to form a concept of self in the early months of life, a clear body image apparently takes shape much later (age 3 to 5 years). The factors which are important in the molding of this concept are significant others (especially the mother), environmental stimuli, and the individual's own physiologic and psychologic characteristics. There is great variation among people regarding the relative strengths of external and internal stimuli. Some individuals are primarily attuned to their own internal cues. In the event of conflicting input from the environment, internal cues override conflicting data. For others, body sensations are readily subordinated to messages from the external world. Most people fall somewhere between the extremes. It is interesting to note that receptivity to internal cues seems to increase with the clarity of the perception of self.[2]

The body image is colored by feelings, attitudes, and conditioning. Some individuals who have suffered traumatic changes in body contour fail to incorporate this change into their body image, as measured by a variety of tests. Also, a number of individuals whose appearance has been markedly improved by weight loss or plastic surgery fail to integrate changes and continue to feel and respond as if no such improvement had occurred.[3-5] The ability to gain satisfaction from restorative and cosmetic procedures seems to be directly related to whether the defect was ever incorporated into the body image. If a person never perceived himself as having a defect, its elimination does not substantially improve him. In fact, though the patient may seek corrective surgery, he may be angered by the results because he had to undergo the pains of surgery for so little benefit.

That body image changes in the course of living should be obvious. The crises associated with puberty, menopause, and senescence are occasionally considered in terms of rapid changes in the body requiring a corresponding change in body image. Indeed what is called "growing old gracefully" may be the obvious congruence between body changes and body image. This is not to imply that it is advantageous at a certain age to "take to one's rocking chair." Rather, a realistic view of the changes which have occurred and their meaning for an individual can bring about new modes of behavior which are more active and indicate a greater zest for life. Energy is not wasted concealing, overcompensating for, and dealing with the discrepancy associated with a body image inconsistent with external reality.

SEXUALITY

Sexuality refers to all those perceptions related to feeling like, acting like, or being recognized as a man or a woman. For the most part, the first differentiation of a human infant, beyond the "I versus non-I" of early infancy, is the assignment of gender. This distinction is evidenced by name, type of clothing, hair style, play activities, and parent and peer interactions. By the age of 2½ years, a child has a concept of gender, and by the age of 4, he possesses a rather structured model of sex-specific behaviors. The school-age boy is very different from the school-age girl. By the age of 8, behavior is quite predictive of adult behavior.[6] Yet at this age only the concrete visible differences between the sexes have been perceived and incorporated by the child. The child accepts the extremes as the norm, ignoring much of the ambiguous area of overlap between sexes in terms of psychosexual behavior and identity. This may account in part for the observation that despite the changes which have occurred in adult female behavior as part of the feminist movement, childhood perceptions have shown little change.[6]

In the United States, it is assumed that males will be dominant, aggressive, and controlled and that females will be passive, receptive, and nurturant. It is currently in vogue to view this as a culturally induced phenomenon, the result of a male-dominated, male-chauvinistic society. However, there is evidence to indicate that at birth there are sex-specific differences. To help illustrate the complexity of developing a sexual identity, one such difference will be considered. At birth girls are more attuned to external stimuli than are boys. The infant girl is more aware of and more affected by the responses of her caretakers. To maintain or attain a state of comfort, she must gratify her internal demands and also minimize the anxiety produced by discord between herself and the "mother." Conditioned responses are begun in the early days of life which help establish the female as receptive, obedient, and passive. On the other hand, the male infant, at this time, is usually less aware of his environment. He responds primarily to his internal cues. Even in the early weeks of his life, he is perceived and reacted to as independent and aggressive. As the infant boy becomes more alert to external cues, he too must incorporate the reactions of his caretakers into the mass of stimulation to which he responds. As the child grows, this small initial variance is magnified by the culture.[6,7]

With very few exceptions, the mother or mother-substitute is the primary caregiver. The growing female child identifies with the mother-figure as "Mother" is perceived by the child in her caretaker-nurturing roles. The young boy is aware that he is not female and, therefore, cannot model himself after the mother figure. His model becomes essentially *anti*mother.[8] It is unlikely that boys and girls will ever be raised so that they are comparable groups. Essentially identical behaviors by the parent seem to yield results in the child which are dependent on sex.[7] If this is true, child-rearing practices will continue to produce boys who behave and respond differently than girls. In fact trying to program child-rearing to assure absolute uniformity seems one step worse than the current process of inculcating conformity to the ideal male/ideal female model. The only model which has relevance considers the known and unknown biologic and experiential variables between men and women and recognizes that there will always be representatives at both ends of the spectrum, with the majority somewhere in between (Fig. 8.2). Patients will very likely conform to or feel pressure to conform to the ideal model concept. The previous information should indicate that such conformity is not essential, nor is it the natural situation of mankind.

The relationship of female sexuality to female body image is quite different from the relationship of male sexuality to male body image. The penis is a concrete example of masculinity. The little girl has a more difficult time recognizing what is inherently female about her body. Her sexual investment in her body is more diffuse. The development of breasts at puberty may serve as an external sign of femininity, and this may account in part for the tremendous importance they assume for many women. This diffuse nature of female sexuality is further reinforced by the cultural values placed on female breasts, legs, hips, and face. At the same time the view of a penis as equivalent to masculinity is reinforced by the popular misconception that penis size is a measure of manhood or sexual prowess.

Ambivalence is part of female sexuality and is reinforced at various stages of development. Female genitals provide sensory pleasure but menstruate. Intercourse is pleasurable, but childbirth is the "worst pain in the world." Boys are always little men, but to become a woman, a girl must bleed, an inherently objectionable occurrence. Punishment for masturbatory acts is externally imposed upon both sexes. For the most part it is a single negative factor in the male's otherwise pleasurable view of his sexual sensations. For the female it is one of a number of negative factors relating to her body and sexuality. Again biologic and cultural factors interact to shape a model of masculinity which is very narrow and limited and a model of femininity which is unclear and ambivalent.

Until recently it has been the popular belief that women were asexual or antisexual beings, and that sexual interest, sexual response, and sexual pleasure

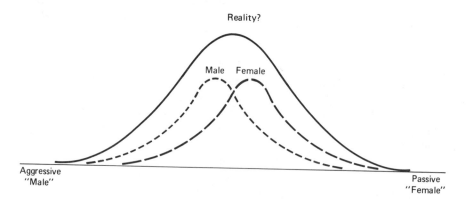

FIG. 8.2.   A model for the distribution of a characteristic by sex. If one had access to a test sensitive enough to measure different modes of expressing the same emotion, it might be apparent that only the larger curve existed and that what was previously viewed as a passive female trait was in fact another mode of an aggressive male trait. (Tests indicate that when verbal aggression is included, the aggression levels of grade schoolchildren are not sex differentiated.)

were the unique province of the male of the species. Recent evidence of the almost insatiable sexual potential of the female points to cultural repression of this potential as the primary cause of the unrecognized sexuality of women.[9] Sexual interest and desire vary in strength as do all human characteristics and needs. The result has been that some women are essentially asexual beings. Their naturally low sex drive has been virtually eliminated by cultural controls. Even the woman with a strong sex drive and unlimited sexual potential may not realize that this is so. The primary sign of sexual arousal in the male, erection, and the proof of sexual release, ejaculation, can hardly be overlooked by men. Vaginal lubrication, pelvic vasocongestion, and myotonia (signs of sexual arousal in the female) are more easily misinterpreted by women.[10] The possibility of misinterpretation is increased by the lack of knowledge of the relationship of these signs to sexual arousal, the cultural factors controlling the recognition and expression of female sexuality, and the tendency to overlook internal cues, a common tendency in individuals with an unclear or ambivalent body image.

Both men and women have been taught to play out their sex-specific roles rather than relate to one another as human beings. Some manage to learn to relate as individuals despite conditioning to the contrary. Identity and sexuality are learned. If the role developed is too narrow for continued acceptance of oneself, one can learn a broader definition. One can break out of the roles and express oneself as a unique human being, with all the attributes and potentials that entails. Indeed much of the information within this text would be valueless if people were not able to learn to put aside roles (if only for a time) for the more honest and meaningful relationships of person to person.

RESPONSE TO BODY IMAGE ASSAULT

That cancer poses a threat to an individual's sense of self, his image of his body, and his sexuality needs little substantiation. Given a moment to reflect on the meaning of a particular cancer should one be told that it had struck him, the reader will certainly be able to think of a number of threats it would pose for him personally. But personal empathy has its limits, which can be minimized by the addition of some empirical data. Very little published material specifically relates to the patient with cancer and the threat cancer poses to body image and identity. However, studies done with individuals who have suffered mutilating injuries or extensive disabilities offer some worthwhile information.

The meaning of a loss is related to (1) the visibility of the loss, (2) the functional loss, and (3) the emotional investment in, or the meaning of, the part affected. Regardless of the objective severity in any of these categories, adaptation relates to an individual's perception of the magnitude of the loss and its meaning to him, its threat to those aspects which form the most stable portion of his identity, the core. A man with leukemia may have no visible loss, he may have lost little function, there is no lost part, yet if he perceives illness per se and leukemia in particular as a sign of weakness and a threat to his role of provider and head of the family, it can have broad ramifications related to his body image. Weakness, a "female trait," may be a direct threat to his masculinity. His identity and sense of self-worth may be shaken by the perceived threat to the goals and roles of husband, provider, father. When roles are in jeopardy, changes are often harder to cope with than one would expect from observing the magnitude of the defect. Most often, however, the threat of cancer and its treatment is related to the organs involved. The fact that over 70 percent of the cancers in the United States affect organs which are given great emotional investment must be a primary factor in the response elicited by the mere hint of cancer.

Expectation and selective attention are very important to the process of coping with a defect. The more negatively an individual perceives a given defect the more likely he is to expect a negative reaction (confirmation of his expectations) and the less likely he is to see positive reactions (contradiction of expectations). The strength of these expectations is dependent on several factors: (1) the frequency and kind of previous confirmations, (2) the lack of alternative expectations, (3) cognitive consequences (special meaning to the patient), (4) motivational consequences (secondary gains), and (5) social consequences (responses of others).[5]

At times, it has been common to view persons who are physically disabled as stigmatized. However, negative feelings about the physically disabled, isolation because of their defects, and feelings of inferiority among the disabled themselves do not universally occur. In fact, studies often indicate that normal persons feel admiration and respect (increased status) for handicapped persons rather than scorn or discredit.[5,11] At the same time, the normal person may perceive that the disabled person feels threatened, guilty, or inferior. (Is this projection??) When negative attitudes of normal persons toward the disabled have been identified, it has been relatively easy to alter the stereotyping with simple factual information.[12] Studies of the disabled themselves do indicate an increased tendency to hypochondriasis, feelings of having been assaulted, vulnerability, and some narrowing of autonomy.[5,11,13] In general, however, the feelings of inferiority anticipated have not been found. Investigation of the effects of various sociologic and psychologic variables on the reaction to disability and eventual adaptation yield even less uniform results. In fact the only conclusion really possible is that there are so many interrelated variables that no *one* can be considered predictive. What a person is like before he had cancer does not predict whether he will be able to cope with the traumas he may face after he has cancer. It does, however, indicate ways he will tend to cope. This yields valuable information about his inherent patterns, so that offers of assistance can be planned to interface with his own psychologic strengths.

Certain identifiable components seem to be part of the process of adapting to a change in body image. These include:

1. Changing one's value system: Physical characteristics become less important as measures of worth, living itself becomes more important and success is redefined.

2. Confining the effect of the disability: Spread of the effects of the defect to aspects of one's self and actions which are not directly affected is a common initial occurrence. Realistic reappraisal and confinement of the handicapping effects of a given defect to those areas unavoidably affected contains the defect and makes adjustment more feasible.
3. Viewing physical factors or functions as assets in themselves rather than as liabilities in comparison with the ideal: The ability to speak is an asset. If esophageal speech is viewed only in relation to normal speech (comparative), it can become a liability.[3,5,11]

There is no doubt that many cancers and their treatment constitute major treats to an individual's sense of self and well-being. Emphasizing and maximizing positive input is one way of minimizing this assault. One factor which has been shown to have a significant effect in terms of increasing the positive input is the reaction of others of importance (usually nurses and the immediate family) immediately after the threat to one's self is realized. These responses seem to be far more important than the visibility or severity of the defect itself. In her book on physical disability, Beatrice Wright states:

> Being brought face to face *for the first time* with one's shortcomings in a hostile and rejecting environment can be such a devastating experience that precautions must be taken to avoid this. . . . It makes all the difference in the world if painful facts about the self are first realized in a friendly and accepting atmosphere. In the former case there is a cementing between the self-core and the negative fact, whereas in the latter case there is a separation.[14]

Thus the man with half his jaw, face, and neck removed, who must wear a prosthesis to prevent a reaction of horror, may be very self-confident, giving only minimal time and energy to his defect, because he has seen that his worth and acceptability to those who matter is not dependent on a handsome face. The authors recall a man who had undergone laryngectomy complicated by multiple infections. He had lost a third of his normal weight and had been hospitalized for several months. He described what for him was the turning point from pessimism and self-pity to hope and feelings of self-worth. "My wife came to pick me up at the hospital. She had arranged for the children to be cared for by a friend. Ten minutes after we entered the house, she had me in bed. Nothing else she could have done could have said to me as clearly, 'You look different and you speak differently, but to me you are the same man.' " Certainly this way of transmitting the message that changes in appearance often do not alter the acceptance of or value of a person to those around him is not appropriate in all cases. The important thing is that the message is transmitted (if it is real) and that it be done in a way in which it is clearly received by that patient. The uniqueness of human beings may require that some effort be spent in searching for and finding the right coding of the message.

THE CHALLENGE FOR NURSING

At the first National Conference on Cancer Nursing, Alice Costello presented the following steps which seem to be necessary in dealing with surgically created alterations in body image. The individual:

1. Accepts the importance of viewing the operative site;
2. Touches and explores the operative site;
3. Accepts the necessity of his learning to care for the defect;
4. Develops independence and competence in his daily care;
5. Reintegrates his new body image and adjusts to a possibly altered life style.[15]

It is a challenge to nurse these patients, and one must develop a positive attitude. As Ms. Costello says so well,

> Even if not all the procedures involved in the treatment of cancer are acceptable to us personally, none of us has the right to communicate his own doubts or fears to the patient. . . . It is not always easy for him to make this choice, and it helps us to gain insight regarding his problem if we try to put ourselves in his position.[16]

Certainly hemicorporectomy or translumbar amputation is the most radical of surgeries. The common reaction among nurses when first informed of the existence of such surgery is shock, horror, and revulsion. Yet if one considers the reasons why this surgery is performed, ie, to help patients whose disease with its pain, odor, and other symptomatology is uncontrollable by more conventional means, and when one sees the courage of those patients who have actively sought this surgery, it should become clear that the response of one who is not facing the situation may be totally unlike one who is facing the very real problems of this particular condition. A nurse may be certain that she/he would never resort to such measures, but until he has suffered as the patient has suffered, feared as the patient has feared, and hoped as the patient has hoped, one cannot know the meaning of such a step nor make such a judgment. No matter how well one knows another, there is always at least one thing which is not known, and that one thing may be vitally important.

The nurse needs to consider a patient's value system, usual patterns of adaptation, and the interruptions of his life style necessitated by his disease when planning the patient's care. The probability of furthur loss, the organ involved, the treatment, as well as the relationship between the patient and the nurse, affect the meaning of this experience for the patient. Recall the model proposed for the development of identity (Fig. 8.1). The more information that the nurse has about the multiple factors operating, the easier it is for her to tailor therapeutic interventions to minimize the negative input and accentuate the positive input.

When a nurse first meets a patient, the patient may be exhibiting a number of behaviors. Early in the process of diagnosis, denial or anxiety to the point of panic is common. Normal defenses can be so effective at this time, however, that the only verbalization of stress may be the revelation of bizarre dreams, and even this information may have to be carefully drawn from the patient. Later a gamut of responses appears. This may include regression, depression, anxiety, hostility, hypochondriasis, counterphobia (overcompensation), obsessions, or schizophrenia. Regardless of which type of reaction a patient is manifesting, two factors aid in establishing a relationship which will be beneficial to the ultimate rehabilitation of the patient. The first of these relates to the nurse's approach to the patient and the second to the involvement of the patient in planning and implementing his care. What has been recommended to make sympathy acceptable to the disabled can be used as a guide to make nursing intervention acceptable as well. Three characteristics are essential to this approach: (1) congruence of mood between the patient and the nurse, (2) respect for the complexity of the situation, and (3) a readiness to help.[5] Another feature of a good approach is the enlistment of the patient as an active team member and as comanager of his care. Giving the patient as much control and decision-making power as possible minimizes the negative aspects of loss of control and feelings of worthlessness and maximizes the positive aspects of self-worth and self-control. And since the patient sets the goals, motivation is less of a problem.

Crisis Intervention

Nursing intervention with patients who are adjusting to changes in body image is essentially crisis intervention. The diagnosis and the treatment and their effects are crises not only for the patient but for the family as well. They are anxious and eager for help, but very little help is available. The patient whose symptoms indicate marked psychopathology may be referred to a psychiatrist. The family which is obviously distraught may be referred to social services. What happens to the other patients and their families? What happens to the vast majority? Nurses trained to use crisis intervention could assist these patients and families. Ruth Murray suggests a very practical reason for employing crisis intervention techniques: "When the patient is in a crisis, he is ripe for help and may be capable of great change in a relatively short time because of the discomfort he feels."[17] The authors hope that the following overview of crisis intervention will serve to illustrate how these techniques could be considered requisite to hospital and outpatient care of the patient with cancer. The principles previously identified throughout this chapter are incorporated in the process of crisis intervention.

A crisis as defined in this context occurs when an individual faces an obstacle to life goals which cannot be handled by his usual methods of coping. A period of disorganization, emotional turmoil, and abortive attempts at seeking a solution ensues (Fig. 8.3). Though a crisis is somewhat self-limiting, intervention serves

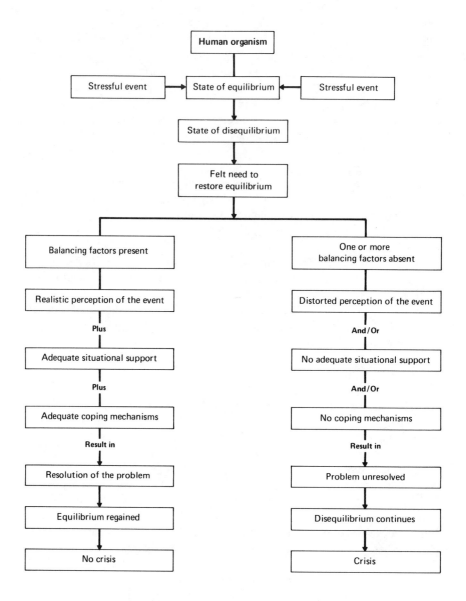

FIG. 8.3.   A. A paradigm: Effect of balancing factors in stressful events—general model.

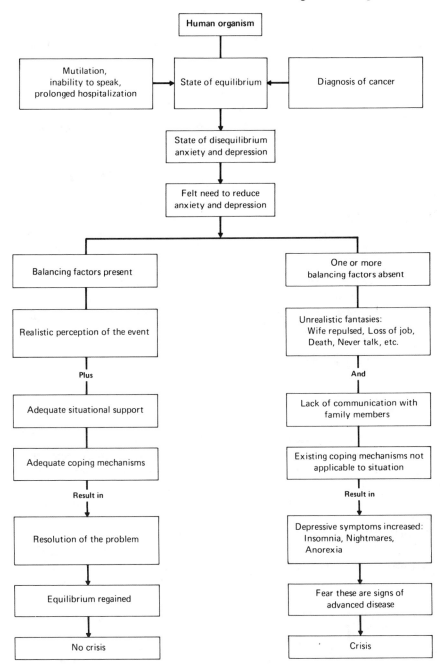

FIG. 8.3   B. A paradigm: Effect of stress on anticipating radical head and neck surgery. (Adapted from Aguilera and Messick: Crisis Intervention, 2nd ed. 1974. Courtesy of C.V. Mosby Co.)

three purposes: (1) to accelerate relief and return the patient to pre-crisis levels of functioning; (2) to prevent development of chronically pathologic patterns; and (3) to help the patient find ways of handling future crises in his life. The steps in crisis intervention, like the nursing process, are a special variation of the scientific method: (1) assessment, with emphasis on the precipitating event; (2) planning therapeutic intervention, with emphasis on strengths, skills, previously beneficial coping mechanisms, and supportive others in the environment; (3) intervention, which may include helping the patient to gain greater intellectual understanding, to express his feelings, to explore his coping mechanisms, and to re-enter his social world; and (4) resolution, with anticipatory planning for future crises.

There are two categories of crisis therapy: generic and individual. Most crisis intervention with cancer patients could be of the least complex generic type. This therapy is based on a good understanding of what generally occurs in response to a particular type of crisis, such as mutilation or cancer. Better understanding of the meaning of the patient's responses, general support to the patient, encouragement of adaptive patient behaviors, environmental manipulation, and anticipatory planning are the foundations of generic therapy. Individual therapy, though it concentrates on the present crisis and how to cope with it, investigates more fully the interpersonal and intrapsychic processes which may be operational. Generic therapy is easily taught to nurses who are not psychotherapists. It requires less time than individual therapy and usually achieves the goals of providing necessary relief and aiding the patient in dealing with the future.[18]

Role Play

Role play has been used with some success as a method of testing how well coping mechanisms will work when patients reenter society. Nurses seem to have a very negative reaction to role play. This is unfortunate, as nurses have the opportunity to utilize this technique in a variety of settings and with patients who would be unable or unwilling to seek help elsewhere. Role play enables the patient to test behaviors in a setting which can provide all of the positive reinforcement which is so important. Esophageal speakers could role play going into a restaurant and ordering a meal, amputees could role play getting onto a bus, and mastectomy patients could role play the first day at the beach. These are only three of an endless number of possibilities. The nurse may be the only other person in the role play, or it can be part of a group experience. Other group members with the same disability, who play normal people, have the opportunity to deal with their fears, prejudices, and expectations as projected in the persons they play. Activities are not the only subjects suitable for role play. Preparing a child for the appearance of her father after radical head and neck surgery could be an ideal situation for a mother to role play to gain confidence. Despite resistance, role play can also be used to advantage in helping nurses test their interviewing and intervention skills.

A certain degree of desensitization to highly charged words and topics can also take place in the role play, as happens often in discussions regarding sexual practices. Despite the technique employed, the purpose of intervention remains the same—to maximize the regulatory and control potentials of an individual so that his defect has the minimal impact on his life, a life which continues to be a satisfying experience.

Problems Related to Sexuality

Identity problems arising from the diagnosis and treatment of cancer can, for the most part, be combined under the headings of sexuality and cosmesis. The authors will attempt to correlate the previous basic information in each of the more specific instances to be discussed with emphasis on more specific nursing care measures.

An individual's sexuality and its expression are a highly individualized aspect of personality. The common narrow view of male sexuality and the ambivalence and denial of female sexuality were mentioned on page 207. Despite the very uniqueness of sexuality, there do exist some common aspects. Masculinity and feminity are core aspects of identity, that is, they are very basic, emotionally charged, and resistant to change. There is also a great deal of ambivalence and guilt or shame associated with sexual feeling and sexual expression in our society. Sex is a very private function, and though it may be joked about and freely discussed in the abstract within some groups, intense feeling is evoked when one's own sexual activity is considered. Sexual expression is more than a biologic activity. It is a form of communication. It is a means of achieving closeness and comfort, of expressing love and concern. It can represent caring, needing, and commitment. It can mean fun, happiness, and relaxation. But it can also communicate control, authority-submission, disgust, or a frantic need to relate in any available manner.

We seem to be in many ways a sex-oriented society. Yet sexual needs and actions are generally acceptable only within certain culturally defined limits. The limits may vary somewhat from reference group to reference group, but unlimited license is virtually unknown. It is generally expected that sexual interest will be controlled and sublimated except at the culturally sanctioned time and place. For instance, at times of crisis, during illness, or with advancing age, an individual is assumed to have no sexual interest or needs. Indeed a patient with cancer may be too ill to assume the active role in any sexual activity. However, a patient in the terminal stages of illness may desperately need the comfort, closeness, and relaxation his mate has previously been able to assure by hugging, petting, and other forms of sexual expression. As a person adjusts to his diagnosis, his needs change. A woman who blames herself, her mate, and their active sex life for her cervical cancer may well avoid all sexually related activities. As she becomes more accepting of her disease and the treatment, she may have a tremendous need for comfort, reassurance of her femininity, and proof of her continued ability to function as a sexual partner. Her interest in sexual activities of all types may increase significantly at this time. In general, depressed individuals are not interested in interchange with others, and this includes sexual interchange. Angry patients do not actively seek comforting, calming, and tenderness. If an angry individual sees and uses sex as a means of control or punishment (of himself or his mate), he may be very aggressive sexually during those phases of his illness characterized by anger. Very weak patients will often be unable to engage in sex, and they may or may not be interested. Once again the meanings of sex beyond its biologic function have great influence when one is interested in seeking out and participating in specifically sexual activities. An example may help to illustrate these points:

> Mr. J is dying from lung cancer. He has withdrawn gradually from all the people, activities, and pleasures of his life but one—frequent intercourse to the extent that his waning strength allows. He and his wife had delayed having children. Impregnating his wife is now something he *must* do before he can die peacefully.

> Mr. L is also dying of lung cancer. He is no longer able to work at his heavy labor job. Ms. T, the young woman with whom he has lived for two years, is now supporting him. Mr. L has no interest in sex. To him manhood means bringing home a paycheck and aggressive male dominant intercourse. Loss of the ability to do the former has eliminated all pleasure from the latter.

Almost any body part or function can have meaning for an individual's femininity or masculinity. Any alteration in such an organ or function can alter one's perception of and expression of his sexuality. These include the breast, uterus, vagina, penis, and testes. A great deal has been written about the meaning of the breast and the effect of mastectomy. Almost nothing has been written about the effect of amputation of the penis or orchiectomy. Certainly this is accountable to some extent because of the numbers of persons involved. While 89,000 cases of breast cancer occur yearly in the United States, only 4,100 cases of penile and testicular cancer occur.[19] However, since prostatic cancer accounts for another 54,000 cases of cancer yearly,[19] and treatment for prostatic cancer often affects male sexual activity, one wonders why the emphasis is on female sexual alterations. Is it possible that physicians (mostly male) find the thought of mutilation of the male sexual organs too threatening to discuss?

VISIBLE ASSAULT–FEMALE.   Because breast cancer represents the most common cancer associated with sexuality, and because there is much written on this subject, the authors will begin with a discussion of the nurse's role in the care of the patient with breast cancer, a visible assault to the female body. Subsequent sections will treat the subjects of visible assault to masculinity (removal of penis or testes), impotence, hysterectomy, vaginectomy, and nonsurgical assaults on sexuality.

Health Teaching.   The most significant activity to which a nurse can devote herself in relation to breast cancer is health teaching. Ninety-two percent of breast tumors are found by women themselves. Whether a woman finds the lump during monthly breast examination when it is small or by accident when it is much larger is a crucial factor. Most women are unaware of the significant facts about breast cancer which place them at risk. They are listed below

1. Over the age of 40
2. Fertility problems
3. Early menarche and long menstrual history
4. Family history of breast cancer, primarily mother and aunts
5. History of prior breast disease
6. History of prior breast cancer

A recent Gallup survey conducted for the American Cancer Society indicates that women "grossly overestimate the prevalence" of breast cancer, assuming that at least half of all breast lumps are cancerous, while, in actuality, only 20 percent of all such lumps are malignant.[20] Forty-six percent of the women answering felt that practicing monthly breast self-examination (BSE) would increase their fears. Only 18 percent of the women practiced BSE monthly, though 77 percent knew of the practice.[20] Three primary factors involved in reasons why this population did not practice BSE were (1) lack of awareness (in 40 percent) that *monthly* BSE should supplement a physician's examination, (2) fear (46 percent avoided BSE because of this), and (3) lack of knowledge about BSE.

Though women were acquainted with the term "self-examination of the breast," 35 percent feared that they would be unable to carry out BSE properly and/or that they would not recognize the presence of any abnormality.[20] The conclusions of this survey are relevant to health teaching:

> Clearly, it would be a great mistake to exaggerate the emotional reactions of women to breast removal. It is unlikely that the strong aversion of women to breast loss could itself account for all fears of women regarding breast surgery. Rather, the fear of cancer appears to be the important deterring factor. If this is so, we can infer that increasing the confidence of women in survival chances after breast removal would contribute significantly in acceptance of extensive surgery. Moreover, a realization of the extent to which early detection increases survival rates could also reduce the inhibiting effort of worry upon the desire for frequent breast examinations.[20]

Hopefully, programs now being implemented which approach women on a more personal basis may increase the number of women who regularly practice BSE by dealing more directly with pessimism, fear, and insufficient knowledge. Beyond these structured programs, the nurse has an opportunity to influence the many people she meets each day. Just the admission that one is a cancer nurse can precipitate a variety of high-anxiety responses and a flood of questions. Far too

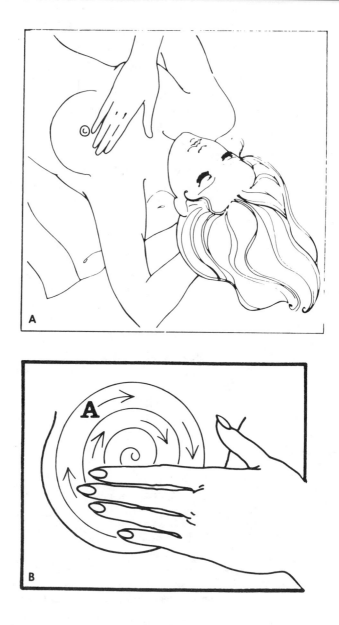

often this opportunity is not recognized for its tremendous worth. In a nonthreatening social encounter, where the anxiety level is not a deterrent, an individual is
more receptive to health teaching and good sound information. The American
Cancer Society booklet on BSE is an excellent teaching aid (Fig. 8.4). Apparently
the most successful method of teaching, however, is for one woman to demon-

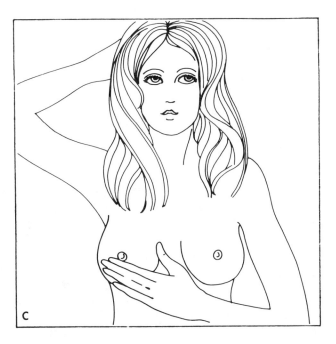

FIG. 8.4.   Instructions for breast self-examination. A. Lie down. Put one hand behind your head. With the other hand, fingers flattened, gently feel your breast. Press lightly. Now examine the other breast. B. This illustrates how to check each breast. Begin where you see A and follow the arrows, feeling gently for a lump or thickening. Remember to feel all parts of each breast. C. Repeat the same procedure sitting up, with your hand still behind your head. (From A Breast Check, 1973. Courtesy of the American Cancer Society)

strate to another the exact technique of BSE. Emphasis is on acquainting the woman's fingers with her own normal breast so that she *will* recognize even a very small lump which, should it be malignant, is likely to be more readily cured than a larger lump.

Health teaching is also needed after a woman finds a lump. The woman may delay seeing a physician. She may be somewhat reassured to know that most lumps are not cancer. And certainly in terms of relieving anxiety (the primary reason for delay), it can be helpful for her to discuss her feelings and fears regarding breast cancer, its treatment, and prognosis. Despite the tremendously difficult controversies regarding the best method of treatment for breast cancer, there will remain some women whose way of coping is to leave everything to the physician (47 percent in the ACS study[20]). There will also be adamant supporters of one form of treatment over another. While the choice of the individual woman must be respected, it is worthwhile to investigate the basis of this choice to determine if all major considerations have been reviewed. If the basis of the decision is not comprehensive, the patient's attitude and rehabilitation may be adversely affected. There will also be women who are very confused about everything they have read in the lay literature. They fear that the wrong procedure will be done, and this fear and confusion need to be dealt with before the woman makes a decision. The woman needs the understanding and guidance of someone who knows and understands the alternatives and will give the time to help the patient come to terms with them. This type of encounter may take place in the course of a conversation before a lump is ever found (causal conversation, when teaching BSE, or in the physician's office before routine examination), at the time a lump is examined, or even in the hospital while a woman is awaiting diagnosis or treatment. It behooves any nurse involved in these situations to be acquainted with the controversies regarding the treatment of breast cancer, to have as many facts regarding all sides of the issues as she can obtain, to be comfortable with this material, and to be open to the variety of women who must face some form of treatment for breast cancer.[21,22]

The significance of the female breast is greater than its physiologic function implies primarily because men and women alike have been conditioned to believe that femininity and sexual attractiveness of females are proportional to breast size. To assume that the stress of mastectomy is related to breast size, however, is an error. The small-busted woman may have invested more of her identity in her small breasts because she was so conscious of her failure in this area. She may also be dealing with a large load of negative feelings regarding her femininity because of her small breasts. On the other hand she may view her femininity virtually isolated from her breasts and be far more fearful of the cancer than the threat to her femininity. Though the effect of mastectomy is not proportional to breast size, it is proportional to the magnitude of negative input which a given woman is receiving about herself at the moment. Because of the age at which breast cancer occurs, the quantity of negative input (realistic or unrealistic) is often high: menopause, weight and muscle changes, major life revisions. Some investigators suggest a causal relationship among negative life experiences, pessimism, and the development of cancer. The continuing research at the University of Washington involving life stress points and predisposition to illness certainly lends credence to these theories.[23,24] Other studies of the personality of women who develop breast cancer indicate a higher likelihood of ambivalence toward childbirth, pregnancy, and marriage.[25] There also seems to have been an inordinate number of deaths of significant individuals in the lives of those who develop cancer.[23,25]

Preoperative Period.   The care that a patient with breast cancer receives, whether she undergoes lumpectomy or extended radical mastectomy, must be directed toward maximizing the positive aspects, not just minimizing the negative ones. Openly acknowledging and discussing the deformity and the resulting emotional response, while at the same time encouraging the maintenance of a hopeful philosophy, shows respect for the difficult present and realistic hopes for a better future.

In most cases a woman faces the possibility of mastectomy without any certainties. She is admitted to the hospital for a biopsy. She is anesthetized, and the biopsy specimen is examined. If malignant cells are found, definitive surgery proceeds without the patient having awakened from the anesthetic. Thus in the case of Betty Ford, the nation knew the diagnosis and the treatment required before the patient herself did. The ambiguity of this situation leads to high anxiety levels preoperatively as well as a high level of denial. Some physicians elect to biopsy breast masses under local anesthetic and schedule definitive surgery for the next day to allow patients some time for preoperative preparation. Some surgeons try to prepare every women for mastectomy. Other surgeons resort to the unacceptable practice of reinforcing the patient's preoperative denial. Unless definitive surgery is delayed, the patient goes to surgery unsure of what she will find upon awakening. The family, equally unsure, retire to a waiting area hoping that a short wait heralding good news is ahead of them. When waiting during surgery is protracted, the family usually guesses that surgery was extensive. An emotional overflow of this buildup of tension is common at the point when a doctor verbalizes what the family has already deduced. Helping the family to deal with their suspicions before confrontation with the physician can help them to assimilate and understand what he may need to tell them. Since this is often the only time that the entire family will speak with the surgeon, maximal use of this time should be assured. The patient may guess the extent of surgery, but fear to ask, soon after she begins to respond in the recovery room. She should be told honestly and with a positive approach what surgery was required. Ideally, the surgeon and family would tell her together. Realizing that this ideal is often not realized, it is certainly more comforting to a patient to hear this news from a nurse she has already learned to trust (eg, primary nurse, clinical specialist) and/or her family than to lie half-awake, fearing what each stranger will say.

Postoperative Period.   After surgery, despite the extent of the procedure, the primary goal is to reestablish maximal self-care as early as possible. Unless skin grafting has been necessary, the woman can brush her teeth, feed herself, and begin hand/wrist exercises the first postoperative day. These do not entail a great expenditure of energy, and the reinforcement that they give to the philosophy that "you are only slightly changed; you can care for yourself and be yourself as before" is essential. Several cancer centers schedule group exercise sessions. These may be similar to the exercises recommended in the American Cancer Society pamphlet, *Help Yourself to Recovery* (Fig. 8.5). The motivating effect of group dynamics should never be overlooked.

The woman with breast cancer needs a careful balance between understanding sympathy and realistic determination to contain the disability. Supervised and guided group interactions often provide all of this for a number of patients in less time than intense personal counseling could provide it for one. Obviously the group leader must be a skilled, knowledgeable, and perceptive person.

Bilateral exercises reduce the likelihood of the complication of curvature of the

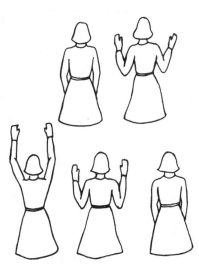

A. Hand wall climbing

1. Start in standard position, facing wall, with toes as close to wall as possible.
2. Bend elbows and place palms against the wall at shoulder level.
3. Work both hands up the wall parallel to each other until arms are fully extended.
4. Work hands down to shoulder level.
5. Return hands to standard position.
6. Rest and repeat.

B. Pulley motion

1. Toss the rope over the rod.
2. Stand directly behind the rope in standard position.
3. Hold the ends of the rope in each hand with knots between your third and fourth fingers and raise arms sideways.
4. Using see-saw motion and with arms stretched sideways, slide the rope up and down over the rod, until the knots in the rope touch the rod.
5. Return to standard position, rest and repeat.
6. Do not bend at the waist. Keep your feet flat on the floor during this exercise.

C. Elbow pull-in

1. In standard position, extend arms sideways to shoulder level.
   In rhythm:
2. Bend elbows clasping fingers at back of your neck.
3. Pull elbows in toward each other until they touch.
4. Return to position (2) with elbows bent—fingers clasped at back of neck.
5. Unclasp fingers and extend arms sideways at shoulder level.
6. Return to standard position. Rest and repeat.

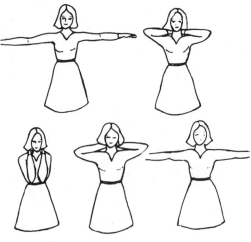

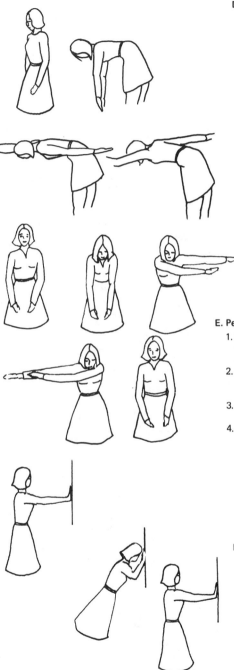

D. Paddle swing

1. Stand in standard position.
2. Bend forward from the waist, allowing arms to hang toward the floor by gravity.
3. In this position, place right arm forward over your head; place left arm back. Do not bend elbows.

   In rhythm:
4. Swing right arm back while left arm comes forward, then allow arms to hang forward as in position (2).
5. Return to standard position. Rest and repeat.

E. Pendulum swing

1. Start in standard position. Bend forward from the waist, allowing arms to hang toward the floor by gravity.
2. Swing both arms together, describing an arc from one shoulder to the other. Do not bend elbows. Keep arms parallel.
3. Return to standard position and allow arms to fall to sides.
4. Rest and repeat.

F. Forehead touch

1. In standard position, face wall at arm's length distance. Place hands against the wall at shoulder level, parallel to each other.
2. Slowly bend elbows, leaning forward until forehead touches wall.
3. Straighten elbows slowly, pushing body away from wall.
4. Return to standard position, rest and repeat.

FIG. 8.5.   Postmastectomy exercises. Top to bottom: A. Handwall climbing. B. Pulley motion. C. Elbow pull-in. D. Paddle swing. E. Pendulum swing. F. Forehead touch. (From Help Yourself to Recovery, 1957. Courtesy of The American Cancer Society)

spine. They also help minimize concentration on the defect. For this same reason, gadgets are discouraged, and upon discharge exercises are translated into an Activities of Daily Living (ADL) program.

The postoperative period remains an extremely stressful period for the patient, her relatives, and her friends. They cannot be counted on to remember much of what they are told. For this reason it is important to devise some method(s) to improve patient assimilation of information. Some hospitals give written directions with pictures to their patients. Some have prepared special booklets or use the ACS pamphlet, *Help Yourself to Recovery*. Memorial Cancer Center, in New York City, has developed a set of recordings for exercise and discharge information as well as for preadmission teaching. The patient can refresh her memory as often as she finds necessary. It is important to incorporate reassuring information and a hopeful, positive attitude in any method used so that each reference is a positive experience for the patient. These do not substitute for human contact. But neither does a single or daily teaching session substitute for a concise, ready reference.

Since its inception in 1952, Reach to Recovery is gaining wider and wider acceptance in aiding in the physical and emotional rehabilitation of postmastectomy women. The Reach to Recovery volunteer is a role model, a woman like the patient who has had a mastectomy and recovered successfully. These women are eager to be of help, but they are not professional counselors. It remains the responsibility of the professional nurse to know her patient and the information she is receiving and to assess the effect this information has on the patient. A buxom volunteer who is exuberant over her lifelike, $85, gel-filled prosthesis may be overwhelming to the shy, flat-chested lady, who would never consider paying even a fraction of that amount for a "falsie" even though she feels conspicuously lopsided. Weighted prostheses have been a boon for the full-busted woman. However, the average or small-busted woman may do well with dime-store falsies sewn into her favorite bra with the addition of an anchor to prevent the bra from riding up on the affected side. (This anchor consists of a piece of elastic sewn to the bottom band of the bra toward the outside of the front; it can be pinned or snapped to a girdle or panties.) The new lightweight all-in-one foundations or a long-line bra can also be adapted with inexpensive padding without riding up.

The first viewing of the surgical scar is a major stress and a major step forward. It is the first unavoidable step on the road to recovery. The earlier the patient views the scar, the more content she usually is with the cosmetic result at a later time. The woman who just cannot look should be assisted in achieving this intermediate goal by systematic personalized steps administered with sensitivity and patience. For example, it could be described to her, then she could touch the area, and finally take just a peek. The constant reminder of the obvious deformity of the chest through a gown and robe does not help anyone. Some form of padding, attached either to the inside of the gown or on top of the dressing, should be worn as soon as the bulky pressure dressing is changed.

The most important single factor in a woman's response after mastectomy is the reaction of the male with whom she is most intimately, and often sexually, involved. Many of these men are very supportive. However, no one helps them in this area. An individual man may feel he must be nonchalant and cheerful at all times even though the relationship may have been in difficulty before the surgery, or he may be very pessimistic about cancer and may already be dealing with the possibility of his woman's death rather than the mastectomy. In accord with the cultural norm which requires all men to be strong, self-reliant, and totally controlled, a man may be reticent to reveal the depths of his distress. Certainly an observant and sympathetic nurse can encourage him to acknowledge his feelings and to express himself. He needs to do this before he can openly and sincerely reassure the patient. The patient generally needs specific reassurance of his love, his support, and his faith in her and in the future. How this is done is an individual matter, but it needs to be done and not just left to chance or passed over because "she knows I love her and it doesn't matter." The male nurse may have a distinct advantage here with the man who must keep up an image for all females.

Helping the patient and her man express their own feelings and then helping them to communicate with one another is a vital task which is seldom attempted. Studies as well as experiences with individual patients repeatedly indicate that cancer, surgery, fears, and feelings become taboo subjects which interfere with open communication for extended periods of time after the initial crisis.[26] Some Reach to Recovery chapters have enlisted couple volunteers. These couples are employed for married patients, usually only when the husband is more verbal, inquisitive, or upset than one has come to expect. It is usually necessary to specifically inform both the patient and her man that this surgery will in no way interfere with their sex life—that, with care not to traumatize the incision, their sex life can be resumed at once. Without this specific information, a male, fearing he will injure his mate, will often refrain from demonstrating even his usual signs of affection. His lady may easily interpret this behavior as rejection of her. Just because most couples eventually work these matters out, one should not be lax about preventing them whenever possible.

To assure every woman that her mastectomy will have no effect on her marriage and that her husband will be understanding and helpful is absurd. One in three marriages is under enough stress to end in divorce. Will a mastectomy heal the wounds of these marriages? Will a mastectomy make a cruel husband kind, a disinterested husband attentive, an unfaithful husband faithful? Many women who have breast cancer are not married to supportive husbands, are not married at all, or do not have a lover or a boyfriend. These women also need support, comfort, and someone to help them face the future with hope.

It is the woman's feelings about herself which are most important to her eventual rehabilitation—psychologic and physical. The easiest and most direct way to provide positive input into the reconstruction of this self-image is through the person most important emotionally to the patient. For some women this is a husband, lover, or boyfriend. For others, the most important person is a child, parent, or friend. And for some patients (married and unmarried), the nurse becomes the most significant person and, therefore, the most influential variable in the patient's development of a positive attitude, a positive self-image, and realistic hopes for the future. This is truly crisis intervention. The coping patterns which have previously been effective for the patient need to be identified and explored, the individual's strengths and the supportive aspects of *her* life style need to be illuminated in an effort to help the patient regain the degree of equilibrium which she possessed prior to this crisis. Mentally unstable patients will generally continue to be mentally unstable, and mentally healthy individuals will generally be able to regain their emotional stability.

Lymphedema, swelling of the arm on the surgical side, can develop after mastectomy. There are things the patient can do to help prevent this swelling: (1) use the arm normally, (2) prevent injury, and (3) prevent infection in the affected arm. Problems of lymphedema and muscle weakness are not uncommon after radical or extended radical mastectomy. After removal of the axillary lymph nodes and after radiation to the axilla, the flow of lymph from the affected arm is reduced. With the current trend to less radical procedures, the need for special sleeves and other unusual measures to deal with these complications is less common. Active full range of motion and prevention of infections in the affected arm will decrease or prevent more lymphedema. Surgical procedures to reestablish better lymphatic drainage or to amputate a totally useless and painful lymphedemic arm are rarely needed. Return to an active normal life soon after surgery (with a few modifications because of strength and endurance) serves not only to improve one's emotional outlook and motivation but also to minimize the number and degree of long-term complications.

The following are some hints for patients to help in arm care after mastectomy to prevent injury and infection.*

> TAKE PRECAUTIONS TO PREVENT BURNS
> > Hold cigarette in the unaffected hand
> > Use padded mitts when using the oven, grill, or fireplace
> > Tan slowly to prevent sunburn
> TAKE PRECAUTIONS TO PREVENT TRAPPING OF MORE FLUID IN THE ARM BECAUSE OF PRESSURE
> > Carry purse, packages, suitcases, and other heavy objects on the unaffected side
> > Wear watch and jewelry on the unaffected arm
> > Avoid clothes with tight sleeves or those with elastic in the sleeves
> > Prevent anyone from taking a blood pressure on the affected side
> > Avoid allowing the arm to hang limply at the side
> > Wear elastic sleeve regularly if your surgeon has prescribed one

*Adapted from Hand Care, *Courtesy of Cleveland Clinic Department of Physical Medicine and Rehabilitation; and Robbins and Markel: The Postmastectomy lymphedematous arm. Courtesy of the American Cancer Society*

TAKE PRECAUTIONS TO PREVENT CUTS, SCRATCHES, AND IRRITATION

Wear heavy gloves while gardening, and avoid thorny plants

Wear a thimble while sewing

Use an electric shaver to shave

Keep hands and cuticles soft with the regular (three times daily) use of hand cream. Gently push cuticle back when applying hand cream; never cut cuticle. If hands become very dry during cold weather, apply hand cream and wear cotton gloves while sleeping

Always wear gloves outside in cold weather

Prevent all injections (flu shots, vaccinations, medications) from being given in the affected arm

Prohibit the taking of blood from the affected arm

Wear lined rubber gloves when washing dishes or doing household cleaning

Use a mild deodorant on the affected side

Immediately wash even the slightest cut and apply a Band-Aid

Call a physician if arm becomes hot, red, or swollen

Carry a card or wear a Medic-Alert tag which indicates *Lymphedema Arm– No Tests–No Hypos*

The value of follow-up visits cannot be overemphasized. The period of hospitalization is frequently one of shock and disbelief, and it takes place in an artificial environment. When the woman returns to her own home, she begins to face her situation in a very different way. The peak of emotional distress is estimated to occur eight weeks after surgery. Jeanne Quint's study indicates that fears of recurrence of the cancer and death continue for at least a year, and that during this entire time no one is helping the patient cope with these fears.[26] Group sessions at three and six months or home visits with a structured goal may be useful in minimizing the threat and disruptive influence of these apparently normal responses. Persistent physical complaints can also be dealt with at these times.

Recurrence of the cancer or untreated breast cancer with open, draining sores is another tremendous assault on one's femininity. Women with these conditions have multiple problems to contend with: the recurrence of the disease itself, fear of death, pain, odor, and repulsiveness. Efforts to deal with body image threat and the resulting emotional distress without an equally vigorous effort to alleviate the physical symptoms of odor, pain, and drainage are destined to fail. Both aspects must be given attention. In the midst of the emotional turmoil which is commonplace in a situation of multiple problems, the premenopausal patient is often called upon to deal with the additional threats posed by oophorectomy. Aging is considered a greater crisis for women than for men because cessation of menstruation is a single event to which are attached all of the feelings and fears regarding aging, dependency, loss, and death. A woman's reaction to menopause seems to be related to two factors: (1) how positive she feels about herself at the time and (2) how rapidly ovarian estrogen levels fall. The premenopausal woman with recurrent or inoperable breast cancer is dealing with an overload of negative input about her self, and surgical or radiation-induced menopause causes a very rapid reduction in estrogen levels. Every effort needs to be made to encourage the patient to express her feelings and fears, and to provide appropriate emotional and physical care based on these individual concerns.

VISIBLE ASSAULT–MALE. Amputation of the penis or orchiectomy, like mastectomy, is a visible assault to sexuality and body image. The small number of men who contract cancer of the penis and its high cure rate seem to relegate it to minimal concern. Cancer of the penis occurs almost exclusively in uncircumcised males and then generally in the presence of a phimotic foreskin, poor hygiene, and chronic local irritation. Hopefully, the current attack on routine circumcision as an unnecessary surgical procedure will not yield a new generation which proves by the rapid increase in this cancer that circumcision was not without merit.

Testicular cancer, which is more common in men under the age of 40, receives more consideration. A variety of histologic types of cancer affect the testes, with virulence, with 10-year survival figures, ranging from 11 percent to 90 percent.[27] The initial therapy of choice for primary testicular cancer is unilateral orchiectomy. However, bilateral orchiectomy is often required for recurrent prostatic cancer. The information obtained from studies of women who underwent mastectomy or hysterectomy which imply that cancer and the fear of recurrence are problems at least as big as the changes in body image and function may or may not be relevant for the male population. Certainly more information regarding patient perception, response, and rehabilitation is needed. In the absence of this information, application of some general principles remains the only basis for planning patient care.

The patient should be given all of the information which *he needs* or wants at such a time and in such a way that he can use it. It is not the responsibility of the nurse to inform the patient of the nature of his disease or its treatment. However, after the physician has acquainted the patient with these basic facts, it most certainly falls to the nurse to reinforce, clarify, and reiterate what was said. The assumption is made that the nurse has the necessary information to do this. This suggests that the nurse takes part in the discussion with the physician, the patient, and the family. This is not the time for modesty. The nurse of the past who said and did nothing without a physician's specific order could hide behind the fact that she had no need to be part of this very private conversation and that her presence would embarrass patient and physician. Such an excuse is no longer valid. The nurse, male or female, is a professional whose expertise can be of assistance to the patient and his family. The sooner this is clarified, the sooner the initial embarrassment is overcome and a therapeutic relationship can begin. The fact that therapy based on the Masters and Johnson model can be effective with very inhibited couples illustrates that very intimate information can be discussed cross-sexually in a professional context to the benefit of the patient/client. Certainly a deep respect for the feelings, beliefs, and mores of the individual and couple is essential. With this it is possible to assist in the process of coping.

Unilateral orchiectomy should produce little long-term effect on the patient. Neither impotence nor sterility should be problems. What having cancer means to the man, how the important figures in his life react, how he feels about himself and his masculinity, the meaning of the missing scrotal contents—all of these have as great an effect on potency as the surgery itself. To alleviate some of the concern with the missing testis, silicone testicular implants have recently been developed.

INTERNAL ASSAULT–IMPOTENCE.   As indicated above, not all men who have orchiectomies are impotent. They are obviously sterile if the surgery is bilateral. What this sterility means, as well as the meaning of masculinity, the reactions of others, and the meaning of cancer, affect a man's potency. That many men are impotent after bilateral orchiectomy seems to be at least partly related to the fact that they expect to be, since after puberty sexual response is a reflex response with much cortical input and very little hormone dependency. If even some of the pelvic nerves are intact and the patient is mentally receptive, erection may occur. Basically, the man and his sexual partner need the best information available regarding the disease, treatment, prognosis, and effect on the future. Given this information in a positive and supportive manner and given the chance to express their specific concerns, the problems of pessimism, isolation, and reduced libido should be largely preventable. Even for the patient with a poor prognosis, an active sex life or the ability to continue to see himself as a man, at least in bed, may be very helpful. Sex is a very personal and idiosyncratic behavior. Its meanings are multiple and complex. Either to minimize or to overemphasize its relevance is to do the individuals involved a great disservice.

Of the 54,000 men who develop prostatic cancer yearly, 90 percent are over the age of 50 when diagnosed. Either of the preferred methods of treatment, bilateral orchiectomy with the addition of estrogens or radical prostatectomy, results in impotence in a high percentage of patients. Castration plus estrogens can also result in feminization with gynecomastia, an additional assault on the patient's masculinity and body image. This gynecomastia can be controlled with small doses of radiation to the male breasts.

Impotence may also result from neuropathies developing from radiotherapy or in conjunction with certain chemotherapeutic agents (specifically vincristine and vinblastine). In conformity with the cultural myth that libido and sexual capacity become negligible past the age of 50, the standard view has been that impotence resulting from treatment in this age group is not a significant problem. This attitude fails to recognize the mass of evidence currently available which indicates that sexual ability and interest do not disappear with age. Certain timing factors change with aging: erection takes longer to occur, ejaculation is delayed, the refractory period lengthens. But the capacity to engage in sexual intercourse, regularly exercised, continues into the 70s and 80s. Chronic illness, not age, is the usual reason for the cessation of sexual intercourse. At any age the magnitude of an individual's sex drive may fall anywhere on a very broad spectrum. There is no evidence for the assumption that at age 55 a man will suffer less from interruption of this function than a younger man would. He may initially be more philosophical about it, he will often repeatedly insist that it is a small price to pay for life; yet weeks or months later, the price looms much larger and the repercussions in other spheres of his life may become evident.

As mentioned previously, sex fulfills many needs, and it is often the necessity of finding outlets or satisfaction for this whole gamut of needs that is so stressful for the individual. At a time when encouragement, comfort, stroking, reassurance, and tension reduction are all needed more than usual, a major method of achieving these is lost. It is often said that a willing couple will find a way. It is a shame, however, that we, who can so quickly create a problem, can offer so little assistance beyond the consolation that sometime in the future they will settle upon a compromise which is at least tolerable for them. For older couples possibly more than for the younger, this problem is difficult to surmount. Sexual practices other than vaginal insertion of the penis with the man on top are often not even known let alone part of a repertoire of lovemaking exchanges. One cannot impose a new set of sexual standards and practices on the couple. However, it behooves the nurse to be aware of the information available concerning the broad spectrum of normal sexual practices which can supplement or replace vaginal intercourse, for example, manual or oral stimulation.[28-31] The simple fact that hugging, kissing, and petting can give pleasure without the orgasmic goal orientation usually associated with sex can be astounding information and food for thought. In fact there is some information that psychologic orgasmic release can occur even when the physiology of orgasm is interrupted.[32,33]

In her preoperative assessment of the patient, a sensitive nurse can usually find the opportunity to suggest that concern over loss of sexual potency is a *valid* concern and that there are ways to compensate for this loss. Having given the patient an opportunity to express himself and having presented oneself as willing to be of assistance, it is up to the patient to proceed as he wishes. The opportunity should also be given to his sexual partner to express her concerns as well. Throughout this section, reference is made to the female sexual partner. There is no reason to assume that some of these patients may not be homosexual. Generally, this situation is extremely difficult for all members of the health team to handle. Denial or retreat from the situation are practiced en masse. The homosexual patient and his mate may need as much understanding, support, and counseling as any other couple. Very little can be accomplished in the immediate surgical period. At this point, *living*, with any restriction, is the all-encompassing goal. The subject can be opened, the importance of the problem agreed upon, and the fact that help is available made known.

The next problem which arises concerns the actual counseling. Were there an ideal situation, it would consist of a surgeon who was comfortable and well versed in matters of sexual relations. He would offer his counsel gradually over time with each contact with the patient. His prestigious position would help overcome the patient's resistance and guilt, stemming from a feeling that gratitude for life should replace any thoughts of sex. Unfortunately, physicians, including gynecologists and urologists, often do not have sufficient sexual knowledge or comfort with sexual matters. Certain psychologists or marriage counselors may be willing to attempt to help a couple reestablish a meaningful sexual relationship without vaginal intercourse, but many of these professionals also have their own hang-ups about cancer, sex, and aging. They all too often resort to the "sex isn't everything" response. Sexual dysfunction clinics have available people who understand the broader implications of sex, who are aware of the many alternative forms of sexual expression, and who are comfortable in discussing sexual matters. They are not geared to treating patients with physiologic deficits but can probably offer more than any other source. The concerned, involved nurse may find that it is very difficult to find professionals willing to work with these patients/families. The nurse may find she has to do it herself. Depending on the background, education, and experiences of the nurse, what can be offered varies. The very least is that (1) the problem can be recognized and respected, (2) dialogue between the parties involved can be encouraged, and (3) appropriate references can be suggested.* Beyond this she may feel the need for and obtain education in sexual counseling and group work. She may arrange for some consistent follow-up of these patients either by the public health nurse or outpatient visits. Should the need for intervention to assist in the adjustment to the altered sexual functioning become apparent, she may offer the appropriate information, suggest some counseling sessions, or form a group for work on similar concerns. She may also become a crusader and canvas the area for malleable counselors in whom she can kindle an interest in trying to help these people so that when she identifies a problem she can follow through with appropriate referral. The only general requirement, regardless of which course is followed, is sensitivity to the feelings and needs of the individuals involved.

INTERNAL ASSAULTS–FEMALE. The woman with cancer of the genital organs faces an essentially invisible assault to her sexuality. Though vaginectomy is the only surgery which precludes vaginal sex, all treatment modalities have a significant effect either psychologically or physically. Studies of the meaning and effect of hysterectomy yield contradictory results. Some indicate that the surgery precipitates major social and psychologic changes, while others reveal no change in the sample attributable to the surgery. Obviously, the effect of the surgery depends on the meaning of the organ, of the disease, and of the treatment to the individual woman. Some grief is to be expected when one's health and perception of self as a whole and vigorous human being are assaulted. Obviously, an additional stress is endured by the woman who loses her reproductive capacity

*References which might be appropriate for couples dealing with alterations in sexual functioning: Brecher R, Brecher E: An Analysis of Human Sexual Response. Boston, Little, Brown, 1966; Comfort A: The Joy of Sex. New York, Crown, 1972; Comfort A: More Joy. New York, Crown, 1973; Gambrell E: Sex and the Male Ostomate. Los Angeles, United Ostomy Association, 1973; Norris C, Gambrell E: Sex, Pregnancy and the Female Ostomate. Los Angeles, United Ostomy Association, 1972.

while she still wishes to have children. Some women attribute a number of nonreproductive functions to the uterus: it cleans the body of impurities, it is the source of femininity, it is the source of strength. The degree to which these expectations and fears exist and interact determines to a great extent a woman's reaction to hysterectomy. Expectations alter perception so that one is predisposed to see and interpret in accord with the expectations. Thus, a woman whose perception is that her uterus is a source of her strength will be reinforced by the usual postoperative weakness and lethargy. For some women, hysterectomy becomes an all-encompassing excuse for their weaknesses and problems. This may be a worthwhile defense for the individual, but it can be extremely harmful to all with whom this woman has contact, for her complaints become the expectations of the listener. Preoperatively, it is important to elicit information regarding perceptions, beliefs, and expectations in order to eliminate as far as possible those which will interfere with maximal rehabilitation. Use of a booklet such as *After Hysterectomy What?*[34] to stimulate discussion is helpful. It can also lead to a discussion of a variety of topics between the patient and her spouse which had been previously overlooked or avoided. This kind of discussion can take place in the hospital, but it is better done by the office nurse or public health nurse prior to admission. Audree Vernon states that the woman anticipating hysterectomy needs answers to the following questions:

> The difference between hysterectomy and oophorectomy?
> Vaginal vs abdominal surgery?
> Results of hysterectomy?
> Routine care: Catheter? IV? Why?
> Why surgery is necessary? Why/why not oophorectomy?
> Results of oophorectomy? Hot flashes? Hormones?
> Relationship to Cancer?
> Sexual drive? Sexual ability? Orgasm?
> Weight gain? Masculinization? Nervousness?
> Insanity? Diabetes?
> Bowel and bladder function?
> How long healing takes? How long incapacited?
> Restrictions? Stairs? Work? Need for help?
> Positive effect(s) of hysterectomy?[35]

After radical pelvic surgery, even without vaginectomy, physical difficulties may arise. Wound healing often takes a considerable amount of time. In a study one author began but was unable to complete, women who had Wertheim hysterectomies for cancer of the cervix often delayed several weeks after they were told specifically that they could resume intercourse. Six months after surgery they continued to report discomfort and lack of satisfaction. This was accompanied by, and probably compounded by, their expressed feelings of vulnerability and fragility. These feelings have often been reported in conjunction with the diagnosis of cancer and the response to a change in body image. A recently published study indicated that at one year after treatment, 90 percent of patients treated surgically for cervical cancer reported no sexual dysfunction, but 25 of 28 who were treated with radiation reported some changes. This seems to be related to the fact that though surgery shortens the vagina, radiation causes loss of elasticity, loss of lubrication, and obliteration of the venous plexuses and arteries around the vagina, all of which produce a greater impediment than a shortened vagina which can still lubricate and expand in response to stimulation.[36] Women who require total vaginectomies are frequently in an older age group. However, the procedure for reconstruction of a vagina is available and, though not promulgated by the medical profession, has gained some recognition in the lay press.[37] It is not a simple procedure; it requires certain surgical expertise. The decision to reconstruct a vagina should be made by the patient and her sexual partner and should not be an arbitrary decision by the surgeon. Even if a woman elects not to have the surgery, the fact that it exists as an alternative saves her from the fate of having had no choice. Of interest in the Abitol study was a report of five sexually active women who had either an ileal bladder or a colostomy. They were asked which they would prefer, their present incapacity with an active sex life or normal excretory function without sexual relations. Four women definitely preferred to be active sexually, and one was uncertain.[36] Regardless of this information, far more concern is shown over forming an ileal bladder or colostomy than about obliterating a vagina. (Furthur information regarding sexuality and diversions of elimination is included in Chapter 7.)

A frank discussion of the problems which may be encountered in first attempts at intercourse after surgery or radiation, with information regarding lubrication, preliminary stimulation, positions which limit depth of penetration, and assurance that difficulties will decrease with time and sexual activity may eliminate some of the mental and physical suffering experienced by these women. This subject must generally be opened by the professional. Patients who have had cancer hesitate to do anything they are not specifically told they can do, especially anything to do with sex. Feelings that sex may be responsible for the cancer or that sex will precipitate a recurrence are not uncommon. Another frequently encountered belief is that any woman over 35 should not be interested in sex, and that certainly at a time like this it should be the farthest thing from her mind. A woman is further inhibited from expressing her concerns by the old cultural beliefs that women are not really interested or should not be interested in sex, that a woman's enjoyment of sex results from pleasing her mate, and that concern regarding sexual function and the right to have the preservation of that capacity considered is unique to the male. These and other misconceptions prevent a patient from discussing the subject openly with her physician. From the beginning it is important to convey the attitude that sex is a normal, healthy, basic part of life, that it is worthwhile and good, not insignificant and evil. Conveying this kind of attitude along with the information that help is available to aid the couple in working out any difficulties they may encounter would be a tremendous step forward. If 50 percent of all physically intact couples have some problems with sexual dysfunction, it can be expected that patients with genital surgery have problems.[38]

The obliteration of a vagina or the diversion of elimination produces obvious changes we can view in terms of threats to body image, identity, and sexuality. Many other less obvious assaults exist in cancer patients as a whole: surgical or radiation-induced menopause, severe leukopenia with prohibitions against vaginal intercourse, and neuropathies resulting from radiation or chemotherapy. Within the sphere of acceptability for a given couple, despite the cause of the impairment, there should be alternatives to vaginal intercourse: manual, oral, anal, interthigh, interbreast. A given individual may or may not know of such alternatives, and any degree of feeling from very positive to disgust may exist toward any specific alternative or to sex in general.

The manner in which physical care is given says a great deal. Urinary and bowel problems are frequent in many patients with cancer and only serve to reinforce the negative input of loss of control. Regimens to regain bladder control and bowel regularity are frequently required after pelvic surgery, radiation, certain chemotherapy, and with prolonged use of analgesics. Evaluation of elimination practices and institution of such regimens should be standard practice. Meticulous cleanliness is essential to minimize the chance of infection. The practice of using a common tub or sitz bath for patients is to be avoided, since the opportunities for transfer of pathogens need to be reduced not enhanced. Seromas develop rapidly in areas of dense lymphatics. After vulvectomy, orchiectomy, and radical lymphadenectomy, the danger of wound dehiscence due to fluid accumulation is considerable. For this reason drainage tubing is frequently inserted under the skin flap and attached to some form of suction. The adequacy of this method is dependent on the patency of the system.

A prepared patient finds it easier to accept routine problems and little setbacks because everything is not a surprise. During these periods of observation, the nurse can impart a great deal of information. She can also have a major impact on the new attitudes and perceptions which are necessarily being formed. Her sensitivity, her concern, and her forthrightness are strongly positive factors at a time when the negative aspects of life can seem overwhelming.

It is often appropriate to involve the mate of the patient during the later period of hospitalization in some of this care. This assumes that the nurse is comfortable in doing this, for her anxiety can defeat the purposes of the action. It also assumes that the nurse knows the patient and partner well enough to determine the appropriateness of this action. Under these conditions both parties can derive a great deal of support from the nurse and can proceed from this first anxious encounter with a basic trust and confidence generated by a positive experience.

The role of the nurse in the realm of sexuality needs to be expanded. Few people are comfortable with or prepared to aid others in this area, and it is one which is so often affected by the diseases called ''cancer.'' Our commitment to rehabilitation and self-care principles should include this aspect of the total human being as well. In terms of the nursing process, a nurse's role in aspects of sexuality should consist of (1) assessment of the total patient and his environment with emphasis on needs, feelings, expectations, and fears related to sexuality, (2) planning with the patient and his mate how best to deal with those aspects which may be problematic because of current life crises of diagnosis and treatment, (3) implementation of the plan in terms of knowledge and expertise of the professional nurse and available resources, and (4) ongoing evaluation of the effect on the patient. The attitude of the nurse is vitally important. Her attitude can say that sex is taboo or embarrassing, or her attitude can say that sex is normal and not to be hidden or feared. She can help the patient to see that sexuality includes more than the ability to perform a particular action, that how one perceives oneself and is perceived by others is equally important. The patient can succumb and become less than before. Or she/he can exert himself as an individual and contain the defect within realistic limits. The prepared nurse can help a couple work together to find a way of relating which is acceptable to them rather then automatically eliminating sex and the related aspects of touch, closeness, tenderness, and sharing from their relationship.

Problems Related to Cosmetic Appearance

By cosmetic problems, the authors mean the effects of the tumor or treatment which result in visible defects. Radiotherapy to visible cancers will produce scarring, which is generally less noticeable than the tumor itself. Alopecia is one very visible result of either radiotherapy or chemotherapy. Hair is tremendously important to some individuals. Generally, women are more upset than men by alopecia. The patient should begin to wear a wig as soon as it is decided to use a treatment modality which produces alopecia. If the individual delays until hair loss begins, depression at the loss of the hair and discomfort with the unfamilar wig frequently interact, resulting in erratic wearing of the wig and progressive depression and disgust with the appearance. Most of the time, however, radiation produces few cosmetic repercussions. The changes associated with radiation therapy are related primarily to changes in function (dry mouth, difficulty in eating) and to the disease, cancer. Chemotherapy can result in a variety of visible defects in addition to alopecia. Severe acne from steroids can be as threatening as some of the results of facial surgery discussed in the next section. Acne, because of its close association with adolescence, can reactivate adolescent conflicts with authority, self, and sexuality. Hirsutism can be a tremendous burden for the woman who is also dealing with the negative feelings about herself related to breast cancer, mastectomy, and oophorectomy. Acceptance by others and open discussion of these problems can lead to increased self-esteem and acceptance by the patient whether or not specific measures, such as the use of makeup or a facial depilatory, are implemented. The most drastic changes in appearance and, therefore, the greatest problems occur in relation to radical surgery for head and neck cancers, amputations, interference with nerve transmission resulting in paralysis, and debility. The following sections will deal with these problems.

HEAD AND NECK PROBLEMS.   It has been said that the face is the mirror of the soul. Whether or not this is true, people do react to another's facial appearance as if certain features were indeed signs of some inner secret or personality trait. The individual with close-set or small eyes is thought to be dishonest or sneaky. The person with a round full face is seen as happy and easygoing. Prior to the recent interest in beards and mustaches, a man who grew either for no identifiable reason (for example, religious custom or part of a celebration) was looked upon with some suspicion. Even adolescent acne, essentially a hormone-induced phenomenon, is viewed by some as representing a dirty person either physically or mentally. Millions of dollars are spent annually to prevent or remove wrinkles or reshape a nose, chin, or face. The face is the most obvious feature of an individual, the thing we are most aware of when we meet someone. For this reason, and because we each know how we withdraw from someone we perceive as ugly or repulsive, treatments which alter the face are wrought with terror. Patients facing surgery for head and neck cancer have no choice but to face this terror.

Preoperative Period.   Certain factors are common to most head and neck surgery: alteration in appearance, radical neck dissection, and tracheostomy. Preoperative assessment and preparation of these patients is vitally important, since communication is often impaired postoperatively. Misconceptions about head and neck surgery, the prosthesis, speech, and prognosis are common among patients and families. Adaptation to a realistic perception of the results of the disease and its treatment is difficult enough without the added burden of fatalistic misconceptions. Since high alcohol consumption and heavy smoking are a common duo in patients with head and neck cancers, preoperative assessment needs to include (in a nonjudgmental manner) a clear determination of the quantity of alcohol consumed daily or weekly and the number of cigarettes smoked daily. It is also important to ascertain the effects of these habits on the patient's family and friends and the relationships which may exist between certain individuals or situations and the forementioned habits. There is evidence that less than two-thirds of these patients significantly change their drinking and smoking habits after surgery despite the life-endangering aspects of continuing.[39] Obviously many factors in the environment interact to perpetuate the need for and continuance of these habits. Hopefully, a clearer picture of these interrelationships may lead to more effective intervention.

A clear idea of the particular job held by the person facing head and neck surgery for cancer is also needed in order to plan for maximal rehabilitation. The patient's drinking may have made him less than the most desirable employee, and cancer, especially that which results in a visible deformity with loss of speech, can be the ideal excuse for replacing the patient. The story of Mrs. Lanpher in *The Climate Is*

Hope tells how one woman returned to a very verbal occupation (language teacher) after laryngectomy.[40] However, statistics indicate that 30 to 40 percent of laryngectomees never speak again.[41,42] Other factors which need to be considered in assessing employment status include the physical as well as the psychologic results of the surgery. For instance, removal of the spinal accessory nerve in radical neck procedures may adversely affect an individual who drives a truck for a living but will be only a slight inconvenience to most others. The anticipated results of the surgery (visible, physical, and psychologic) and the specific life style of the individual need to be considered together. Social service departments and vocational counselors are usually better equipped than nurses to evaluate this area in depth and intervene constructively to help the patient overcome the disabling effects of his treatment. The nurse is in the best position to identify the potential problem. She is also needed in assisting the social worker, patient, and vocational counselor in defining the extent of the disability and planning realistically.

A great deal of special and confusing equipment is attached to the patient after radical head and neck surgery. During the preoperative period, the patient should be introduced to this equipment, its function, and its manner of use. Some specialists suggest that preoperatively the patient learn to do the procedures (eg, suctioning) he will be required to do postoperatively. The authors are hesitant to subject a very anxious patient to this degree of concrete additional stress. It behooves those involved in the preoperative care to do everything possible to allay the patient's anxiety. Acquainting the patient with the routines can help to relieve some of the anxiety related to the unknown, but a minimum of learning can be expected to occur at this time. Learning how to do those things which will directly affect the immediate postoperative course—coughing, deep breathing, exercises, and turning—is probably all that one can reasonably expect from a patient preoperatively. These patients do not seem to be in any better position to learn procedures preoperatively despite the fact that pain and medication will decrease learning ability postoperatively. In fact, motivation to learn, often the principal variable, may only be achieved and the patient has learned that suctioning provides relief.

As with many things in medicine, a debate rages regarding the relative merits of prostheses versus plastic surgery for cosmetic and functional defects after radical head and neck surgery. Often a prosthesis is seen as a temporary measure until the surgeon can succeed in correcting the defect by grafting. Unless grafting is part of the original procedure, a prosthesis should be used to provide a cosmetically acceptable appearance, to allow for function, and to relieve the patient and family of the grief of a period of visible horror. There are indications that a prosthesis may actually speed healing by protecting the wound.[43] If at a later date plastic repairs are carried out, the patient has been spared weeks or months of loss of function and visual repulsiveness. For the patient with a poor prognosis or in whom more surgery is contraindicated, lifetime use of a prosthesis is recommended. The preference surgeons have for corrective surgery may not be good for patients who, given no choice, follow only what their physician advises. It requires some skill to learn to apply an extensive prosthesis. On the positive side, a prosthesis can be removed to evaluate healing and to examine the area for signs of recurrence, and the cosmetic results can be very good. In fact a prosthesis may provide a better appearance than will corrective surgery. The decision whether to submit to plastic surgery or to rely on a prosthesis should be the patient's decision based on the best information the surgeon can provide. This information needs to include the relative merits and drawbacks of each, the skills involved, the long-term costs, and the availability of alternatives. If the patient will need assistance in securing a prosthesis or in underwriting the cost of the surgery, state rehabilitation agencies must be contacted preoperatively. Contacted later, these agencies can be helpful, but they cannot assume financial responsibility for any procedure or commitments which antedate their involvement.

Communication will be impaired for most of these patients, at least temporarily, and methods to assure an open line of communication must be devised. It is necessary to consider the results of the surgery and the abilities of the patient when evaluating the appropriateness of a form of communication. The patient with a tracheostomy cannot speak; after radical neck dissection he has difficulty shaking his head, and denervation of the trapezius may interfere with writing. The patient with arthritis and an intravenous infusion may be unable to write; the patient who cannot wear his glasses because of facial grafts may be unable to see to write; the patient may be illiterate, deaf, or blind. Magic slates, eye blink codes, lip reading, hand signals, or flash cards (picture or words) may be required. The method must be agreed upon and practiced by the patient, family, and nurses preoperatively. The terror of being unable to call for help is graphically related by many patients who have been deprived of their voices. The nurses providing postoperative care need to understand the previously arranged method of communication to be able to effectively alleviate this terror. The family must understand and be comfortable in using the method of communication to be able to provide the loving acceptance and support so vitally needed by the patient after surgery. Certain behaviors are common when a patient's ability to speak has been temporarily or permanently interrupted. People, the family included, tend to yell at the patient. They frequently answer for him. Family members need guidelines to help them avoid these pitfalls and to be able to communicate effectively with the patient.

A speech therapist should visit the patient who is to have a laryngectomy to evaluate his preoperative speech and to assure him of the availability of help to regain his ability to speak postoperatively. The merits of a visit from someone who uses esophageal speech are questionable at this time. Most healthy persons view their voice, as well as other capabilities, comparatively. Before laryngectomy, even with full knowledge that it is imminent, esophageal speech sounds like a poor substitute for one's own voice. Some people are repulsed by their first contact with esophageal speech. After surgery when the patient needs to communicate (in *any* way), esophageal speech can more easily be seen as the asset it is.

Family members need as much preparation as the patient. They need to understand the nature and extent of the disease and the surgery. Possibly more than the patient, they need to recognize that as mutilating as the surgery is, the tumor unchecked would be worse. They need to be carefully prepared for the patient's postoperative appearance. This includes not only telling them of the tubes, dressings, and tracheostomy, but also giving them a clear image of what will be missing and the appearance of what remains. A description of what a patient looks like after a radical neck dissection may be sufficient. It is hard to conceive that any one not previously associated with head and neck cancers can imagine what a person actually looks like after, eg, a commando procedure (hemiglossectomy, hemimandibulectomy, radical neck dissection, tracheostomy). Desensitization in an individualized way can be helpful. General description followed by specific description, pictures with and without corrective surgery or prosthesis, and introduction to another patient who is recovering from a similar procedure may be necessary. None of this can be attempted without first knowing the strengths and weaknesses of all the individuals involved. A family member can also benefit from an opportunity to speak with the speech therapist. Should the mate or other important figure seem unable to face or accept the results of the surgery or any of the other stresses which are present, referral of the family member to social service, psychiatry, or other appropriate assistance should not be overlooked. Since the responses of people who are emotionally close to the patient are so vitally important, it behooves the nurse to be sure that the people most significant to the patient have all the information, guidance, and support available so that they in turn can fulfill the expectations of this important role.

Postoperative Period. Immediately after surgery, maintenance of an adequate airway, prevention of infection and hemorrhage, assurance of a patent drainage system to prevent fluid accumulation and wound slough, and protection of the graft assume priority. In this period of critical physical need, one should not forget that the patient recovering from anesthesia calls out for help. The patient with a tracheostomy cannot call, yet his basic need for comforting still exists. Frequent reassurance needs to be given from the very beginning. The planned method of communication should be implemented as soon as the patient is coherent.

High-humidity oxygen is usually required to reduce the tenacity of the mucus produced after a tracheostomy. Meticulous attention needs to be given to this equipment as well as to tracheostomy-suctioning equipment and wound care supplied. The incidence of hemorrhage increases with the incidence of wound infection. Therefore, measures to prevent infection serve the dual function of prevention of infection and prevention of hemorrhage.

Most patients have placed in a semi-Fowler's position after head and neck surgery to facilitate drainage. Because of grafting, interruption of nerve transmission, or bulky dressings, the patient may be prevented from turning or doing certain activities. Environmental manipulation can assure ready access to the call light and personal articles, as well as providing the most interesting aspect of the limited view. Ambulation and passive or active range of motion exercises (dependent on the extent of the surgery, tension on the suture lines, and the existence of a skin graft) should begin the day after surgery. The early employment of physical therapy and occupational therapy helps the patient compensate for nerve and muscle loss and aids in the prevention of complications secondary to inactivity. Immediately after a radical neck dissection, some patients, especially if they are obese, may need a sling to support the arm on the affected side due to trapezius denervation. Other muscles soon strengthen and compensate for the defect. The patient to whom this occurs will undoubtedly be fearful that this loss of the use of his arm is a permanent loss compounding all the other losses he has had to face. As in other learning situations, it is helpful if the patient receives some written directions explaining exercises he must do to help regain and strengthen the involved muscles. Environmental manipulation, ambulation, exercise, and the preplanned communication allow the patient some measure of control and independence even in the early hours after surgery.

Laryngectomy is not the only problem involving speech. Loss of facial expression and difficulties with speech may occur as the result of damage to cranial nerves during the course of surgery. Surgery of the oral cavity, especially glossectomy, interferes with articulation. Speech therapy should begin immediately. If the surgeon does not wish the patient to attempt speech until suture lines have healed for several days, the therapist has a definitite role in reassuring the patient of his interest and of the forthcoming efforts to assist the patient in regaining the ability to speak. Statistics indicate that 30 percent of laryngectomees cannot learn esophageal speech.[42] One can validly ask whether the nonspeakers were nonverbal people who do not need to speak. Did their first attempts go unnoticed and unrewarded? What secondary gain is there for silence? What does esophageal speech mean to them? Despite a number of studies there seems to exist no variable which can predict who will succeed and who will not. Each individual is assumed to be able to speak again; if after 60 to 90 days, no intelligible speech is evident, a patient should be helped to explore alternative methods of communication. The nurse and therapist need to be very careful that they do not react to the patient as a failure if he must use an artificial larynx or other alternatives to esophageal speech. Attempts to isolate those factors which aid in or impede the acquisition of intelligible speech need to be continued. Timing, motivation, and environmental factors may become evident as information accumulates about both the patient who succeeds and the patient who fails. Lost Cord Club visitors are a tremendous asset postoperatively. They serve as role models and can give concrete reassurance that success is possible. Most Lost Cord Clubs also offer continued assistance in developing and maintaining esophageal speech.

Dysphagia, drooling, disorders of olfaction, and disorders of taste may all occur and interfere with adequate nutrition. Nasogastric feedings or hyperalimentation may be employed immediately postoperatively. With the use of throat lozenges, the patient with dysphagia may be able to progress to liquid or soft foods. Wicks to drain the saliva, spitting frequently, and the use of bibs reduce the mess of drooling, but the drooling itself remains a demeaning experience. The nurse and family need to exert every effort to enhance the patient's sense of self-esteem while ingeniously devising ways to minimize the demeaning characteristics and to protect the patient from hostile and rejecting experiences. Surgical procedures to divert the saliva can sometimes be performed. For the patient whose senses of taste and smell are impaired, a concerted team effort to find attractive, palatable foods served in a socially supportive situation is required. Patients may be able to eat as a social action even when the rewarding aspects of the taste and smell of food are absent. Furthur information regarding the problems of nutrition can be found in Chapter 6.

Long-term Rehabilitation.   The day before discharge is not the time to begin to teach self-care. The patient needs to learn more than the basic how-to. He needs time to practice and feel comfortable with the procedure, be it nasogastric feedings, tracheostomy care, or application of a prosthesis. During the first days after surgery, the patient can begin to learn some of the techniques he will need to resume self-care. He may initially be responsible for removing the oxygen-humidity adaptor prior to suctioning and for coughing and disposing of his own contaminated tissues. Eventually, if the tracheostomy is to be permanent, he will need to learn suctioning and care of the tracheostomy. The procedures followed should be written out in a number of simple steps. Daily the patient can assume supervised responsibility for a new step(s) of the procedure. Day-to-day progress need not be an orderly progresion from step 1 through step X. Individual needs, fears, and abilities determine the teaching plan. For one patient, the critical step of inserting the catheter into the tracheal stoma may best be learned first—"get it over with." For another it may be essential to develop confidence and courage by graded successes with the least anxiety-producing steps first. Certain steps, such as tying the tracheostomy tapes (in a surgeon's knot rather than a bow) are both nonthreatening and challenging.

The patient with a prosthesis must learn to apply, remove, and care for the prosthesis. He must also learn to care for the area covered by the prosthesis: to examine, clean, and prepare the area. This requires not only that the technical skills be learned but also that the patient be able to tolerate looking at himself without his prosthesis. He also needs to be prepared for mishaps which are likely to occur and how to handle these. For example, is his prosthetic eye likely to come out at certain times? How can this be prevented? If he bumps his head or glasses will his entire facial prosthesis shift? What if the dental attachments are not fastened securely? Listing all of the possible problems that could arise without positive suggestions for avoidance or coping serves no purpose. Preparation can often prevent the occurrence of many little happenings which could easily be construed as crises by the patient in these early weeks of rehabilitation.

One member of the family should take part in this training as well. The willingness to learn and the doing of the procedure serve as a sign of acceptance. A knowledgeable family member (or friend) can be an invaluable aid in cases of illness, memory lapse, or sudden panic. For some patients and families, this period of time is too soon to demand this degree of unveiling. It is the rare situation when other methods of assuring acceptance, support, and emergency care cannot be substituted. In other cases, the family member assumes total responsibility. If this is in accord with the wishes of the patient and the family, it is difficult to progress toward patient independence. The patient should be encouraged to assume more responsibility and become more independent with time. The family needs to be counseled regarding the merit of the patient's becoming independent—self-worth, long-term plans. However, no decision is so binding that changes cannot be accomplished in the future. People change, needs change, and motivational factors change. If someone is available to help at later times, adaptation and self-reliance may be increased at any time.

Certain matters regarding adaptation to the home situation need to be considered. The esophageal speaker may need a phone amplifier. All patients with permanent tracheostomies will need to provide intermittent regular tracheostomy and stoma care. If they shower rather than bathe, they will need a stoma shield. Humidification equipment may be necessary in areas of low natural humidity. Arrangements for the supplies or at least information regarding their acquisition must be provided the patient prior to discharge. State vocational rehabilitation services which have been consulted previously may be helpful at this time. The excitement, exhaustion, and general anxiety of the discharge day make it a poor time to plan and shop for supplies. A kit composed of the supplies the patient will need for care during the first few days should be provided to aid in the transition. Plans for the acquisition or rental of equipment should have been made in advance so that it is in the home and operational before the patient's homecoming. Despite his level of competence before discharge, written instructions and a phone number to be called for advice, reassurance, and assistance should be given every patient. The need for outpatient or home nursing, at least for evaluation and reassurance, should be anticipated and arranged in advance. A predischarge home visit by the public health nurse may be worthwhile. In some cases it is essential.

Role play, occupational therapy, and social contacts within the hospital will help the patient gradually expand his relationships and abilities. Since many of these individuals have been heavy drinkers, psychotherapy or referral to Alcoholics Anonymous may be indicated. Obviously, the patient and not just the nurse or the family must recognize this need. Industry continues to function on the premise that a patient with cancer is already dead. Return to gainful employment is especially difficult when the therapy has produced a visible defect concomitant with the stigma of cancer. Resources which may be helpful are the various social service agencies, groups for the disabled, counseling services, and vocational rehabilitation services. In addition to the state vocational rehabilitation agencies, there now exist various rehabilitation programs sponsored by insurance companies for their insured, such as International Rehabilitation Associates, Inc., a company which provides rehabilitation consultation to private insurance companies. Cancer patients have historically been exempted from these services. Survival statistics do not support the logic of this practice. Indeed, facts indicate that the cancer patient may be easier to work with and be a better client from the points of motivation and use of the training than those whose mutilation is the result of trauma. The cancer patient can frequently be expected to outlive the cardiac, diabetic, and stroke patients commonly served by rehabilitation programs. Policies within these agencies have been changed in recent years to allow for more involvement with the cancer patient. The attitudes of people toward cancer and those who have had cancer has not kept pace with administrative changes. As one rehabilitation counselor stated, "They've been through so much, you hate to pressure them to become involved in retraining programs and everything that goes with it when you don't know what else might happen."

Healing and rehabilitation are long-term goals. The patient who expects to feel like "his old self" in a few days will be disappointed. The expense of hospitalization, surgery, and the loss of income for a number of weeks or months is compounded when furthur corrective surgery or expensive prostheses are needed. (The initial cost of a prosthesis is high, and periodically the prosthesis must be repaired or replaced. The multiple hospitalizations often required for plastic repairs are even more expensive.) Ongoing counsel—social, financial, and psychologic—must occur in conjunction with this long-term treatment.

AMPUTATION. Amputation for cancer is a major rehabilitation problem. The population is essentially youthful; 50 percent are under 29 years of age. Despite the fact that the average survival regardless of extent of disease is greater than three years (and that the first prosthesis generally must be replaced in two years), prostheses and rehabilitation services in general have not been readily available to cancer patients. The recent surgery of young Edward Kennedy, Jr., and the publicity given his rehabilitation may help the process of change.

Preoperative preparation is essential. The fact and cost of rehabilitation depend on it. Referral to the state rehabilitation agencies is necessary preoperatively if they will be expected to assume any financial responsibility for the hospitalization or rehabilitation. Such an agency can generally arrange to assist in the payment of surgical cost, prosthesis, and rehabilitation programs only if they are notified before the debt is incurred. Preoperative exercises and crutch walking give the patient a head start after surgery, strengthen the unaffected extremities, maintain range of motion, and reduce pain. The patient needs to understand the nature of his surgery and what he can expect of his prosthesis.

In 1965 a surgical procedure was introduced which allowed the use of an immediate postoperative prosthesis (IPOP). This has significantly reduced the disability effects of lower extremity amputations. In this procedure, the muscles are sutured to the bone through holes drilled in the distal end. A cast is applied over the dressing, and the prosthetic unit is attached to this cast. Conditioning exercises started before surgery are resumed within hours after surgery. The patient is ambulatory within 48 hours.[39,42] Edema and pain are reduced, and phantom limb sensations are less bothersome, possibly because other sensations are being received from the amputated area. When phantom limb sensation does occur, it can aid in gait training. Lower limb prostheses are both cosmetic and functional to the level of hemicorporectomy. The patient with a hip disarticulation receives a prosthesis which approximates the inferior bones of the pelvis so that weightbearing is done by the pelvic girdle. This is a useful and stable prosthesis. Hemipelvectomy and hemicorporectomy prostheses allow standing and ambulation, but since they approximate soft tissue only, they are inherently unstable. The patient will require some additional stability in the form of a walker or crutches. Most of the time these patients remain in a wheelchair, which is less tiring and easier to manipulate. Upper limb prostheses are far less satisfactory. The more proximal the amputation, the less functional is the prosthesis. The prosthesis after shoulder disarticulation provides for some function. However, after forequarter amputation (transscapulothoracic), the arm is only cosmetic. The reality of prosthetic wear includes the forementioned variables regarding the functional capacities of various prostheses. It also includes some facts regarding comfort and cosmesis. A prosthesis cannot be expected to be an exact replacement for the lost extremity. There is always an awareness of its existence; formerly automatic acts require thought and effort. It is more tiring to perform a given activity with a prosthetic leg than with a normal leg, though the new lighter materials are reducing the energy expenditure associated with manipulation of a prosthesis. The prosthesis will be cosmetically as close as possible to normal, but it will always be possible to determine by scrutiny which is the artificial part. Patients' expectations may be very different from reality. The patient who expects that after a short time he will be able to forget he has a prosthesis will have a difficult time increasing his activity when this automatic state does not occur. He will continue to view the prosthesis in comparison to the integral body part rather than as as an asset in its own right. The patient who expects to be an invalid after surgery may resist all attempts at rehabilitation because they "cannot help me anyway." Every effort needs to be made preoperatively to bring the patient's and his family's expectations into close approximation to reality.

Many of these procedures are uncommon and unacceptable to a healthy person. The nurses involved in the care of the patient may be shocked and repulsed. They need preparation to understand the rationale for the surgery, to work through their feelings, and to determine the role they can play in helping the patient cope with a very difficult period of his life.

Postoperative Consideration.   Self-care and ambulation are begun as soon as the particular procedure will permit, usually within 24 hours. Minimizing the period of bed rest minimizes complications and decreases the tendency of the disability effects to spread to areas which need not be affected by it. Stump care is important. The specifics are related to the exact surgical procedure performed and the preferences of the surgeon. The newer procedures have eliminated much of the tedious dressing changes and conditioning previously needed to prepare the stump for a prosthesis. However, the need to observe the area for color, temperature, and fit remains essential. Before a patient is ready for independent care, he must learn how to apply, wear, and care for his prosthesis in the activities of *his* life style. This can be accomplished by allowing him to experience graded expansion of his environment and social contacts. A discussion group of Vietnam veterans with lower extremity amputations proved worthwhile in terms of improving the outlook of the participants.[44] Role play, group excursions, and weekend passes give the amputee an opportunity to test his skill and emotional responses gradually.

Long-term Rehabilitation. Long-term rehabilitation must consider architectural modifications, dietary counseling, vocational rehabilitation, and financial assistance. The patient, family, physician, nurse, social worker, and other rehabilitation specialists will need to work together to evaluate the need for change of residence, mobility aids, and how these will be obtained and financed. Addition of a ramp, removing or widening a doorway in the home, or conversion into a bathroom of a small closet on the main floor may mean the difference between self-care and dependency. A doorway too narrow to accommodate a wheelchair may be the only impediment to an individual's return to gainful employment. Recently attention has been given in the news media to the problem of discrimination against the disabled in the form of restricted access to public buildings, schools, drinking fountains, phones, and restrooms. Legislation has been introduced in all levels of government to help overcome these problems. State rehabilitation services, private rehabilitation organizations, organizations for the disabled (eg, Easter Seal Society), and certain schools (eg, with rehabilitation programs or engineering or architecture courses which deal with this subject) can be valuable sources of information and advice for the newly disabled.

The patient who must depend on a prosthesis, whether an artificial limb, a breast prosthesis, or an ostomy appliance, is dependent for adequate comfort and function on a good fit. The fit depends on the skill of the person fitting the prosthesis and on the body contour's remaining stable. Any significant weight gain or loss will necessitate refitting of the prosthesis. Certainly an emaciated patient should be encouraged and helped to gain weight. The obese patient should be counseled regarding the loss of some weight. In anticipation of these changes, plans can be made to minimize the expense of remaking the prosthesis. One way to minimize the expense is to delay construction of the final model until a stable weight is achieved. Food and its ingestion are so closely tied to emotions that in times of stress, it is not uncommon for individuals to become anorexic (even without a recurrence of their disease) or to overeat. Patients who do not need to gain or lose for medical reasons need diet counseling to maintain their weight to minimize fitting problems.

Vocational rehabilitation may be required not only because of an actual inability to perform the previous job but also because of the unwillingness of an employer to rehire a patient with cancer and/or a handicapped person. The age of many of these patients is such that they do not have seniority in the job market. At this time, it may take a crusade to find the retraining services outside of the cancer centers which are anxious to assist the patient with cancer. Certainly there have been improvements in this area in recent years. The American Cancer Society's emphasis on quality of survival and rehabilitation has helped accomplish these changes. Much work is yet ahead to implement these concepts so that they are more than mere words or dreams which only approach reality in the major cancer centers which treat only a small percentage of cancer patients. The development of regional cancer centers can help bring rehabilitation to the cancer patient. Community involvement, referral of patients, and a more positive attitude toward cancer are also needed.

Aside from the financial problems which will obviously arise if a patient is unable to return to work, productivity itself is a very important quality to Americans. If no form of employment can be obtained for a patient, some activity needs to be discovered to which he can devote himself. This can help occupy his time and be a rewarding experience. Use of the prosthesis and activity are closely related. Increased use of the prosthesis improves one's sense of self-esteem and leads to an ever expanding scope of activity, which in turn requires increased use of the prosthesis. On the other hand, minimal activity requires minimal use of the prosthesis, resulting in a view of oneself as an invalid, which in turn leads to a reduction of activity. The degree to which even the most disabled can be rehabilitated is illustrated by the following report on one of the first patients to undergo hemicorporectomy.

> Rehabilitation was started with bed exercises for strengthening the upper extremities. The patient was prepared for eventual sitting in a prosthetic jacket, wheelchair propulsion, independence in activities of daily living, and ultimately he was provided with a full prosthesis in which he was trained to stand and ambulate. Finally he received driver training and obtained his driving license, after passing his road test. He is active, out and about at the present time, ten years after this surgery.[45]

DISORDERS OF NERVE TRANSMISSION.   Neuropathies may result from the tumor or from the treatment (surgery, radiation, or chemotherapy). Indeed a neuropathy or myopathy may be the first sign of a malignancy. There is generally less residual damage after treatment for a brain tumor than after cerebral vascular accident. The long-term difference is a function of better rehabilitation for the stroke patient. Rehabilitation must begin at once, even during the process of diagnosis. The goals of rehabilitation are set by the patient's desires and the impairment involved. What he wants to do will affect what he can do. When repetitive, boring procedures, such as range of motion exercises, are done with a specific goal planned by the patient, they have a meaning beyond their mere repetition, and the patient is more cooperative.

Dependent on the impairment, therapeutic success, and the individual rehabilitation may be (1) restorative—oriented to restoring normal function, (2) supportive—oriented to maintaining maximum function by minimizing the loss through training and supportive aids, or (3) palliative—oriented to inhibiting the progression of the disability. Basically all rehabilitation starts out as palliative. Range of motion exercises, turning schedules, control of pain, and maintenance of nutritional status are directed toward preventing any furthur loss while definitive therapy is employed to allow higher goals to become feasible. The real failures in rehabilitation are failures in this area of preventing progression of the disability in the early hours and days of the impariment. This is equally as true for the patient who develops a radiation neuropathy 12 months after treatment as it is for the patient who is as yet undiagnosed or who develops paralysis after craniotomy. The effects of bed rest and immobility so rapidly occur and so slowly abate that it behooves all involved in the care of the patient to fight diligently to prevent their development. It is believed that routine stretching of a muscle is essential not only to maintain strength but also to prevent the formation of denser, shorter muscle fibers in accommodation to the shorter, flexed length which results in contractures. Active range of motion exercises twice daily will significantly reduce this in most joints. To maintain a mobile hip, it is almost mandatory to stand or ambulate the patient daily. It is extremely difficult to obtain full extension of the hip while the patient is bedfast. Isometric contractions for a few seconds four times daily will prevent nearly all of the 10 percent loss of strength per week which normally occurs during inactivity. After three weeks of bedrest, it may take several weeks to fully regain normal orthostatic reflexes and an equal period of time to regain preimmobility cardiac reserve. Demineralization of bones due to immobilization is measurable in healthy individuals after two weeks. This is compounded by the calcium loss associated with bony metastasis. Decubiti occur because of interference with oxygenation and nutrition of cells. In the debilitated patient, *hourly* turning may be essential. An alternating pressure mattress may increase the interval to two hours, but there is no alternative to turning. If the area of erythema caused by pressure does not subside within 10 minutes after turning the patient, the length of time he was in the previous position was too long. Improvement of nutritional status with high-protein, high-vitamin B complex, and high-vitamin C diets is helpful but cannot substitute for mobility and turning. The wheelchair-confined patient must be taught to relieve the pressure on his ischial tuberosities by raising himself on his hands every 15 minutes for one to two seconds. Urinary tract damage results from hypomotility and hyporeflexia compounded by the high calcium excretion. The damage may be irreversible. Susceptibility to infections, specifically urinary and respiratory infections, increases with the length of enforced immobility. Mental alertness and emotional stability are impaired with prolonged rest. Confusion and lethargy are common and interfere with motivation and cooperation. Mental activity, social contacts, occupational therapy (activities of daily living), exercises, and ambulation beyond the confines of one room are essential just to maintain the status quo.[46,47] Specific regimens to help overcome the residuals for any tumor must be individualized. Often a hospital geared to rehabilitation is required. Assuring that the patient is in the best condition to use the services of such a specialized center is the responsibility of those who have cared for him in the intervening days or months.

The rationale for these various programs needs to be explained to families in such a way that they understand and are eager to participate. Consider the patient with brain metastases receiving radiation and chemotherapy. A devoted spouse might well object fiercely to all of the pushing and pulling that range of motion and ambulation entail. His cooperation and help is dependent on his understanding and support of the goals and the methods employed to attain these goals. The patient with a residual handicap often returns home where rehabilitation depends on the family. What role is expected of various family members? Can they fulfill these expectations? What needs have they which will help or hinder the care of the primary patient? Public health nursing assessment of the home situation can be invaluable in answering some of these questions. The public health nurse can also aid in planning for and implementing actions to facilitate the readmittance of the patient into the family unit, their adjustment, and the quality of their lives in the future. Whether the patient is cured, controlled, or dying, he deserves the best of humane care. He deserves to be able to be himself as long as possible. His perceptions, those of his caretakers, and their collective needs will influence his care as much as any specific treatment measures.

DEBILITY.   The debiliated patient (or for that matter the edematous patient) is facing a change in body image sometimes as great as that of the patient facing radical surgery. It certainly has occurred more gradually, but adjustment is not always such a gradual process. Adjustment rarely keeps pace with such changes, and the patient's response depends so much on the responses of others. He may be continually confronted by the surprise on the faces of those who come to visit who have not been exposed to the gradual change. This can be especially traumatic if physical attractiveness has been an integral part of the individual's core self. Every effort to provide positive input via support of the individual's control factors, concern and respect for the individual, and good preventive rehabilitation help offset these negative aspects.

Functional interference with sight, smell, hearing, and taste occur with many therapies and tumors. They obviously interfere with an individual's enjoyment of certain aspects of living. They accost an individual's positive feelings about himself to varying degrees. What has been said throughout this chapter can be said of these defects as well. In fact, though certain facts or interventions are included in one section, there is great overlap; information and areas to be considered should be applied wherever they seem relevant.

In summary, one cannot guess the meaning of a given defect to an individual, but one can learn the meaning and the attendant needs. Planning of intervention is based on the patient's needs and the principles of providing maximal positive input while minimizing negative aspects. The role of education, the necessity of training in self-care techniques, and the role of the family and health-care personnel are central to the provision of this positive input. Caring, listening, planning, implementing and evaluating—these are both the process and the skills required.

References

1. Gale RF: Developmental Behavior. New York, Macmillan, 1969
2. Wapner S, Werner H: The Body Percept. New York, Random House, 1965
3. Garrett JF, Levine ES: Rehabilitation Practices with the Physically Disabled. New York, Columbia University Press, 1973
4. Norris CM: The professional nurse and body image. In Carlson CE (ed): Behavioral Concepts and Nursing Intervention. Philadelphia, Lippincott, 1970
5. Wright B: Physical Disability—A Psychological Approach. New York, Harper & Row, 1960
6. Cohen MB: Personal identity and sexual identity. Psychiatry 29:1–14, 1966
7. Bardwick JM: Psychology of Women. New York, Harper & Row, 1971
8. Vincent CE (ed): Human Sexuality in Medical Education and Practice. Springfield, Ill, Thomas, 1968
9. Sherfey MJ: The Nature and Evolution of Female Sexuality. New York, Random House, 1966
10. Masters WH, Johnson VE: A pictorial review of the stages of sexual response in women. MAHS 4:11–17, 1970
11. Goffman E: STIGMA—Notes on the Management of a Spoiled Identity. Englewood Cliffs, NJ, Prentice-Hall, 1963
12. McDaniel JW: Physical Disability and Human Behavior. New York. Pergamon Press, 1969
13. Orbach CE, Tallent N: Modification of perceived body and of body concept. Arch Gen Psychiatry 12:126–135, 1965
14. Wright: Op cit, p 161
15. Costello AM: Supporting the patient with problems related to body image. Proceedings of the National Conference on Cancer Nursing, Chicago, September, 1973. American Cancer Society, 1974, p 40
16. Ibid, p 37
17. Murray RLE: Principles of nursing intervention for the adult patient with body image changes. Nurs Clin North Am 7:698, December 1972
18. Aguilera DC, Messick JM: Crisis Intervention, 2nd ed. St. Louis, Mosby, 1974
19. Silverberg E, Holleb AI: Cancer statistics, 1974—Worldwide epidemiology. CA 24:2–21, 1974
20. Women's Attitudes Regarding Breast Cancer—Summary. Code No. 0501. American Cancer Society, 1974
21. Crile G: Operable breast cancer: In defense of conservative surgery. CA 23:334–338, 1973
22. Anglem TJ, Leber RE: Operable breast cancer: The case against conservative surgery,. CA 23:330–333, 1973
23. Le Shan L: An emotional life history pattern associated with neoplastic disease. Ann NY Acad Sci 125:780–793, 1966
24. Rahe RH: Life change measurement as a predictor of illness. Proc R Soc Med 61:1124, 1968
25. Gorman W: Body Image and the Image of the Brain. St. Louis: Green, 1969

26. Quint J: The impact of mastectomy. Am J Nurs 63:88–92, November 1963
27. Maier JG, Sulak MH: Radiation therapy in malignant testis tumors. Cancer 32:1225, 1973
28. Brecher R, Brecher E: An Analysis of Human Sexual Response. Boston, Little, Brown, 1966
29. Comfort A: The Joy of Sex. New York, Crown, 1972
30. ———: More Joy. New York, Crown, 1973
31. Masters WH, Johnson VE: Human Sexual Response. Boston, Little, Brown, 1966
32. Comarr AE; Sex among patients with spinal cord and/or cauda equina injuries. MAHS 7:222–238, 1973
33. Hohmann GW: Considerations in management of psychosexual readjustment in the cord injured male. Rehabil Psychol 19:50–58, 1972
34. Curtis LR: After Hysterectomy, What? Bristol, Tennessee, Beecham Laboratories, 1966
35. Vernon A: Explaining hysterectomy. Nurs 73 3:36–38, September 1973
36. Abitol MM, Davenport JH: Sexual dysfunction after therapy for cervical carcinoma. Am J Obstet Gynecol 119:181–188, 1974
37. Keiffer E: Brink of tragedy. Good Housekeeping p 85, July, 1974
38. Masters WH, Johnson VE: Human Sexual Inadequacy. Boston, Little, Brown, 1970
39. Rehabilitation of the Cancer Patient. Chicago, Year Book Medical Publishers, 1972
40. Ross W: The Climate Is Hope. Englewood Cliffs, NJ, Prentice-Hall, 1965
41. Gardner WH, Harris HE: Aids and devices for laryngectomees. Arch Otolaryngol 73:145–152, 1961
42. Healey JE (ed): Ecology of the Cancer Patient. Washington DC, Inter-disciplinary Communication Associates, Inc., 1970
43. Higher cancer "cure" rates create human problem—Rehabilitation. JAMA 222:418–421, 1972
44. Anders RL, Purol RM: Amputee discussion program. J Psychiatr Nurs 10:12–15, July 1972
45. Dietz JH: Rehabilitation of the cancer patient. Med Clin North Am 53:607–624, 1969.
46. Kottke FJ: Deterioration of the bedfast patient. Public Health Rep 80:437–450, 1965
47. Stryker RP: Rehabilitative Aspects of Acute and Chronic Nursing Care. Philadelphia, Saunders, 1972

Bibliography

A Breast Check. American Cancer Society, 1973
Adsett CA: Emotional disfigurement from cancer therapy. Can Med Assoc J 89:385, 1963
Ammon LL: Surviving enucleation. Am J Nurs 72:1817–1821, October 1972
Amster WW, Love RD, Menzel OJ, et al: Psychosocial factors and speech after laryngectomy. J Commun Dis 5:1–18, 1972
Corbeil M: Nursing process for a patient with a body image disturbance. Nurs Clin North Am 6:155–163, March 1971
Crile G: What Women Should Know about the Breast Cancer Controversy. New York, Macmillan, 1973
Cuica R, Bradish J, Trombly SM: Range of motion exercises, active and passive: A handbook. Nurs 73 3:25–37, December, 1973
Dlin BM, Perlman A: Sex after ileostomy or colostomy. MAHS 6:32–43, 1972
Dorpat TL: Phantom sensations of international organs. Compr Psychiatry 12:27–34, 1971

Drellich MD, Bieber I: The psychologic importance of the uterus and its functions. J Nerv Ment Dis 126:322–335

Drellich MD, Sutherland AM: The psychological impact of cancer and cancer surgery. VI. Adaptation to hysterectomy. Cancer 9:1120–1126, 1956

Ervin CV: Psychologic adjustment to mastectomy. MAHS 7:42–65, 1973

Facial Disfigurement—A Rehabilitation Problem. US Department of Health, Education, and Welfare, Vocational Rehabilitation Administration, 1963

Foss G: Breaking the architectural barrier with crutches wheelchairs and walkers. Nurs 73 3:17–31, October 1973

Gallagher AM: Body image changes in the patient with a colostomy. Nurs Clin North Am 7:669–676, December 1972

Gardner WH: Adjustment problems of laryngectomized women. Arch Otolaryngol 83:31–42, 1966

Gould R: The phases of adult life: A study of developmental psychology. Am J Psychiatry 129:521–531, 1972

Help Yourself to Recovery. American Cancer Society, 1971

Huffman JW: Sex after hysterectomy. Sex Behav 3:42–43, 1973

Hugos R: Living with leukemia. Am J Nurs 72:2185–2188, December 1972

Human Sexuality. American Medical Association, 1972

Jordan HS, Kavchak MA: Transfer techniques. Nurs 73 3:19–22, March 1973

Jordan HS, Cypress RM: All-around Care for the leg amputee. Nurs 74 4:51–55, April 1974

Katchadourian HA, Lunde DT: Fundamentals of Human Sexuality. New York, Holt, Rinehart and Winston, 1972

Katz J: Biological and psychological roots of psychosexual identity. MAHS 6:103–116, 1972

Klinger H; Acceptance among alaryngeal speakers. J Commun Dis 4:273–278, 1971

Leonard B: Body image changes in chronic illness. Nurs Clin North Am 7:687–695, December 1972

Macgregor FC: Some psycho-social problems associated with facial deformities. Am Sociol Rev 16:629–638, 1951

Malin JM: Sex after urologic surgery. MAHS 7:245–264, 1973

Maslow AH: Toward a Psychology of Being. New York, Van Nostrand, 1961

Masters WH, Johnson VE: A pictorial review of the stages of sexual response in men. MAHS 6:78–83, 1972

McCorkle MR: Coping with physical symptoms in metastatic breast cancer. Am J Nurs 73:1034–1038, June 1973

Merlino AF: Decubitus ulcers. Geriatrics 24(1):119–124, 1969

Moolten SE: Bedsores in the chronically ill patient. Arch Phys Med Rehabil 53:430–438, 1972

Murray RLE: Body image development in adulthood. Nurs Clin North Am 7:617–630, December 1972

Owen ML: Special care for the patient who has a breast biopsy or mastectomy. Nurs Clin North Am 7:373–382, June 1972

Rannalls J: Crutches and walkers. Nurs 72 2:21–24, December 1972

Raven RW (ed): Rehabilitation of the Cancer Disabled. London, William Heinemann Medical Books, 1972

Robbins GF, Markel WM: The Postmastectomy Lymphedematous Arm. American Cancer Society, 1973

Schilder P: The Image and Appearance of the Human Body. New York, International Universities Press, 1950

Schwab JJ: Body image and medical illness. Psychosom Med 30:51–61, 1968

Staples R: The sexuality of black women. Sex Behav 2:4–15, 1972

Terry FJ, Benz GS, Kleffner FR, et al: Principles and Technics of Rehabilitation Nursing. St. Louis, Mosby, 1961

Trowbridge JE: Caring for patients with facial or intra-oral reconstruction. Am J Nurs 73:1930–1934, November 1973

Welty MJ, Graham WP, Rosillo RH: The patient with maxillofacial cancer. I. Surgical treatment and nursing care. Nurs Clin North Am 8:137–152, March 1973

———: The patient with maxillofacial cancer. II. Psychologic aspects. Nurs Clin North Am 8:152–164, March 1973

Wolf ES: Nursing care of patients with breast cancer. Nurs Clin North Am 2:587–596, December 1967

Yachnes E: Some mythical aspects of masculinity. MAHS 7:200–215, 1973

Zalewski N, Geronemus D, Siegel H: Hemipelvectomy—The triumph of Ms A. Am J Nurs 73:2073–2077, December 1973

Zavertnik J: Emotional support of patients with head and neck surgery. Nurs Clin North Am 2:503–510, September 1967

Zeissler RH, Rose GB, Nelson PA: Postmastectomy lymphedema: Late results of treatment in 385 patients. Arch Phys Med Rehabil 53:159–166, 1972

Index